SARAH'S LAST WISH

A chilling glimpse into forced medicine

Eve Hillary

Sarah's Last Wish

Permission requests or general correspondence to:

sarahslastwish@gmail.com

Eve Hillary, PO Box 5165, Chittaway, NSW, Australia, 2261

Or visit: www.sarahs-last-wish.com

First edition 2010

ISBN 978-0-9806629-0-0

Biography, literary non-fiction, health, integrative medicine, child protection, human rights, children's rights, crisis management, end-of-life care, institutional abuse.

Edited by J.G.

Front cover design and graphics by David D. Back cover and author's photo by Kim and Alex. Images inside book and of Sarah on front cover, courtesy of the Westley Family.

In Memory of Sarah

ACKNOWLEDGEMENTS

I dedicate this book to my family, with love and appreciation for their caring and support. I thank them for often asking me how I was travelling during this three-year book-writing marathon. They have freely donated their legal and scientific expertise, and when the going got tough, they generously gave me enough encouragement and practical assistance to nudge this book across the finish line.

Mark and Dianne, the subjects of this work, have navigated a course that few would find the strength to endure, let alone so courageously. I thank them for sharing their journey with me and for trusting me to tell their story and Sarah's story. I am grateful to Sarah's siblings, Hannah and Laura for their significant contributions to this book and to Clara, Leah, and Joshua for their joyful innocence. My thanks extend to Ruth and Jim and to other family members. I will always be thankful to Sarah, whose invincible dignity and courage is a constant source of inspiration to me and to countless others.

I thank my editor for recognising the magic in this story and for polishing and strengthening it with her professional expertise until it proudly stood on its own. I am grateful to the graphic artist for creating the cover design and to others who contributed to it.

I am also grateful to the two world-renowned medical experts who generously gave their time and expertise to this project. One of them is a professor of paediatric oncology, while the other, a prominent professor of medicine, authored some of the definitive sources about the rare condition that Sarah had suffered from.

Thank you to all my friends for their loyal support, even though I saw too little of them over the past few years. Thanks to my close friends for still believing in me, even after reading the early drafts.

My thanks and admiration to all the ethical professionals who allowed me to interview them; this includes doctors, nurses, social workers, child protection workers, and law enforcement personnel.

Finally, thank you, Suzi, for sitting at my feet and keeping them warm over three long, but productive, winters.

Eve Hillary
Sydney, December 2009

READER'S NOTE

This book portrays a true story, told in a literary narrative form, which is based on over 1000 legal, government and medical documents, dozens of interviews with the Westley family and witnesses – as well as this author's own experiences and recollections of the depicted events. In this book, I have used the real names and identities of the immediate family members, with their permission. Nearly all other persons mentioned in this book, except actual scientists listed in the references, have been given pseudonyms, out of courtesy, and in some cases, their physical characteristics, (but not necessarily their conduct) have been deliberately disguised. The names of most hospitals featured in the story have not been revealed. The intention of this book is to tell the family's story, which clearly highlights the need for reform to the current health and child protection system, rather than to identify the specific individuals or institutions involved.

The scenes and dialogue play an important role in conveying the story. Often I used the dialogue verbatim from available records, and at other times, I reconstructed dialogue from interviews and recollections. Occasionally, scenes and dialogue have been reconstructed, based on what is known, on the record, to have occurred. The feelings and thoughts expressed in the narrative are based on the family's recollections of what they thought and felt and on their impressions of the events at the time, or at a later date. Some of the internal and external dialogue is based on what is plausibly self-evident in the circumstances.

The Westley family graciously allowed me unlimited access to all available records, documents and information, while setting no limitations on me at any time during the writing of this book.

The reader can find more information at the end of the narrative in an extensive medical reference section. Most references are listed in-situ, while some are featured as footnotes – all scientific content is fully referenced at the end. The information in this book is not intended to diagnose, treat, or cure any diseases. The author and publisher are in no way liable for any misuse of the material.

TABLE OF CONTENTS

The Wish...1

Paradise Lost 5

Worse Than Pregnant 27

For My Eyes Only 43

Getting Very Messy 65

The Whole Box of Frogs..89

Storm Warning...103

Dark Nights 115

Sarah's New Parents 135

The Department Wants Your Spleen 149

Brute Force 171

Psycho-profiling 193

How Could They Do This to Her? 215

In The Public Interest 243

A Snake at the Door 265

A Cry for Justice 277

The Clinic..287

Terminal Betrayal 299

Last Flight to Freedom...319

Going Home 337

Home At Last...343

Epilogue 346

About the Author...349

References 351

THE WISH

**A selfless wish made by an innocent child
Has the power to work miracles.
Anon**

In mid-October 2004, the Melbourne Royal Children's hospital cancer ward was nearly full. A fresh shift of afternoon nurses came on duty at 2 pm. Some dreaded working in the side rooms reserved for children with terminal cancer. In one of those rooms was Sarah Westley – a tall, lean girl with legs a fraction too long for the paediatric bed. Six weeks before, she had celebrated her thirteenth birthday. At that age, she was still a little girl, but the terrifying things she'd experienced over the past year made her look older than her seventeen-year-old sister Laura.

Sarah's favourite paediatric nurse came into the room carrying a sterile dressing pack. After rubbing Sarah's back and washing her face and hands, the nurse deftly removed the narcotic IV from the Sarah's forearm and placed a brightly coloured band-aid over the puncture. She then carefully peeled back a piece of plastic film from an adhesive patch and placed it on to Sarah's skin just under her collarbone. Finally, she readjusted the girl's hospital gown and smiled. 'The patches should take care of the pain now', she said. 'You'll be able to go home soon'.

Sarah looked gloomy because she knew that would never happen. She was a long way from home, and would probably never again see the farm in New South Wales where she had lived all her life. 'I'm not going home', she explained sadly. 'I'm going to my Aunt's and Uncle's house at Yarra Junction'.

The nurse sensed a story there, especially since Sarah was terminal and did not have long to go. 'Oh, that's nice. Will your family be there?'

Sarah struggled to sit up. 'Not all of them. Just Mum and Dad, my sisters and brother and a few others'.

'Here, let me help you, honey'. The nurse smiled and gently propped pillows behind her back. She was feather light, but her distended abdomen made it difficult for her to sit up straight. When she'd finished, the nurse went to the hand-basin and pumped the soap dispenser. 'There you go; I'll tell your Mum she can come in again', she said as she dried her hands with a paper towel.

Sarah strained to shift her swollen legs. The fluid had settled in the tissues and left dents in her skin. 'Mum's upstairs resting. She just came out of the hospital a few days ago'.

The nurse gave such a pitying look that Sarah noticed it.

'Do you know what?' asked Sarah.

'What'.

Sarah looked wistfully out of the window. 'I like this hospital more than all the others'.

The nurse smiled warmly. She sensed Sarah's pain, but could not know the real meaning of what the girl had just said. She waited for Sarah to elaborate.

Instead, Sarah gazed out the window across the Melbourne city business district. Lately, she didn't bother to explain any more. What had gone on over the previous two years would take far too long to tell, and most people would not believe it anyway.

When Sarah's father, Mark, appeared in the doorway, the nurse waved him in and left them to enjoy each other's company.

Mark's solid muscle came from hard work on the family's country property rather than from the gym. He was a traditional Australian country-bred man; gentle and slow to rile but ferociously protective if anyone threatened his family. In his hand, he clutched a bottle of Sarah's favourite ginger ale. She had not been able to keep much down and he hoped it would lift her spirits. He settled back into his chair beside her bed. She seemed preoccupied.

'What's up Jogue?' he asked, using the nickname he had given her as a baby.

Several times Sarah moved her dry lips before giving up. Finally, she wet them and closed her eyes. Mark thought she'd fallen asleep again. He rested his leather boot on the wheel of her bed before picking up the Melbourne Age and leafing through it.

'Dad?' murmured Sarah.

'Yes Sarah?' He put down the paper. She had his full attention.

'I want you to promise me something'. Sarah held down the corner of her pillow to see him better.

'I'll try my best', he said, as leaned forward to hear. In the past few days, her voice had become faint.

Sarah was wide-awake. 'Seriously Dad, I want you promise me this'.

Mark only hoped he could give her what she wanted. 'What is it?' he asked gently.

'Remember what they did to me?' she asked. '...those people in suits and the other doctors?'

Mark tensed. He knew very well what they had done to his daughter, and he would never rest until he found out why it happened to her.

Sarah gave him a piercing look and asked him to grant her a wish so enormous that he did not know if he could ever make it happen – but he promised it anyway.

Sarah relaxed the instant Mark took her load on his shoulders. When she drifted off to sleep, he planned to go downstairs to the cafeteria for a bite to eat. He had to get out for a while and think about what his daughter had asked him to do.

After dinner, he planned to go to the upstairs parents' accommodation to find out how his wife was feeling. They'd all had a rough time over the past 16 months, but Dianne had collapsed with a seriously inflamed leg and spent a few days at the hospital down the road.

An hour later, Mark balanced the meal tray in one hand, while opening the door with the other. Di was just waking up and looked fragile. Her long chestnut hair had come down from the loose roll she usually had it swept in.

Mark put the plate of cold roast beef on the table and sat on the bed beside her.

Di looked gloomy. 'Mark. Could I ask you something?'

'You can, but I'm pretty well all out of answers', he replied. The session with Sarah earlier had his mind reeling.

'Do you think she would have lived longer if –'

'Yes I do', he interrupted. 'If they hadn't done what they did'. Mark felt the bitterness again. He reached over to the bedside table and transferred the plate to Di's bed. 'You'd better eat something', he said, offering her the cutlery. 'We have to stay strong for Sarah over the next few days'.

PARADISE LOST

Ah, to think how thin the veil that lies between
The pain of hell and Paradise.

George William Russell

Sarah Westley was the third of Mark and Di's six children. She grew up in a homestead built by her great-grandfather which stood on the land her forebears had carved out of wilderness in the days when Australia was still an English colony. Few children had such close links to their heritage.

Sarah came from sturdy stock, descended from the earliest European pioneers who settled Australia's eastern regions. Her English ancestor, George Westley, lived in Victorian England until the late 1800s when his sense of adventure led him to Australia. After a long and treacherous sea voyage to what was considered the ends of the earth, George found his way to the one horse town of Gloucester, in a scenic corner of New South Wales. The region was within sight of the Barrington Tops mountain ranges and criss-crossed by pristine rivers. There he bought a parcel of freehold land in 1890 and put down his roots into what was still untamed wilderness. The time was ten years before Federation when Australia was preparing to close the chapter on its colonial incarnation and renounce its convict past. Moves were afoot to draft a Constitution and Australia was on the way to becoming a nation, which finally occurred when Britain passed the Commonwealth of Australia Constitution Act (UK) on 5 July 1900. The official proclamation of the Commonwealth of Australia, made on 1 January 1901, founded Australia's nationhood as a free country.

Over the next years, George hand-cleared his land and bred up a dairy herd. His own family grew almost yearly and before too long he and his wife were raising eleven children. Meanwhile the town of Gloucester expanded from the timber industry, farming, and mining in the region. In 1905, local businessmen built two hotels to water thirsty locals. Country pubs always proved a financial success and a reliable sign the town was there to stay. In 1906, the Barrington Butter Factory opened as a co-operative. Before too long, cultural patrons financed the School of Arts. The town's first newspaper, the Gloucester Advocate, followed, and proved so successful it still circulates today. The railway finally opened the town to tourists and commerce, and from 1913 onward Gloucester was on the map as a thriving regional centre.

In the ten years after Federation, George Westley's clan thrived and, despite the lack of modern conveniences, the family was robustly healthy and prolific. His son went on to produce five children; one of them became the father of Sarah's grandfather, James Westley.

Sarah's grandfather preferred to call himself Jim. Like his forebears, he was a tall hardworking lad, who could cut a tree into firewood in no time – even before the advent of chain saws. In keeping with the Australian country tradition, he carried on working the family dairy farm for his parents and, like most dairy farmers; he took few days off and no holidays. In the mid 1960s, he met Ruth. It took a family occasion to get them together – the wedding of Jim's youngest sister and Ruth's brother.

Ruth was a natural beauty who always managed to look neat and tidy, even in a gale. She had the common sense of two people and seemed to come up with a sensible solution to any problem. She'd grown up on her family's dairy farm at Murwillumbah in northern New South Wales and shared Jim's family values.

After their wedding, Jim brought his new bride to the family homestead. By then Jim's forbears had built a couple of cottages on the original parcel of land. Jim and Ruth started married life in their own home, but the drought year kept them both busy ensuring the stock had enough food and water. Fortunately, the cows still gave enough milk for their own needs and in those days the bush and streams were full of game, fish, and bush tucker. No one went hungry then – provided they were a half-decent shot with a .22. Before too long the young couple was self-sufficient; Ruth had planted a vegetable garden and Jim bought a truck, and started his own business-carting cattle around the district. They both welcomed children and did not have long to wait.

The couple's first-born was Mark, who would grow up to become Sarah's father. By the time he was six; young Mark already had five siblings, including a set of twins. Mark and his siblings grew up during the 1960s and 1970s. The family produced and grew much of what they consumed and it gave the kids a sense of freedom and self-sufficiency. By the time Mark was 12 he could cut firewood, farm, hunt rabbits, and fish – and he knew enough about carpentry to build houses. From his father Mark learnt to gauge if someone was telling the truth. Jim taught him to find out all the facts before making an agreement. In the bush, a deal done on a handshake was firmer than any paper contract, and it had no backdoor clause. Country folk had a tradition of honouring their promises, or their reputation was spoilt. In small towns, people had long memories.

Like his father, Mark never took up going to the pub. He grew up to be a quiet, dependable type, who wasn't afraid of hard work. Before his 21st birthday, Mark enrolled in a welding course at the Taree Community College.

Mark's sister had already enrolled at the school and was enjoying a horticulture class. She had befriended Dianne, a shy fellow student, and the two girls hung out together.

Mark soon noticed his sister's friend, but was too shy to ask her on a date. Instead, Di invited him home to meet her family. Dianne and her family had moved up to New South Wales from Melbourne and her parents started a business in the NSW country town. They liked Mark at first sight and after getting to know him, they accepted an invitation to meet his parents. From then on, Dianne and her parents went on holidays to Gloucester and camped on the river at the Westley property. There, the respective families got to know each other, while the young couple eased into a courtship.

Dianne had a wholesome, innocent beauty with piercing blue eyes and fine chestnut hair that she swept back and held in place with pins. She valued economy of words and shortened her name to Di. Under the surface lay talent in handicrafts, photography, and music, which she was too shy to show off in her younger years. Her vulnerability made Mark want to protect her and soon Di overcame her shyness around Mark – while her smile captivated him.

In January 1987, Mark and Di were married at Wingham, a charming old-world country town in the Manning valley. The day turned out one of the hottest days on record with temperatures soaring up to 46° C, but nobody seemed to mind. Dozens of guests from both families mixed happily. The young couple enjoyed the banquet, and left the festivities radiant, fully expecting a wonderful future.

Like his father before him, Mark eventually brought his bride to the homestead. They moved into the main house while Ruth and Jim shifted into a smaller cottage about 8 km away on the family allotment. The young couple also welcomed children and soon were blessed. Their first child, Laura, was born nine months later. A placid baby with an English complexion and a thatch of untamed hair like her father, Laura was an early talker and a born nurturer who mothered any creature, whether it needed it or not. As soon as she was old enough, she dressed the farm cat's kittens in her doll's clothes and paraded them around the yard in her toy pram.

With Laura's arrival, Di started her hobby of quilting, smocking, and sewing, and proudly wheeled her firstborn around town in a pram while grocery shopping, with the baby dressed to the nines in hand-made dresses.

Laura was two years old when Mark and Di's second daughter was born late in 1989. Clara was the image of Di; a classic beauty with naturally rosy cheeks, she was shy but good-natured. She rarely complained and easily gave in to stronger personalities for the sake of peace. Laura was delighted to have a real baby around for a change. She gave up dressing the cats and wheeled Clara around instead.

Each child's arrival increased Mark's enthusiasm for fatherhood. He relished time with his children and instinctively recognised their individual personalities. Before they were out of nappies, he gave them each a distinctive nickname. For Clara it was 'Tiger', while he nicknamed Laura 'Laula'.

Since the young couple already had two placid little girls, Di was sure she was tempting fate when she announced that number three was on the way.

On the first day of spring, September 1 1991, Mark drove Di to Gloucester hospital when her labour started with their third child. He stayed with Di throughout the labour and birth, as he did with all their children. However, soon after the baby girl was born, she looked cheekily around as if she was ready to take on the world, before becoming frustrated at having to learn the most basic skills first. For a week, the little girl had no name, while the parents deliberated. Finally, when Mark took Di and the baby home, they walked into the homestead with her, and it came to them that her name was to be 'Sarah'.

From the beginning Sarah was the most healthy and robust of the children, rarely down with coughs or colds. Long before she was old enough to know about pecking orders, Sarah asserted natural leadership, even over her two older sisters. While Clara didn't seem to mind, it predictably caused some struggles between Sarah and her eldest sister, Laura.

Mark soon gave Sarah the nickname of 'Rogue', a label she'd earned with her unconventional and fearless approach to life. When Clara couldn't pronounce the letter 'r', Sarah became known as 'Jogue'. She not only kept her parents busy but also her two older sisters, who could hardly keep up with her as she set out to explore the world in record time.

When Sarah was two, Hannah was born. Her father nicknamed her 'Grub'. At first, the two sisters looked nothing alike. Hannah was blonder with chocolate brown eyes and a slenderer face. Being Sarah's younger sister, Hannah became Sarah's apprentice prankster in the early years and the more time they spent together, the more similar they looked. In later years, Hannah's talents shone in writing and art. She had her first poetry published at the age of 13.

Leah was next. A quiet but determined child, Leah was small, almost fragile and she caught every sniffle going round. As the youngest girl, her father nicknamed her 'Tot'. She loved art and music but was never partial to housework. In time, she made a mockery of her nickname. Tot loved playing rough sports and wasn't shy about tackling boys twice her size on the football field.

Just as Mark and Di had all but given up on having a boy, Joshua arrived in 1997. He quickly earned the nickname of 'Dude' and turned out a miniature version of Mark. From the time baby Dude was old enough to stand, he stood like his father, with feet square apart and planted to the ground. The two were inseparable and went on outings in the utility together from the time Joshua was still in nappies.

Once the two older girls started school, they were away from home most of the day. Sarah was lonely at first, but soon discovered the joys of spending time with her grandparents, Jim and Ruth. By the age of three, Sarah was Ruth's helper in the dairy. Jim kept a Jersey cow in the house paddock for the family's own use, and she needed milking each day. That meant creaming and butter churning every afternoon. Sarah learnt early on that cows didn't take a day off and neither did dairy farmers.

One day Ruth had just scalded a large bowlful of cream and set it aside to cool while she went off to do other chores. Sarah was curious about what was in the bowl. She up-ended a bucket and used it as a step to peer over the kitchen counter. Just when she caught a glimpse of the cream, she overbalanced – toppling off the bucket and up ending the bowl. The cream splashed up the tiles, ran over the counter, and dripped to the floor, forming a large puddle on the old linoleum. As usual, Sarah had a guardian angel who must have stepped in at the crucial moment, buffering her fall.

When Ruth returned to investigate the commotion, she saw Sarah dangling by her pinafore, which had caught up in the kitchen sideboard's handle. Sarah was suspended over a creamy yellow puddle by nothing but a thin, perished elastic band– with not a drop on her. By 4 pm, Ruth was usually relieved to take Sarah home again, but Sarah was still full of beans and ready to take on her sisters Clara and Laura when they came home from school.

Over the next ten years, Mark and Di's growing brood outgrew the old farmhouse. The children each wanted their own bedroom when they got older, and Mark's building skills came in handy when he had to build on additions. He gutted the bottom floor and rebuilt it with timbers from his land, adding on several bedrooms and a study. When he'd finished the ground floor, he raised the roof and fashioned a cathedral ceiling, spanning an open hardwood beam across the living room ceiling to support the upstairs floor. Next, he built several upstairs bedrooms for Joshua and the girls. Inside a year, Mark had transformed the old cottage to a rambling two-story homestead with a pair of French doors leading out to a wide veranda where the kids could play on rainy days. To save on power, Mark equipped the living room with a wood stove and installed a wood-fuelled boiler into the country kitchen to heat the never-ending water supply pumped up from the river. For years, life was idyllic. Mark put up a swing in the yard for the girls and built a tree house in the Jacaranda tree for Joshua. On sunny days, the kids played in the yard and when it rained, they played under the veranda. Mark and Di had trained a grapevine around it, which sprouted thick bunches of Shiraz grapes each autumn.

The family's main income came from Mark's work at the local mine where he drove heavy earth-moving equipment, but he preferred to spend time on his farm. He constantly studied sustainable agriculture until he succeeded in raising organic crops without chemical fertilisers or pesticides. In return for Mark's careful husbandry, the land rewarded the family with a constant supply of fresh organic food almost year-round. To Mark land conservation made perfect sense when he learnt the Aboriginal people also believed the health of the land directly affected the health of the people living on it.

The young Westley family, like the generations before them, had a good reputation in the district. The children did well at school, regularly winning art and music prizes. The family had never caused any trouble and no local cop ever had reason to come to their door. By all accounts, they were solid citizens with sober habits.

For a decade, the six Westley children grew up in unfettered freedom without fear of anyone. They knew nothing of stranger danger and chatted with anyone. School friends, neighbours, and relatives dropped in to share meals with the family. Sometimes Di fed over a dozen people at the dinner table. She did her own home cooking and always found time to bake birthday cakes for the kids.

Sarah's eleventh birthday fell on Sunday September 1. It was the first day of spring and the laughing Kookaburra outside her bedroom window woke Sarah up early. She rubbed her eyes, threw back the covers, and rushed to the window for a glimpse of the culprit. The speckled bird sat on the railing fence with his bill wide open as if he'd just laughed at his own joke. Sarah thought he looked like a stand-up comic and burst out giggling.

From her upstairs window, Sarah could survey her own private world of changing seasons. She loved the springtime best. Mauve blossoms hung like ripe grapes from the Jacarandas. The Bottlebrush trees along the fence line were laden with orange pollen. Her father's winter oats were ripening down on the river flats. The farm cat dragged her new litter to a sunny place to keep warm, when they still had their eyes closed. Sarah always kept an eye on the winding gravel road that led to the rear of the property, in case her grandparents' car appeared over the rise; she couldn't wait to run out to greet them when it did. On the far side of the road was the river. After a heavy rain, the water roared, and turned foamy white. Loud storms and thunder excited her, especially when they rattled the windows. She loved propping herself on the windowsill and gazing outside for hours. Even in the pouring rain, there was always something to see.

This particular morning a movement caught Sarah's eye in the backyard below. She pressed her face against the window for a better look and saw Brutus, her Black Angus pet calf, stomping around the garden. He had pushed through the open gate and was eating her mother's petunias again. Di had only just freshly replanted them after the calf had devoured the last batch of marigolds a few weeks earlier. Sarah knew her mother would be angry with her. The kids were told to keep the gate shut. Her sister Laura had reminded her just last night and she'd forgotten. She would have to sneak downstairs and get him out of there before anyone noticed.

Sarah didn't get very far before she saw her youngest sister and brother in her doorway.

'Happy Birthday!' yelled five-year-old Joshua as he jumped on Sarah's back and tried to wrestle her to the floor.

'We've got a present for you!' added seven-year-old Leah as she landed a tackle on her sister.

Sarah worked hard at keeping a straight face. 'Get off me, you two', she yelled as she told the little ones off while trying not to laugh. 'I've got things to do'.

'Can we come?' they asked.

'No way', said Sarah as she freed herself from their grasp and escaped through the doorway. She flew down the stairs in her nightie with the two youngest kids in pursuit.

The commotion woke up Hannah who'd been fast asleep in her downstairs bedroom. She wandered out of her room with her hair standing up. 'What are you duffers doing?' she muttered sleepily.

At the foot of the stairs, Sarah met another surprise. Her mother and two older sisters, Laura and Clara, were already preparing her favourite pancakes. Brightly wrapped presents lay on the table and purple balloons bobbed around the kitchen and dining room. Sarah had tried to be quiet, but it was too late now; her entire family had already spotted her. Even her father – who'd worked the night shift – had woken up and stood in the hallway.

'Happy Birthday, Jogue!' came a chorus of voices.

Fifteen-year-old Laura sprinted to the piano and started a jazzed up rendition of 'Happy Birthday'. Sarah was just beginning to enjoy the attention when through the living room window she spotted the black cow face of Brutus who had paused from his flower eating to see what the fuss was. Something told her he might even walk up the veranda steps and come into the house as he'd done before, a stunt that would land her in even bigger trouble. For a while, Sarah looked like a rabbit caught in the headlights – hoping her 200 kg pet would stay out of sight. For now, she would have to act normal and blow out the candles.

When Di went to get a knife from the kitchen to cut the cake, she discovered the calf in the garden and made a terrible fuss about her ruined flowerbeds. To appease her parents, Sarah promised after breakfast to lead him far away from the house into the top paddock where he would cause no more trouble. She promised in future to always close the gate. Mark and Di looked at each other amused; neither had the heart to tell Sarah off on her birthday.

After breakfast, Sarah made good on her promise to take the calf to greener pastures. When Hannah begged to go with her, Di sensed trouble and sent Clara to supervise.

'Watch out for snakes. It's spring and they're just waking up', warned Di as Sarah set off with Brutus and her two sisters.

The kids giggled and fobbed off their mother's warning.

Di shook her head. 'How many times do I have to tell that girl to wear shoes', she muttered as she closed the door and went back to washing the dishes with Laura.

Sarah liked to walk barefoot on the property all year around. It didn't bother her that on the first hot day, poisonous brown snakes and black snakes came out of winter hibernation cranky and looking for food.

On their way up the hill, nine-year-old Hannah stayed close to Sarah, hoping to cook up some fun with her older sister, while Clara lagged behind looking worried. She wasn't so sure she could handle the two younger ones – especially if Sarah had one of her bright ideas. She needed some backup, but Muttley and Pooch; the black cattle dogs were on their chains, waiting for Mark to work cattle with them later that morning.

The three girls and Brutus ambled up the hill past the two dams their father had dug out that winter. The recent rains had filled them to the brim and they were swimming with wild ducks.

'We should catch some of those ducks', said Sarah.

Hannah thought it was a great idea.

'What for?' asked Clara, trying to prevent another one of Sarah's ideas from getting out of hand.

'So they could lay us some eggs', answered Sarah.

'Yea!' agreed Hannah as though struck by a sudden revelation.

When Brutus continued his way up the path, the girls forgot about their plan and followed him up to the hill where they sat down to take in the distant mountain view of the Barrington Tops. Sarah lay on the soft grass with her eyes closed. The sun was warm on her face and she loved the cool breeze coming off the mountain ranges. Hannah copied Sarah in mock enjoyment, while Brutus stood sniffing the air before scooping up a bunch of wild daisies.

'How come you like it up here so much?' asked Clara

'I just do', said Sarah. 'Because it's my mountain', she giggled.

'No it's not', insisted Clara.

'Yes it is. Don't you know – it's called Sarah's Hill and this is my horse'. Sarah pointed to Brutus.

'Rubbish', murmured Clara.

With that, Sarah got up and took a running leap onto the calf's back. She missed and fell heavily to the ground. For a time she lay there in pain holding her belly, while the calf patiently waited for Sarah to try again.

'What do you think you're doing?' asked Clara.

'I was going to ride Brutus over to Grandma Ruth's', said Sarah as she dusted herself off. 'But I think I'll walk instead'.

The other sisters were not thrilled about walking 8 km across the paddock to their grandparent's house, so they headed back home.

An hour later, Ruth and Jim weren't at all surprised to see barefoot Sarah walking up their path. She had run the distance many times before and could have found her way there at night with her eyes closed, without getting lost. They drove Sarah back home just in time for the family lunch.

That night Sarah went to bed early. It wasn't like her to be the first one down.

During the next six weeks, Sarah went to school and was up to her usual pranks, but Muttley behaved increasingly oddly around her. Di could not even tell Sarah off occasionally without Muttley growling at her. The dog even tried to keep Sarah's siblings away from her. With strangers, he was fierce, and when no one was around, the dog stayed by Sarah's side as if protecting her from invisible enemies. It seemed strange, since the family had never made enemies. The children felt perfectly safe; they had scores of acres just to themselves, where no one had ever bothered them. Meanwhile, Muttley for reasons of his own stepped up his watch. He was an ugly brute, but he and Sarah had an understanding.

In late November, Sarah seemed under the weather for a few days. Di worried when she came home from school with a nosebleed, and kept her home. The following day was Saturday and Mark worked outside in the afternoon, digging another dam. A rural doctor shortage made it difficult for Mark to get an appointment on short notice and the local surgery was mostly closed on Saturdays. Sarah rested quietly at home for the day, but late that evening Mark and Di noticed her abdomen seemed distended. Mark tried several times to contact the family doctor that night and finally arranged to take Sarah to the small community hospital at Gloucester, some distance away. Meanwhile Di had no choice but to stay home with the other five children. By the time Mark changed out of his work clothes and showered, it was past 11 pm and Sarah had fallen asleep. With Sarah seemingly comfortable for the time being, the parents decided to wait until morning rather than take the long journey over rough gravel roads in the dark. Overnight, they took turns getting up to check on Sarah – who slept through the entire night, though somewhat restlessly.

Early next morning Sarah's tummy was still distended with what looked like an irregular lump. Her skin felt clammy, and she complained of pain around both sides of her upper and lower abdomen. Around 7 am, Mark drove Sarah over winding unsealed roads to the community hospital. They arrived at 8 am and were met by their family doctor, who examined Sarah and told Mark he suspected a distended or blocked bladder. He sought Mark's permission to catheterise Sarah, which Mark agreed to immediately. Sarah had never experienced an examination on a private area of her body, but the female nurses carried out the procedure efficiently, and were respectful of Sarah's modesty. The catheter produced no significant amount of urine drainage, and the problem lump remained. The family GP was puzzled but not concerned enough about Sarah's condition to call an ambulance. However, he did advise Mark to drive Sarah to the next large hospital, a better-equipped facility over an hour away.

Mark left the community hospital and rushed Sarah to the next hospital, using the most direct back road connecting the two townships. Mark took each bend carefully and checked Sarah often. She was slumped in the front seat with her eyes closed. He checked her seatbelt and tipped her seat back a fraction before flicking on the car air-conditioner. It was only midmorning, but already the sun was as hot as high noon. An unsettling northwester from the outback swept hot winds across the road, carrying debris in its path. Already November 2002, was becoming one of the hottest on record. As a volunteer fire fighter, Mark had spent the past week putting out spot fires in the district. Between fire fighting and working at the mine, he was starting to feel worse for wear. With Sarah sick, he was running on raw nerves.

In the seat next to him, Sarah was unusually quiet. Whatever she had in her belly was knocking her flat. Occasionally she opened her eyes and smiled a little, but Mark knew she was only trying to reassure him and it made him feel even worse. The poor kid needed to be in the hospital. Mark put the gearshift into overdrive and stepped on the accelerator. If the police stopped him, he would ask them to escort them with their sirens on, so he could flatten the pedal.

An hour later, Mark carried Sarah into the emergency department (ED) of the larger district hospital. The desk clerk stared at the sick child and took down a volume of personal information and medical details from Mark, including their family doctor's contact number. Mark handed over the GP's letter, and before too long the clerk called a nurse and asked her to show them to a cubicle. Sarah climbed on to the emergency room trolley and curled up under the sheets.

After a few minutes, a young looking male doctor parted the curtains and came into the cubicle to take Sarah's medical history. When Mark told him about Sarah's abdominal lump, he called over a female doctor to conduct the physical examination. Both doctors were involved in taking a medical history, noting that Sarah had a temperature of 38.4° C on arrival and that she had been vomiting that morning. The female doctor examined Sarah's abdominal area and chest while the young male doctor stood in the background. Mark noted the name on his hospital ID was Dr. Blake. Despite the female doctor's gentle approach, Sarah winced with pain when she examined the lump. She then asked Sarah if she'd started her menstrual periods or if she had had any discharge. Mark wasn't sure how much sex-education Sarah had received from Di or from the school and he wanted Di to be there before they went too much further with their line of questioning. By now, all eyes were on Sarah. It was obvious no one had asked her these questions before, and after a short explanation about what those words meant, Sarah answered 'No'.

Both doctors conferred in the cubicle's corner for a moment before the female doctor returned to question Sarah about boyfriends.

Despite feeling desperately ill, Sarah was annoyed by the question. 'No! I've never had a boyfriend!' she growled, before pulling up the sheets.

The female doctor exposed Sarah's chest and abdomen again to check her development. She noted that the child had no signs of puberty, before both doctors retreated to the staff office for further discussions.

When they were gone, Mark noticed that Sarah looked bewildered. He pulled the sheet up and sat on the chair beside her. Sarah put one corner of the sheet into her mouth like a comforter. She had never been inside a hospital before and warily looked at the array of tubes and wires leading from the wall.

Sarah took the sheet corner out of her mouth. 'Hey Dad, what are they asking me that stuff for?' she whispered.

Mark tried to sound reassuring for Sarah's sake. 'They need to know these things to find out how to help you', he explained.

In the ED office, Blake took charge and wrote up the clinical records. He noted that Sarah 'looks lethargic', and had a 'palpable mass in the lower abdomen', with tenderness over the left kidney area. The mass 'feels like uterine fundus at umbilicus'. It meant he suspected Sarah of being pregnant. After this entry, the doctor noted that Sarah had no discharge or bleeding. He further noted she had no signs of puberty or adult development, an observation that made a pregnancy unlikely or even physically impossible.[1] He ordered blood tests including a βHCG (beta human chorionic gonadotropin) test. A positive result is both an indicator for pregnancy in women of childbearing age and a tumour marker denoting a germ cell tumour – a class of tumours that can arise from ovarian or testicular tissue in children. After he had recorded his pregnancy suspicions, the doctor ordered an abdominal ultrasound, a test that would discover the exact nature of Sarah's lump. Unfortunately, it was Sunday afternoon and no

---

[1] Cases of pregnancy in young girls have been documented in the medical literature, but all have been associated with precocious puberty – a condition clearly absent in Sarah.

one was on duty at the imaging department to carry out the scan. Most hospitals have technicians on call that are available for urgent cases, but in Sarah's case the doctors chose to wait until the imaging department reopened at 9 am Monday morning.

Mark had just calmed Sarah down when Dr Blake returned and summoned him to a quiet corner.

'Is your daughter sexually active?' asked the young doctor unexpectedly.

Mark was appalled. 'What? No! What do you mean?'

'Does she have a male friend?'

'No of course not – she's only a child!' Mark felt outraged at such a question.

'Are you sure?' the doctor persisted.

'Of course I'm sure. She doesn't leave our supervision, except to go to school'. Mark was starting to want some answers of his own. 'What on earth makes you suspect that? What have you found?' he asked.

'Nothing – yet', replied the doctor.

Mark forced himself to keep his voice down for Sarah's sake. 'Listen', he said struggling to remain calm. 'You're the doctor – but aren't there some tests you need to do before we go off in the wrong direction? Is there someone else I could talk to?'

'I'm the senior doctor on today', replied Blake. 'And we'll be keeping your daughter here to run whatever tests are needed'. With that, the doctor headed for his office.

Mark watched Blake retreat down the hallway. The doctor looked barely in his late twenties and he did not seem very experienced, but he was clearly on a mission and it made Mark uneasy. Was there something they weren't telling him? Wasn't there a supervisor he could talk to? Didn't senior doctors usually handle these matters? He returned to Sarah's cubicle visibly shaken and leaned on the bedside chair to steady himself.

Sarah squinted at her father. Her fever had spiked again, and the fluorescent light hurt her eyes. 'What's wrong Dad?' she croaked.

'I have to ask you something and I need you to tell me the truth', said Mark somberly.

'Sure Dad'.

'And I promise not to get angry with you. Okay?' he added.

Sarah sat up a fraction. She had not seen her father this serious before.

Mark took a deep breath. 'Have you ever had a boyfriend...or has anyone ever touched your private parts?'

Sarah burst out laughing. 'No. Never! I hate boys. They're too silly'.

'It's no laughing matter Sarah'.

'Dad, now you're starting to sound as weird as everybody else around here. I've never had a boyfriend in my life'. Sarah curled up again. Her stomach was hurting and she ached for some rest.

Moments later, a different female intern arrived and made several unsuccessful attempts to draw blood. Sarah became so annoyed by the fourth try that the young doctor called in a more senior doctor who drew the sample at the first go and sent it to the lab. While the doctors waited for the results, the ED got busy with accident patients arriving, and two nurses arrived to wheel Sarah into another cubicle farther away where it was calmer.

Two hours later the lab faxed Sarah's blood results to the ED staff office, where they immediately captured Dr Blake's interest. The βHCG test was elevated, denoting a germ cell tumour in a child. In a woman of childbearing age, the test could also denote an early pregnancy. Immediately the doctor discounted the childhood tumour markers and presumed a pregnancy, even though Sarah had no signs of puberty.

According to the medical literature, in prepubertal girls, a mass arising from the pelvic cavity (an adnexal mass) has an 80 per cent likelihood of being a tumour and warrants prompt ultrasound evaluation and immediate referral to a surgical specialist.[2] In Sarah's case, the pelvic mass had arisen from the ovary to become sizeable tumour, which was already causing symptoms of torsion or twisting. This accounted for Sarah's severe pain, vomiting, sweating and fever. These late signs indicate that pressure from the tumour is impairing blood supply to the pelvic organs and to the tumour itself, leading to tissue death (necrosis) and infection [3] – a fact that was confirmed later. In a prepubertal girl, an adnexal mass of such enormous size, causing these symptoms, constitutes a surgical emergency where best practice involves an immediate ultrasound or scan, and a surgical assessment. While waiting for specialist intervention, the usual ED protocol includes intravenous rehydrating fluids and sufficient narcotic medications to achieve pain relief.[4] If the hospital is une-

---

[2] Curtin 1994, Russell 1995, Brooks 1994, Morrow 1993.
[3] Adams, Hillard. Obstetrics and Gynecology Consult, Lippincot 2008.
[4] Juretzka 2008

quipped to handle this urgent condition, the patient is normally airlifted or otherwise urgently transferred to a larger hospital with specialist facilities.

Instead, Dr Blake discussed his pregnancy suspicions with other ED doctors and decided to order a Doppler to detect the baby's 'foetal heartbeat'.

Before too long, two nurses moved Sarah back to a cubicle closer to the central nurse's station. They then brought in the Doppler machine, pulled down the covers and swept the wand over Sarah's exposed abdomen. The Doppler is designed to detect the weakest foetal heartbeat from as early as 10 weeks gestation. In Sarah's case, the machine was silent. There was no sound from the mass, which had, if anything enlarged since the examinations and palpations. Despite finding nothing resembling a baby on the Doppler, Dr Blake wrote the next entry in the clinical notes: 'Most likely an intra-uterine pregnancy, βHCG-producing tumour unlikely but possible'.

With Sarah now in significant pain from the tumour, Dr Blake contacted the New South Wales child protection department (DoCS). [5] To the caseworker on the phone, the doctor reported that Sarah was an 11-year-old girl likely to be pregnant. The doctor's report to the department, before waiting for the scan results, would prove to have far-reaching effects.

Next, Blake phoned Dr Little, the paediatric ward registrar. Little was older and more experienced, but appeared to accept the pregnancy idea and told the resident he would come down to ED for further discussions.

Meanwhile in Sarah's cubicle, the constant flow of staff walking past and peering through the curtains disturbed Mark, but he was even more concerned about Sarah's condition. Her face felt hot and her mouth was so dry, she could hardly speak. She had vomited several times that morning and he was worried she was getting dehydrated. He had asked a nurse on the morning shift to bring her a glass of water, but it was now late afternoon and nothing came. Finally, a nurse arrived with a glass of water and a paracetamol tablet. Sarah took it and Mark waited for it to work, but after half an hour, she was still feverish and in pain. He was afraid Sarah was getting worse.

Meanwhile Dr Little walked across from the children's ward to the ED and briefly glanced into Sarah's cubicle on the way to the staff office. He met Dr Blake and the two doctors had a lengthy discussion about Sarah. The doctors agreed to conduct further pregnancy related tests. Instead of calling in a radiographer to carry out an emergency scan confirming whether there was in

---

[5] DoCS is an acronym for the New South Wales Department of Community Services, also known as Child Protection Services (CPS) in other countries.

fact a pregnancy, the doctors thought Sarah should be tested for venereal diseases, including HIV. Dr Blake wrote these orders in Sarah's clinical notes while Dr Little returned to the paediatric ward to conduct further research into Sarah's history.

It was nearly six o'clock on Sunday evening when the Westley's family doctor received a call on his mobile phone. Dr Little from the hospital introduced himself to the GP and told him that Sarah was pregnant. After waiting for the GP to get over his initial shock, Dr Little asked him to help identify the possible 'perpetrator'.

The GP had only that morning examined Sarah and not even suspected a pregnancy. Now a hospital registrar told him this was so and the GP assumed all the necessary tests had been done to confirm the diagnosis. The registrar wanted confidential information from the family GP.

In 2001, the Federal Privacy Act came into effect, preventing anyone from obtaining a patient's medical information without the patient's written permission. This also prevented anyone from legally handing over a patient's medical or personal information, without the patient's consent – or in Sarah's case, the parents' consent.

However, without obtaining the parents' consent, the family GP gave out personal and medical information about Sarah, the parents and the entire family.

The GP told Dr Little that he had delivered the family's children but had not seen much of them since they weren't sick very often. He claimed the family belonged to a particular religion and that Di had suffered from mild postnatal depression after giving birth to the youngest child, for which she chose natural medicine remedies. Since both doctors were discussing the family in the context of Sarah's purported pregnancy, over the course of the discussion, the family's most innocent activities seemed to take on a sinister façade. From the discussions flowed several untrue and unfounded stories: the family was part of a religious fundamental sect, Di's postnatal depression was more like a psychosis, and a sexual perpetrator was on the loose and needed to be identified. In fact, the family belonged to no church or organised religion, Di was not and had never been psychotic and Sarah was not pregnant. However, various medical staff subsequently recorded these unfounded rumours as facts into Sarah's permanent clinical record as well as into the discharge summary document. These tales would turn out to have tragic and far-reaching consequences for the family as they followed them through the hospital system.

Downstairs in the ED, Mark looked around the cubicle for a washer to wet Sarah's face but couldn't find one. He was disturbed that no one offered Sarah any practical help. He tried his best to help her, but she was more lethargic by the hour, and lay curled up in the foetal position. Mark glanced at his watch. He had brought Sarah in six hours ago and so far, doctors had only asked them questions about sex. He had a mind to take Sarah and walk out. He thought about driving her to a large Sydney hospital. It was a 300 km drive that would take four hours, but surely, there was some place with a scanner in the city, where the doctors could find out what was causing Sarah's lump. Mark was about to get Sarah ready to leave when Dr Blake and the female ED doctor returned with a third doctor in tow. They called Mark out of the cubicle and into the far corner of the unit for another discussion. This time Mark braced himself. From the looks on their faces, he expected to hear something unpleasant.

'Your daughter is about 14 weeks' pregnant', announced Dr Blake.

'What?' exclaimed Mark. 'Are you sure about that?'

'Yes, and we are going to have to question Sarah about it', said the other doctor.

'And we have a duty to call the social worker and child protection', added Blake, who had already made the call from his office.

Mark was speechless. 'You want to interrogate my daughter again? And call child protection?'

'We're required by law to report these things', insisted Blake.

Mark wondered if any of these doctors had any common sense. 'What things? You haven't even done an ultrasound! None of you know what that lump is – even I know that and I'm not a doctor!'

'We're just doing our job', said the female doctor.

'Your jobs are not to go off half cocked', said Mark. 'And I won't allow it'.

The doctors were shocked. 'What do you mean?' they asked.

'I won't give you permission to question Sarah again until she has the ultrasound and we know what the lump really is', said Mark. 'And if the test shows she's pregnant then call your social workers and everyone you want. But until then, stop with the weird questions and do something to help her. Can't you see how sick she is?'

The three doctors discussed it among themselves before heading back to the office where Blake wrote an addition into the clinical notes:

Father aware of all results and implications, has requested Sarah not be told of results or questioned regarding sexual history until results of ultrasound confirm a pregnancy, father will discuss with Sarah's mother. Father understands need for social worker/DoCS involvement if pregnancy confirmed.

With the doctors gone for the time being, Mark frantically tried to place another call to Di from the public phone in the hospital lobby. He'd been attempting to reach her most of the day on their home phone but there was no answer. He knew she was trying to organise a baby-sitter for the other children and borrow a car for the one-and-a-half hour journey to the hospital. On deciding to try his parents' number, Di picked it up immediately.

'I was waiting for you to call'. Di sounded anxious. 'What do they reckon is wrong with Sarah?'

Mark hesitated. 'They think she's pregnant'.

'What?' shrieked Di. On the other end, Mark heard the phone drop, and then Di called out to Ruth: 'They think Sarah's pregnant!'

After a minute, Ruth's voice came on the line. 'I'm sorry Mark. Di went white and I had to put her head down to stop her fainting. She was just leaving for the hospital when you called. Your father and I lent her our car and we'll take care of the kids tonight. I expect she won't be too long getting there'.

'Thanks for taking care of things Mum', said Mark wearily.

'Mark, listen,' said Ruth in an urgent tone, 'I don't know what's going on there, but promise me, you'll take that little girl to somebody that knows what they're doing'.

'I wish it was that easy, Mum', replied Mark before hanging up.

Mark returned to Sarah's cubicle to find her surrounded by doctors again. At first, he thought something had happened and they were reviving her, before realising they were leaning in to talk to her. He arrived to find the same group questioning Sarah again.

Normal clinical practice standards require doctors to obtain consent from parents before examining or questioning a child about alleged sexual abuse. Only senior clinicians trained in assessing child sexual abuse normally perform such examinations. In Victoria, specially trained doctors from the Victorian Forensic Paediatric Medical Service handle all such cases (available 24 hours 7 days a week). Team members do not report allegations of sexual abuse until reasonable grounds exist and all other possible causes for the symptoms are eliminated. This service is not available in NSW.

Mark shook with anger as he waved the doctors away. 'That's enough,' he snapped. 'I said I wouldn't give you permission to do this again until after the scan. 'Now leave her alone'.

The group scattered, and Mark waited for them to disappear into the staff office before he could check to see if Sarah was all right.

She was lying on the trolley sweating and distressed. Her hair clung to her face in damp curls. She looked worse than before with dark hollows beneath her eyes. The day's probing had made the lump more prominent and Sarah clutched her abdomen protectively. Mark rushed to the cubicle's washbasin and turned on the water. He cupped his hands and rinsed his own face before tearing off a length of paper towel and moistening it for Sarah. He returned to the trolley and ran the moist towel over Sarah's face and hair.

'Why aren't they helping me? Sarah asked drowsily. 'You said they would'.

Mark stood helplessly clenching his hands while searching for an answer but could find nothing to say.

'Dad, I want to go home', whispered Sarah. 'Please get me out of here'.

With that, Mark had an unpleasant realisation that leaving the hospital was no longer an option. Things had gone too far. Since the doctors had contacted the authorities claiming Sarah was pregnant, he wasn't free to leave or find another doctor, or go to another hospital – at least not until the scan was done. For all he knew they might suspect him as the perpetrator. It was anybody's guess what could happen from now on.

Mark tried to sound encouraging for Sarah's sake. 'Honey, I think we just have to be patient for a while longer and besides, your Mum will be here soon'.

Sarah looked at him sceptically.

Mark looked at his watch; it was nearly seven. He rolled the wet paper towel into a ball and chucked it in the waste bin. Then he sat down next to Sarah. There he would stay without leaving his daughter alone for one minute until Di came. He'd never dreamed he would one day have to protect his daughter from doctors in hospitals.

Di arrived shortly after ED staff had transferred Sarah to the children's ward. Nurses had settled her into a more comfortable ward bed. With both parents nearby, Sarah allowed herself to lapse into an exhausted sleep. She was dozing when Dr Little arrived. He introduced himself to Mark and Di. By then Mark had his own suspicions that Sarah might have some kind of a tumour and he hoped this doctor would soon help.

'I'm going to have to do an examination on your daughter', Dr Little told Mark and Di.

This woke Sarah up and she looked pleadingly at her parents, but the doctor pulled the curtains around and carried out a detailed examination anyway. He asked the same personal questions the other doctors had, but now Sarah was giving no more answers.

When he had finished, Dr Little returned to the ward office and wrote an entire page into the clinical notes. He observed Sarah had a 'notable tan' and added that she was 'Presumed pregnant'. Though Sarah had never had a menstrual period, he noted: 'LMP [last menstrual period] – pregnant – biological father currently unknown...'

Without the benefit of an ultrasound, the doctor added: 'Not a surgical abdomen'. It meant he did not consider Sarah's problem would require surgery, though he made no mention of having discussed the matter with any other professional colleagues such as a paediatric surgeon or oncologist. Nor, evidently, did he match Sarah's abdominal mass to the tumour markers it was secreting. Instead, he wrote: 'Must exclude sexually transmitted diseases'. This meant the nurses were later required to take specimens from Sarah to test for a range of sexually transmitted diseases.

Finally Dr Little wrote of his plan to take a 'history' from Sarah and her father 'separately' – presumably to find the perpetrator. Perhaps he planned to do this with Sarah's parents out of the room – in any case, he did not ask for their permission to interview or examine Sarah in their absence. Of the extensive entries the registrar made into the clinical notes, he made no mention of the word *tumour*, nor did he attempt to explain why germ cell tumour markers were in Sarah's blood.

After the doctor finished his examination, Sarah found it difficult to settle for the night. Di changed Sarah from her street clothes into her own pajamas from home. For the next hour, Di held Sarah until she was calm enough to fall asleep.

When Di had settled Sarah into bed, a nurse approached. 'I've arranged for you to stay at a motel tonight', she said to the parents. 'Of course, you'll have to pay for it'.

Di was disappointed to hear the nurse asking her and Mark to leave since she had only arrived not long before. 'I thought the hospital let the parents stay overnight', she protested. 'It says so in your pamphlet'.

'Sarah has never been in the hospital before', added Mark.

'Usually that's allowed, but it's better you stay in a motel tonight', replied the nurse. 'I'll get you the address', she added as she headed back to the staff office.

The parents looked at each other anxiously. They felt uncomfortable about leaving Sarah alone at the hospital.

After Mark and Di left, Sarah woke up distressed to find her parents had gone. The nurse came to gather specimens to test for sexually transmitted diseases. The hospital procedures confused Sarah and when the staff asked her probing questions, she refused to answer them. In the clinical record, the night nurse described Sarah as a 'Very quiet young girl' – unaware that 'quiet' was not a word that anyone had ever used before to describe Sarah.

Meanwhile, precious time was being lost. As yet another night passed without doctors making the correct diagnosis, the highly malignant tumour in Sarah's abdomen continued to spread, casting off malignant cells throughout the region. The enormous mass compressed Sarah's internal organs, making it difficult to sleep. When the nurse offered Sarah another paracetamol tablet, Sarah recalled that the previous one had not helped the pain and declined the pill. Staff offered her no stronger analgesic and Sarah had to stick out the pain for the rest of the night.

The night nurse wrote: 'Sarah awake several times when observed during the night...'

WORSE THAN PREGNANT

Social workers oppose prejudice and negative discrimination
Against any person or group of persons, on any grounds.
Social workers challenge views and actions that vilify
Or stereotype particular persons or groups.

Australian Social Workers' Code of Professional Ethics

The next morning was Monday 25 November. Mark and Di had not slept well in the motel the nurse had advised them to stay in. It was on a noisy interstate highway, the room smelled of stale cigarettes and toilet deodoriser, and they worried all night about Sarah. At 7 am, they woke up early from a restless sleep only to have the worries from the previous day flood back. No tea bags were in the room and without a heart starter; they dragged themselves back to the hospital. They wondered how Sarah had fared overnight.

When the parents walked into Sarah's room, the nurse gave them a sideways glance and continued taking Sarah's blood pressure. Before leaving, she carefully drew back the room's curtains to open a direct line of vision to the nurse's office.

'It looks like they think we're terrible parents'. Mark whispered to Di.

Sarah looked sick and miserable curled up in bed, still dressed in her own pink pajamas. When Di sat down, Sarah climbed on her lap and refused to budge. Mark asked her how she was but Sarah was mute.

From where he stood, Mark glanced into the nurse's office; there was no one he recognised from last night and no sign of Dr Little. Instead, another doctor sat writing at the desk. Now it seemed that yesterday's events were surreal.

At 11 am, a nurse walked in with Sarah's case notes. She said there were no wheelchairs available but offered to walk Sarah to the Imaging and X-ray department, and Mark and Di could come if they wanted. The family followed the nurse, who walked ahead of them through a series of corridors. After a short distance, Sarah was too sick to walk any further, and Mark carried her the rest of the way. The nurse left them with a receptionist while she disappeared into the office with the notes and sat down there to wait. Moments later a male ultrasound technician emerged from one of the rooms and showed the family to a darkened cubicle with a bed surrounded by ultrasound equipment. Sarah resisted Di's efforts to put her on the bed and clung to her anxiously.

'What are they going to do to me?' Sarah asked fearfully.

Mark wrapped his arms protectively around his daughter and locked his gaze on the technician. 'This gentleman here is going to find out what the real problem is. That's right, isn't it', he glared.

The technician gave a friendly nod and pointed to the imaging bed. 'That's absolutely all we're doing right now', he affirmed and then patiently waited for the parents to coax Sarah onto the bed.

Sarah pulled the sheet up and peered over it cautiously. The technician gently explained what he needed to do, asking Sarah if it was all right for him to put the wand on her tummy. When she weakly nodded, he gently exposed Sarah's abdomen. He went on to explain that he would need to put cold blobs of lubricating jelly on her skin so the machine could see inside better to find out what the trouble was. The technician apparently had no preconceived ideas and was intent on finding out the cause. When he did not question Sarah, she relaxed – as did the parents, who took up the technician's offer to watch the screen.

The technician had barely placed the device on Sarah's abdomen when a large dark mass appeared on screen. The ultrasound showed the mass taking up most of the abdominal space, while fluid from it had filled up the pelvic cavity. This was no pregnancy, but rather an enormous tumour consisting of both solid portions and fluid filled cysts. It was likely there were haemorrhages into the cysts as well. The tumour had originated from left pelvic region and grown high enough into the upper abdomen to compress the left ureter, the tube carrying urine from the kidney to the bladder, which explained Sarah's left flank pain.

Mark and Di saw the technician's expression change from surprise to shock and then to pity. He turned the screen toward them more and outlined with his pen the black shadow that took up the entire view. Then he turned to them looking gloomy. 'I'm sorry – but this doesn't look like good news', he said.

Sarah looked from one parent to the other. Di gripped Sarah's hand.

'So it's not a pregnancy', said Mark.

The technician shook his head. 'Oh heavens no', he said. 'This is much worse news – it's as serious as it gets – a rather large mass that doesn't belong there, and I'm afraid you'll have to go to a better-equipped hospital as soon as possible to have your daughter treated'.

With Sarah on Mark's arm, the family walked out of the X-ray department in shock. When they arrived on the ward, the registrar called the parents aside and told them Sarah would have to go; either to a larger regional hospital or to a Sydney hospital for treatment. The parents chose the regional hospital since it was close enough for Sarah's siblings and family to visit. Despite Sarah's serious and deteriorating condition, staff told the parents that an ambulance would not be available until late that evening and gave them the option of driving Sarah to the regional hospital themselves or waiting all day for the patient transport vehicle.

The NSW patient transport service operates vehicles to transfer patients with non-urgent conditions to hospitals or between hospitals and nursing homes. However, for patients with life threatening conditions like Sarah's, the NSW ambulance service operates hundreds of emergency response vehicles including ambulances, fixed wing aircraft, and helicopters. Eleven helicopters alone, with pilot, crew, a doctor, and paramedics are based in eight locations throughout the state and available 24 hours a day. These hundreds of emergency medically equipped vehicles are available to patients with serious or life threatening conditions, and particularly to those living in rural and remote communities like Sarah. Sarah needed to be urgently transported to a hospital 170 km away – only half an hour by air ambulance. The same trip by road ambulance would take two and a half hours. For a family vehicle with a critically sick child on board, the risky trip would take far longer.

It is not known why hospital staff did not call on an urgent transport vehicle with paramedics to deal with Sarah's deteriorating condition. However, this gave the parents only two choices – either Sarah would remain in pain for another day or they would have to drive her 170 km to the next hospital themselves. The parents chose the latter. They realised they had to rush their daughter to the next hospital urgently, and did not feel they had time to get into long discussions with the staff as to why Sarah could not have an immediate ambulance transport. However, they still had two cars; Mark's utility and his parent's sedan were both in the hospital car park.

While waiting for a ward doctor to write a discharge summary outlining Sarah's condition for the doctors at the regional hospital, Mark tried to phone his brother-in-law to ask him and his wife to meet him as soon as possible in the hospital car park to collect his utility and drive it back to the farm. Unfortunately they weren't home, which meant that Mark and Di had to do the job. Once relieved of the extra car, the parents would be able to leave with Sarah in

Ruth's sedan. On their return, Di removed Sarah's pajamas and dressed her in fresh clothes from home to prepare her for the trip.

By 1 pm, the hospital faxed the discharge letter to the regional hospital; it would be waiting at the ED when they got there. The parents had no idea what the doctor had written in the letter, or what had been discussed between their GP and Dr Little the previous day. But even with the pregnancy notion thoroughly discredited and the tumour diagnosed, it seemed the family's troubles with hospital staff were far from over. The letter contained enough innuendos and unfounded materials to red flag them at their next port of call.

When the parents left the ward with Sarah, staff made no apologies for the humiliating pregnancy debacle and expressed no concerns about the devastating tumour diagnosis.

By 2 pm, the family set out on the perilous trip with Sarah to the next hospital. The temperature had already climbed above 40° C, setting an all time heat record for that month. Mark turned the car air-conditioner on full, but it still made little difference to the heat inside the car. Sarah was stretched across the back seat looking over heated and only half-conscious.

On the road, Mark faced risky driving conditions. Heat mirages danced over the asphalt and a furnace hot westerly buffeted the car around the road. He had to focus on driving while Di watched Sarah.

About 50 km into the trip, gagging noises came from the rear seat.

'Pull over', said Di. 'She's choking'.

Mark veered to road shoulder and braked hard on the gravel. He bolted out of the driver's side and opened the back door just in time to hold Sarah's head while she vomited yellow bile onto the ground.

Di handed Mark a tissue from the front seat. Mark cleaned Sarah's mouth with it but couldn't remove the vomit stains from her top. With the car doors open, the heat was oppressive and Mark helped Sarah back into the seat. He tried to put her seatbelt on, but he realised Sarah had become too weak to sit up and she was in too much pain to have the belt around her abdomen. He hoped he could get her there in one piece without a seatbelt. When he stretched her out across the back seat, he noticed how floppy she seemed – as if the life was oozing out of her.

Di managed to find a bottle of water and offered Sarah a drink, but she refused, mumbling that she felt so sick she would only bring it up again.

During the rest of the trip, Sarah had to vomit again around every half an hour. The frequent stops expanded the normally two and a half-hour trip to four hours. On the last stretch, Sarah seemed difficult to rouse. The parents could do nothing but carry on. They had no mobile phone to call 000 in those days, and in any event, there was no network coverage in the area.

Di looked panicked. 'What are we going to do if she...'

'We're nearly there', interrupted Mark. 'This was no job for us. She needed an ambulance – if anyone ever needed one'.

Di noticed Mark had clenched teeth and tight jaw muscles. She had never seen him this tense before. 'Are you all right, Mark?' she asked. 'You look terrible'.

'I'll feel a whole lot better when we get her to that hospital', he answered.

Di thought silently for a while before lowering her voice to prevent Sarah overhearing. 'If trained doctors can come out with all that pregnancy nonsense about a little kid who's not old enough to have babies – what else can they get wrong when they treat her for that tumour?'

The same idea had occurred to Mark earlier, but he did not want to make Di feel worse. 'We just have to hope for the best', he said grimly.

The family arrived at the regional hospital emergency entrance by 6 pm. The weather was still unbearably hot, but the afternoon shadows had lengthened. The main hospital building stood in the shade of tall gum trees, making the entrance look like a gaping mouth. Mark passed the main building and swung into the parking lot near the emergency department (ED).

Sarah felt limp and sweaty when Mark scooped her out of the back seat. He carried Sarah across the car park and rushed toward the ED while Di ran ahead to activate the automatic doors. Inside, the receiving room was packed with walk-in patients, but once the triage staff found the letter from the previous hospital, they immediately admitted Sarah to the children's cancer ward.

Once in the ward, the nurse showed them to a two-bed room. The parents settled Sarah into one of the beds, while the other empty bed gave them extra privacy and space for their overnight bags. Sarah was too weak to make any objections. Her skin was pale and sweaty, and her hair matted into a nest. None of the hospitals had provided toiletries over the past two days. After the nurse carried out her admission paperwork, Di searched the room and found a face washer and comb to freshen Sarah up. The cool washcloth over her eyes shielded Sarah from the bright light, allowing her to doze off.

After she'd settled Sarah, Di joined Mark at the window. They were both still shaken from their horrific four-hour ordeal of rushing their critically sick child to the regional hospital in the car by themselves. Both gazed out over the grove of trees to the regional city beyond; relieved to know there were doctors in this hospital that could help Sarah.

Sarah woke up with a start when the door opened. Dr Harry Kotz came in wearing expensive European shoes and clutching a clinical folder.

'I'm Doctor Kotz', he announced. 'A paediatric oncologist – you probably don't know what that means. I'm a specialist and I deal in tumours and those kinds of very serious things in children'.

Mark held out his hand in greeting when the doctor's mobile phone rang. He answered it and talked for several minutes.

When he hung up, he went to examine Sarah's abdomen. She yanked up the covers when he'd finished. The oncologist retreated to the washbasin where he pumped the soap dispenser and lathered his hands.

'We do not know what is causing the mass yet', said the doctor. 'But I'm going to order some more tests and a surgeon will see you later'.

When the door closed, Di hurried across the room and felt around the window's metal edges.

'What are you doing?' asked Mark.

'I'm trying to get this cologne smell out of here'.

'I think you'll find the windows don't open here', said Mark. 'Otherwise they might lose a lot of dissatisfied customers'.

Di was happy to hear Mark had regained some of his humour.

A few minutes later, a tall, older man peered through the doorway. 'Okay if I come in?' he asked.

'Sure', said Mark.

The man entered the room. 'Hi there, I'm your surgeon, John Gilbert. I'll bet you've already had a rough day – so I'll make this short'.

Next, he sat next to Sarah and crouched down to her level. He talked with her in an ordinary way; asking about her favourite things before coming slowly around to her symptoms. He asked her about what had happened over the last few days. Then he checked her vital signs and finally Sarah allowed him to examine her abdomen without fuss. This he did in a light and easy manner – while trying not to betray his true concerns. Gilbert was an experienced paediatric surgeon with a large practice in the region, but in his long career, he had not felt anything like this tumour mass before. This was as serious as a problem could get and he needed to see a CT scan before the day was over. After chatting to the family a while longer, the surgeon hurried back to the staff office. There, he filled out a request for an urgent abdominal CT scan and told the nurse on duty to call in the after hours radiographer immediately.

Just on 11 pm that evening a nurse wheeled Sarah to the hospital's X-ray department for an emergency CT scan. Sarah had been in severe pain for three days and any slight movement was now agonising. Getting on and off the CT table was impossible without help. After an hour in X-ray, she was relieved to return to bed. Sarah was about to spend another disturbed night in pain, but this time she had the comfort of her mother who sat in an armchair all night beside her. Meanwhile, Mark retired to the outside accommodation the hospital provided to parents.

The next morning was Tuesday 26 November. Around 10 am, the oncologist and surgeon invited the family into the ward's conference room to discuss Sarah's CT scan. The doctors pulled up the scanned images on a computer screen and pointed out the shape and position of Sarah's tumour. They both agreed that according to the chemical markers given off by the mass, Sarah almost certainly had a germ cell tumour, which arose, from her ovary, but it needed to be confirmed by biopsy taken at the time of surgery.

Neither doctor mentioned to the parents that there are several types of germ cell tumours – and while some are almost harmless, one or two are as deadly as tumours can possibly be. The surgeon, Dr Gilbert, explained about tumour torsion and why part of the tumour was dying off and setting up an infection, which accounted for Sarah's fever and pain. Both doctors agreed that Sarah had an acute surgical abdomen and that the tumour needed to be removed immediately.

If that was the case, Mark wondered, then why had the other doctors left her to suffer for days? And why did he and Di have to drive Sarah hundreds of kilometers around three hospitals in search of help? Couldn't someone have arranged for an ambulance?

He glanced down at Sarah who was sitting on his lap barely alive. She seemed to have become increasingly dehydrated over the past three days, and on top of this, the nurses were fasting her for the surgery. Her mouth was so dry she could hardly speak.

Dr Gilbert asked Sarah her opinion about having surgery.

She tried unsuccessfully to wet her lips. 'I want it out', she said hoarsely.

Di was still in shock and wondered aloud if some simple remedy existed for the problem. Mark gave Di a sympathetic glance and signed the consent form while Di made no objections. The paperwork was complete at around 1 pm. Sarah was resigned to the operation.

Half an hour later Mark accompanied Sarah to the anaesthetic bay, adjacent to the operating room (OR). The anaesthetist placed a mask of nitrous oxide near Sarah's face while Mark held her hand until she slipped under the anaesthetic. From there the anaesthetist carried Sarah into the OR where he inserted an intravenous cannula and started IV fluids. Then he passed a breathing tube into her trachea and hooked her up to a ventilator, which took over her breathing function.

Outside the OR suites, pacing the length of the hospital corridor, Di cut a lonely figure waiting for her husband to return. She'd felt nervous around hospital equipment and thought Mark would be better around Sarah when she was having needles, but Mark turned out to be more than a little squeamish.

Adjoining the OR, John Gilbert was already masked and standing at the sink. As he scrubbed up to his elbows, he wondered what he would find in Sarah's abdomen, and he hoped whatever it was had not spread too far. Judging by its size, however, he did not want to bet on good news.

A few minutes later Gilbert stood gowned and gloved at the OR table. He made a lateral incision, just above the pubic bone, and spread the abdominal muscle layers apart. With his surgical assistant, Gilbert tied off the bleeders and spread the retractor until the abdominal organs came into view. Before the retractor was fully opened, the massive tumour bulged out from the abdominal cavity where it had been tightly contained. The dark fleshy mass was even larger than the surgeon had imagined. As he traced it to its origins, he discovered the malignancy had begun in the left ovary, before growing large enough to escape from the pelvic cavity and up through the abdomen to the height of the diaphragm – the muscle that separated the abdomen from the chest. The monstrous growth was the size of a small football. Gilbert hoped he could safely remove it and that it had not spread too far. At best, it would turn out to be a relatively low-grade tumour that wasn't virulent or prone to spread. On the other hand, a virulent and aggressive tumour of that size was a worst-case scenario, and one he did not want to think about just at that moment.

The surgeon spent the next few hours dissecting the massive tumour away from the surrounding organs and tissues, painstakingly freeing it by increments until he could lift the tumour – along with the left ovary and fallopian tube – out of Sarah's abdomen. The scrub nurse placed the sizeable mass into a bowl of saline. It weighed a hefty 1 kg – but the surgeon's job was only half-finished.

34

For the next hour, he meticulously searched Sarah's internal organs for secondary tumours. Around the intestines, he found and removed nine suspicious looking clumps of tissue and several lymph nodes, which he sent to the lab for (histopathology) careful microscopic examination. Finally, he washed out the abdominal cavity with saline solution and sent some of the fluid to the lab in search of malignant cells.

When the surgeon finally closed Sarah up at 4 pm, the anaesthetist still had further work to do on Sarah in recovery. She would need several hours there, until she was stable enough to return to the ward. She was still dehydrated and required more IV fluids – then her pain had to be managed with narcotics after the anaesthetic wore off.

Gilbert finished his postoperative paperwork at 4.30 pm. While still in his scrubs, he rushed downstairs to talk with Sarah's parents. For him, it was never easy to tell parents bad news and he debated with himself about how much to tell them at that early stage.

For the past four hours, Di had been sitting in Sarah's hospital room armchair while Mark paced the floor, occasionally looking up to watch the afternoon sun disappear below the treetops.

When the surgeon walked in, the parents searched his face for clues. He put them at ease with a quick smile, but they could see he hadn't had an easy time; his scrub top was wet with perspiration and his hair stuck to his scalp.

'Sarah came through the surgery well', said the surgeon gently.

Di covered her face and sobbed with relief.

'What did you find?' asked Mark.

'A tumour, but we'll have to wait three days for the biopsy results to tell us what kind it is and what, if any, treatment might be necessary'.

'Did you get all of it?' asked Mark anxiously.

'All that I could see', he admitted. 'It was as big as a small football, and starting to break down. I took some other tissue around it for biopsy as well'. The surgeon did not go into the meaning of the suspicious looking lesions – the parents looked worried enough. 'I'll look in on Sarah tomorrow'. The doctor gave a nod and turned to leave.

'Excuse me, Dr Gilbert', Mark called out.

'Yes?' Gilbert nudged his head back through the doorway.

'You saved our little girl's life today and my wife and I will always be grateful. Please accept our deepest thanks'.

The surgeon gave an embarrassed smile. He'd always felt shy about compliments and he wasn't convinced he had saved her life if the tumour turned out to be malignant. 'You're very welcome', he said as he closed the door.

Mark stopped pacing and flopped into the visitor's chair with relief. He glanced over to Di, who was drying her face with a tissue, and went over to give his wife a reassuring hug.

The anaesthetist kept Sarah in recovery from 4.30 pm until 10.45 pm. Since she had been dehydrated and in poor condition, it took five hours to stabilise her after surgery and she spent nearly twice as long in recovery as she had in the OR. In addition to pouring IV fluids into Sarah, the recovery staff had inserted an intravenous patient-initiated narcotic pump. When Sarah woke up, she could self-administer doses of morphine whenever she needed pain relief, simply by pressing a button.

At 11 pm, Mark and Di were delighted when recovery nurses wheeled Sarah back into her room. She had an intravenous drip inserted into her right forearm and an in-dwelling urinary catheter draining into a bedside bag. Sarah now had light pink cheeks, and looked better than she had before the operation. The nurses explained to Sarah that she needed to press the morphine button when she felt pain, or ask the staff to do it for her.

With the hospital staff so helpful, Di and Mark felt they could relax a little and try for some much needed rest. Di spent another night sitting at Sarah's bedside, while Mark returned to the hospital's external accommodation.

The following morning was Wednesday 27 November. A nurse gave Sarah a bed-bath while Mark and Di searched the parents' room for a cup of tea. They had been through the worst stress of their lives, and it looked like Sarah was presently in better shape than her parents were. Three tense days lay ahead before they would know more about the tumour. Meanwhile they intended to keep up a cheerful front for Sarah, though inwardly they felt overwhelmed. Mark and Di were experiencing the sense of unreality that people typically feel when going through intense, life-altering trauma.

At 10 am, a nurse notified the parents that the hospital social worker, Caitlin Grimes, wanted to see them. They followed her instructions to the end of the corridor until they found the door marked 'Oncology Social Worker'. Di felt slightly embarrassed. She hadn't packed nearly enough fresh clothes to get them through the days ahead. After several days without amenities and sleeping for two nights sitting up in chairs, she felt ragged around the edges. Di smoothed her cotton skirt and checked Mark, who seemed to be holding up well in his neat trousers and shirt. Neither had any idea why a social worker wanted to see them. They weren't even sure exactly what social workers did, but thought it had something to do with helping them over a bad patch.

'I sure could use a comfy bed, a hot shower and a cup of tea', murmured Di.

'The social workers will probably organise that for us, along with accommodation and things like that', Mark replied, before knocking on the door.

Caitlin Grimes opened the door. She was in her early twenties and smartly dressed in a tailored suit and a red pair of high heel pumps. To Di it seemed the young woman was only a few years older than her daughter Laura.

The social worker offered them a seat and surveyed them for a while before questioning them. 'How do you feel about further treatments for Sarah?' she asked. A cup of hot tea sat steaming on her desk.

'Alright I suppose', answered Mark. 'We haven't been told anything – they said they'll talk to us when the results come back'.

'Do you have a problem with Sarah's treatment?' she probed.

Mark gave Di a puzzled look and she shrugged her shoulders in return. 'No, we don't have a problem. We're very happy with Dr Gilbert'.

'Maybe you could tell me a little about your alternative lifestyle', prodded Caitlin as she sipped her tea.

Mark was taken aback. 'We don't have an alternative lifestyle', he told her. 'We're just ordinary people'.

Caitlin picked at her blouse in mild frustration. She turned to Di. 'Maybe you could tell me about your belief systems', she asked.

Having no idea what the social worker wanted from her, Di squirmed. 'I don't know what you want me to tell you. I'm just an ordinary Mum'.

With that, the social worker wrote something in the clinical notes. Mark wondered what he and Di had said that anybody could find so interesting. He thought the social worker might herself be interested in alternative lifestyles, since she seemed so preoccupied with the subject.

Caitlin had spoken with Dr Kotz and had read the clinical notes from the previous hospital as well as the discharge summary, and she wanted to find out what this family was all about. So far, they weren't saying much, but if she persisted with her questions, they might be forthcoming.

When the young woman carried on with her previous questioning about lifestyles and belief systems, Mark got the impression that she was searching desperately to find something wrong with them. 'Listen', he said, trying to keep a polite tone after the exhaustion and worry of the past few days. 'We're just ordinary people. All we know is that we're waiting on the test results – nobody has talked to us about it yet – and when they do, we'll have to make the next decisions based on what they tell us. You can see we haven't even been home yet to tell the rest of our family'.

Caitlin could think of no more to do and told the parents they could go. On their way out of the social worker's office, they noticed she lifted her phone's receiver to call someone.

Once out of the office the parents walked back to the ward. Mark's arm closed protectively around Di's shoulder.

'What was that all about?' asked Di. 'She looked right through me as if I'd done something wrong!'

Mark searched for a logical explanation. 'No idea. It might be a routine they use on everybody. Maybe they think they're helping'.

'They could start by offering a cup of tea', countered Di. 'We have to go back now and phone the rest of the family feeling like death warmed up'.

Sarah's first postoperative day was busy. Physiotherapists came in and put her through deep breathing and coughing exercises to expand her lungs, which she did despite her painful incision. Nursing staff encouraged Sarah to push the pain pump button, but Sarah told them the drug made her itchy, dizzy and headachy, and that she preferred to be without it. These symptoms are signs of sensitivity or allergy to morphine and standard practice requires staff to substitute another (usually synthetic) narcotic painkiller. Though there were other drugs available, staff did not offer Sarah an alternative pain-killing narcotic that did not cause these side effects. Instead, Sarah simply didn't push the button; she put up with the pain. Despite this, Sarah's first post-op days went uneventfully. By the second day, she was strong enough to sit out of bed and after Dr Gilbert stopped by that afternoon and gave the okay, she was able to eat a light supper for the first time in four days.

On Thursday 28 November, nurses stopped Sarah's morphine infusion. She still complained of incision pain, but the dizziness, itch and drug headache were gone, and gradually she felt better. That evening a nurse removed her catheter and she was able to walk around the room.

Dr Gilbert visited each day and was clearly delighted with Sarah's progress.

On Sarah's third postoperative day, Caitlin Grimes sent for Mark and Di into her office again to re-explore their 'belief systems'. It had been only two days since the previous interview about the same issues and nothing had fundamentally changed. There were no test results yet and the parents knew nothing more. Even more than before, they felt bewildered.

'How do you see medications fitting in with your lifestyle?' asked Caitlin.

Mark was perplexed about these questions. They had never said anything about medications and were perfectly happy with the treatment and medications Sarah was getting, except maybe the stuff that made her itchy, and they hadn't even complained about that to anyone. Mark could see no bearing these questions had on their situation, but he thought that perhaps a longer explanation would help settle the issues that seemed to bother the social worker so much.

'We have no problem with medications'. Mark began. 'We're very happy with Sarah's treatment. At home, for simple problems we try home remedies first. For things that are more serious, we go to our GP. If he gives us a prescription we like to know what side effects come with the drugs, and whether they're going to work or not. It's all common sense. To be honest, our family has been so healthy up to now; we didn't need to go to the doctor that often'.

Caitlin wrote extensive notes before taking some time to carefully frame the next question. 'In view of your belief systems and in view of Sarah's illness, what are your views on chemotherapy?'

Mark drew a blank and had to take a moment to think. 'We don't have any particular view on it. To be honest, we've never given it much thought. The doctors haven't told us anything yet about any sort of treatment. Is there something we should know?' Mark looked baffled and scratched his head. He would rather people just speak their minds instead of playing these head-games.

Caitlin turned to Di. 'And what about you?' she asked.

Di shrugged her shoulders, 'How can I have any thoughts about it if we haven't been told anything?'

The social worker scanned them both before writing a long paragraph in the notes.

Mark felt restless and rose from the chair. 'Look, maybe after we're told something we can tell you what we think, but we just can't help you right now'.

Di followed Mark out the door. Outside in the hallway both parents were speechless.

'This is getting a bit weird', said Di.

'I know what you mean', replied Mark.

Inside the office, the social worker finished her phone call to the oncologist, before writing up the rest of the clinical notes. Her entry, dated 28 November 2002, stated:

> *[Name of social worker] questioned parents re. [sic] belief systems around alternative treatment options and how Sarah's diagnosis has changed these beliefs by questioning their alternative lifestyle & chemical free living. Mark stated that they were waiting for further results before decisions about chemotherapy treatment are made...social worker also noting that issue of risk of harm to Sarah if parents refuse necessary medical treatment & social worker has consulted with Dr Kotz Paediatric Oncologist re. [sic] this. If standard medical treatment refused and this is deemed life threatening then notification to DoCS required to be made on medical grounds. Social worker is requesting all professional staff to clearly document any barriers to patient care &/or any refusals of treatment by patient or parents. Plan: social worker to follow-up & Dr Kotz and family Monday 2nd December re. [sic] treatment planning...*

When the parents returned to Sarah's bedside, it never occurred to them that the social worker had just issued an alert to the staff that included a surveillance order to watch and report all their movements. They were to be reported to the child protection department if they so much as questioned anything. They couldn't even imagine anyone could suspect them of refusing treatment for their daughter, since they were genuinely happy with the staff, the doctors and all the life-saving medications she was being given. They had rushed their daughter to no less than three hospitals within 36 hours in order to have her condition treated and they had never once refused any treatment, drugs, tests, or operations to treat her tumour. They were absolutely delighted with Dr Gilbert's help and grateful to all the staff for their care. They were even polite to the social worker who had asked intrusive and repetitive questions about their lifestyle and belief systems.

When the parents returned to the ward, a nurse rushed to greet them with the news that Dr Kotz wanted to see them in his office. In the interim, they had forgotten about him, since they hadn't seen him since the night Sarah was admitted.

A few minutes later, the parents entered the conference room at the end of the corridor. The oncologist sat at a desk waiting for them. Mark and Di greeted him before looking around for Dr Gilbert.

'There's no one else here. I'm the oncologist – I've taken Sarah over now', he said.

Mark and Di sat down and steeled themselves. They were dreading this moment when they would learn the results of the biopsy.

The oncologist began by telling the parents their daughter's tumour was rare and malignant – a germ cell tumour (GCT) of the ovary of a type he had not previously encountered.

He did not mention that of the many kinds of germ cell tumours, Sarah's type was extremely rare and highly lethal. Nor did he inform the parents about the tumour's spread around the intestine, which further decreased Sarah's already low chance of survival. Most importantly, the oncologist neglected to tell the parents that Sarah's tumour had in fact already advanced so far that few victims survive for five years – even with the heaviest chemotherapy treatments. To make matters worse, tumours of that type are prone to recur, even with surgical removal and all other known treatments. These patients typically have a poor prognosis and are therefore given the option of choosing what treatment, if any, they prefer. They are usually supported in living out what is left of their lives in any way they wish.

The oncologist ended up on a friendly note. 'Your daughter can be cured', he told them with a smile.

Mark could hardly believe their luck. 'Cured?' he echoed.

'Yes, cured', repeated the oncologist. 'She can expect to die of old age and not of her tumour'.

Mark and Di grinned at the good news. They were even more amused by the doctor's smile, which they had not seen before.

'With chemotherapy', said the oncologist, 'Sarah has a better than 87 per cent chance of a total cure'.

The parents still smiled from the good news. 'How does the treatment work?' asked Mark.

'We will be using three different chemotherapeutic drugs over three days – to be repeated four or five times at 21- to 28-day intervals', explained the doctor.

'What does it actually do?' asked Mark, while Di listened carefully.

The oncologist sounded more guarded. 'To be honest, it's actually a poison that kills healthy cells, but destroys cancer cells more so. Besides, we don't have to start it now, it can wait four or five weeks – we should all get the holiday season over first and we'll see you in the new year '.

Mark was happy to hear the news. 'We could use the time. All of us need a bit of a rest', he agreed. 'It'll give us a chance to learn more about chemo'.

The doctor's smile disappeared. 'What's to learn? I've told you all you need to know'.

Mark was surprised at the frosty change. 'My wife and I haven't had anything to do with cancer before and we need to know more – that's all I'm saying. Do you have any more information for us?'

The oncologist clicked his pen in frustration several times and started writing in the notes. 'I'm discharging your daughter from this hospital tomorrow. Bring her back Monday of next week for a check-up'. He looked up at both parents. 'Or there will be – consequences', he added ominously.

Outside in the hallway the parents were both dazed. 'What just happened?' asked Di. 'First he was smiling – saying Sarah can be cured and there was no rush to start treatment, then everything went pear shaped when we asked about the drugs'.

Mark could not hide his own misgivings. 'I think we're going to have to do some research'.

When they returned to Sarah's room, they saw that Dr Gilbert had just come and gone. Sarah sat in bed playing with a toy koala the staff had given her. 'Guess what!' she shouted happily. 'I get to go home tomorrow!'

For the rest of the evening, Sarah insisted on going for walks with her parents up and down the hallway. After Sarah went to bed, Mark and Di retired to the external parents' accommodation for a good night's sleep. They planned to be back in the morning to take Sarah home.

In the room next to Sarah's, a pale girl of about Sarah's age was hooked up to an IV. All night Sarah heard the girl retching. Her whimpering and crying kept her awake most of the night. The next morning Sarah peeked into the girl's room but found it empty. She thought maybe the girl had gone home, and that was where she wanted to go as well.

She was relieved when her parents came to collect her. She couldn't wait to see her two dogs, the calf, and her siblings.

FOR MY EYES ONLY

Refrain from using coercion or unconscionable Inducements as a means of obtaining consent.

AMA Doctors' Code of Medical Ethics

It was the first day of December when Sarah returned home from the regional hospital. She had missed a week of school and in another week, the school year would be over. Then the summer holidays started and in February next year, she would begin Year 6. Meanwhile, Sarah looked forward to a long, six-week summer holiday playing with her siblings.

For now, Sarah was happy to be home and gaze out of her own bedroom window again. From the second floor, she noticed the recent rains had swelled the river and filled the billabong to the brim. She wanted to go down to her favourite swimming hole – a rock pond extending from the stream's main channel, overhung by willows with soft branches she used as a rope to swing on. But her mother had told her to stay around the house because she was just a few days out of hospital. For a while, Sarah tried to be good, until she could stand it no longer and changed into her swimmers, grabbed a towel and charged out the door.

Hannah watched to see which way her sister was heading. 'Hey, where are you going?' she shouted. 'Wait for me!'

Down at the swimming hole Sarah sat on a rock with Muttley while Hannah pulled rank on her older sister. Only rarely did Hannah have the upper hand, but this day she thoroughly enjoyed splashing around in the billabong. 'You aren't allowed to swim and I am!' she taunted.

For a while, Sarah sat on the rock looking grumpy until she gave in to the urge and headed into the pool. Muttley, who hated water, waded in for Sarah's sake.

Don't get your stitches wet!' shouted Hannah. 'I'll tell Mum if you do'.

Sarah immersed herself completely in the water. 'You just try it and I'll tell Dad you broke Grandpa's rocker', she retorted. 'Anyway, the river will make me better', she muttered.

'As if...' grumbled Hannah.

Sarah regained her confidence and splashed around exuberantly. 'You'll see', she answered.

After a few minutes, Muttley pricked his ears up and gave two warning barks. The girls looked up to see their grandparents' car inching up the gravel drive toward them. They looked almost identical as they waded with wet hair from the rock pool. Jim stopped the car on the grass beside the stream while Ruth rolled the window down. She frowned when she saw Sarah's wet swimming costume, while Jim just shook his head.

Sarah peered into her grandparents' car and saw a freshly roast chook in a baking dish sitting on the back seat. 'Grandma, you haven't done that cocky black rooster in!' Sarah scolded.

Ruth could tell when Sarah was trying to change the subject. 'Mind. You'll be in worse shape when your mother sees you've got those stitches wet!' warned Ruth. 'You girls come up to the house for tea now. That rooster will be on the table as soon as your mother makes the trimmings' she added, before Jim carried on driving to the house.

The girls returned to their house a few minutes later. Grandpa Jim had settled into the old rocker on the veranda where he sat telling the little ones, Joshua and Leah, stories about the cattle duffers that passed through the district in the old times. The kids sat enthralled by the old man's stories while Sarah and Hannah giggled – they had heard it all before.

Inside the house, the oldest girls, Laura and Clara, were in the kitchen helping Di prepare the vegetables while Grandma Ruth carved the roast chicken.

The girls sneaked into the house looking for some last-minute fun before dinner. From the living room corner, they surveyed the kitchen and dining room – even the study where their father sat at the computer desk. Fresh out of ideas, Hannah retreated to the shower while Sarah slipped unseen under the dining room table. There, she was well hidden by the tablecloth, but could still see Clara's feet as she set the table. Sarah lay in wait there until the coast was clear and she was ready to make her move.

A few minutes later Di called everyone to dinner. As the family members arrived from various locations, they noticed Sarah swinging from the hardwood beam above the table like a chimp, looking delighted with herself.

'Get down right now, or you'll bust your stitches', shouted Di. 'You've got to see the doctor tomorrow and have them out – what *will* he say?'

Mark watched in dismay but had no heart to tell Sarah off. Ruth and Jim smiled and shook their heads.

Finally, Sarah descended from the beam onto various articles of furniture before ceremoniously taking her place at the table. 'See, I told you that swim made me better', she announced.

The family said Grace before piling their plates with baked veggies, and Ruth's homegrown chicken and gravy. Joshua prepared his favourite mashed potato sandwich appetiser before tucking into his main meal. Sarah helped herself to a second and then a third helping. The mood was happy and hopeful – Sarah's recovery seemed a sure thing.

Late that evening, Di returned from putting the last child to bed and sat next to Mark on the couch. He seemed eager to talk.

Mark showed Di a few pages he had printed off the internet from the website of a world-renowned cancer hospital in the USA.

'You might want to see this information before we go to the hospital with Sarah tomorrow', said Mark. 'It says a lot can be done for people with cancer'.

Di read the first page. 'This says that sometimes there are risk factors for certain kinds of cancer', she said.

Mark agreed. 'Maybe we can ask the doctor about them so we can prevent more problems'. He then enthusiastically showed Di the next page. 'And this is about an anti-cancer diet and lifestyle. It says some nutritional supplements can support the immune system and actually protect against cancer. And just look at the number of clinical studies that support this stuff!'

Di was starting to feel enthusiastic about the idea that things could be done to help Sarah and her other children as well.

Mark showed her more pages. 'Right here it says treatments can be integrated. That means medical treatments can be used with complementary treatments like acupuncture, diet, and supplements to get an even better result'.

'That sounds just what we need'. Di grabbed the paper and read for a moment. 'But look here, it gives a warning to always ask your health practitioner for clinical studies to show their recommended treatments are evidence based', she said.

Mark stretched out on the couch. For the first time he could relax in over a week. 'We'll just have to ask the oncologist tomorrow', he said sleepily. 'These doctors are knee-deep in research. So he shouldn't have any problem giving us some studies to show us his treatment will work on what Sarah's got'.

On Monday 2 December, Mark and Di drove Sarah 130 km to the regional hospital for a scheduled check-up with Dr Kotz. The visit included blood tests and a further discussion about treatment options.

With pots of homemade chicken soup in her tank, Sarah seemed intent on enjoying each minute, even more than before. She swung from the disability aid rails in the hospital waiting room and Di had trouble keeping her in a chair. Before too long a nurse noticed Sarah's high jinx and called Di and Sarah to a treatment room to remove Sarah's stitches and draw a blood sample for pathology.

While Sarah and Di were gone, Dr Kotz invited Mark in to his office. The oncologist got down to business. 'Have you and your wife considered the advice I gave you last week?'

'Yes', said Mark, 'and we have just a few more questions'.

The doctor looked wary.

Mark tried to recall clearly, what he had read on the US cancer hospital's website. 'I read about risk factors for cancer. Do you think anything in the environment or in the water could have contributed to Sarah's ...?' asked Mark.

The oncologist interrupted. 'Absolutely not!'

Mark persevered. 'What about diet and supplements? In addition to your treatment, I read these things can help'.

The oncologist became frustrated and leapt to his feet. 'These are all unproven therapies! Absolutely without foundation'.

Mark steadied himself. He had never seen a doctor become so angry and he wasn't sure what had set him off. 'But I saw dozens of studies that said these other things can help when combined with your treatment'.

'Nonsense', retorted the doctor as he paced around the room. 'Nothing else has any merit. Nothing'. His face turned red.

Mark was alarmed. All he had asked was whether they could avoid any risk factors and add some supplements to the treatment he wanted to give Sarah. A few tense moments passed between them until Di knocked on the door. She wanted to join the meeting while the nurses looked after Sarah. Dr Kotz let her in and composed himself before returning to his desk.

Mark continued cautiously after Di sat down. 'Are there any more treatment options you can give us for Sarah?'

The doctor had collected himself. 'There are none. Nothing else has ever worked – except what I told you'.

Mark wondered why it was so difficult talking with the oncologist, when they'd never had this problem with the surgeon. 'All right then', said Mark, 'could you show us some evidence or some studies showing the treatment you are recommending would work?'

The doctor seemed shocked that someone had asked him to provide this information. He leant over to fossick around his desk. After opening and closing a few drawers, he shuffled a few papers around and then picked up a fist full of loose sheets, waving them in the air. 'These are the studies. It's all I have. You'll just have to accept it'.

When Mark reached out to take the papers, the doctor withdrew them, placed them back in the drawer, and slammed it shut.

Mark was shocked that the doctor had gone through this charade with no intention of showing them anything. He thought this showy gesture was patronising – he and Di were being treated like two naughty children just for asking these questions. If the oncologist's treatment was evidence based, why then wouldn't he let them see some studies to show it would work?

'With all due respect, doctor', said Mark, 'this is an important decision for us, and if you have information there, we would need to see it to help us make the right decision for our daughter. Could my wife and I take those studies home to read?'

The oncologist looked offended. 'They're for my eyes only', he snapped, as he made sure the drawer remained tightly closed. After taking a moment to compose himself, the oncologist reached into the clinical notes folder, removed a consent form, and pushed it across the table for Mark and Di to sign.

Mark glanced at the legal document and then over to Di. She looked anxious and he was becoming uneasy himself. Without the full facts and a useful discussion, they could make no sensible decisions about Sarah's treatment. So why then were they expected to sign a legal document without having their concerns or questions answered? He had a gut feeling things were not adding up.

Mark took a deep breath. 'I'm sorry but my wife and I will need more information before we're able to sign this'.

With deliberate restraint, the oncologist took a blank paper and wrote the names of the chemotherapy drugs he intended to use, and some illegible words, which Mark could not decipher when he read them later on. When finished, he handed it across his desk. 'This is all the information you will need. I will be away overseas for a week and we will talk again when I come back – I'm sure you and your wife will make the *right* decision'. To ensure the parents had understood him, the oncologist added an ominous warning; '...or things could get very messy'.

Mark and Di felt intimidated and uncomfortable. They didn't know what the doctor would do to make things 'messy' for them but, for the moment, Mark decided not to challenge the oncologist until he could get his bearings and think about what to do next. From the way the doctor was talking, there was no telling what kind of powers he could call on. Mark noticed Di wanted to leave, while the doctor clearly had nothing more to say and was already writing up his clinical notes. The parents collected Sarah and left the hospital in a hurry.

On the way home, they avoided discussing sensitive issues in front of Sarah, who was in the back seat. They were both shaky after feeling they'd been threatened. Neither had ever been coerced to sign a legal document before, and it rocked them to the core.

It was nearly dark when the family reached the outskirts of Gloucester. As Mark turned onto the gravel road leading toward the Barrington Tops, Di checked Sarah in the back seat and found her fast asleep. 'What are we going to do now?' she whispered to Mark.

Mark tightened his grip around the steering wheel. 'There's only one thing we can do'.

'What?'

There was no hesitation in Mark's voice. 'We've got to get a second opinion'.

Di studied Mark's profile in the fading light. He looked as resolute as his father. Jim also insisted on finding out the facts before he made decisions. Right now, being part of such a strong family made her feel safe.

It was dark when they arrived home but Mark immediately logged onto the internet. There he found a group of doctors in Melbourne who treated cancer. He thought they might be able to give them a second opinion and answer their questions.

The following day, he called the doctors' clinic and scheduled an appointment for Sarah. Next, Mark made their travel arrangements to Melbourne. Following that, he went to town to buy a mobile phone. He wasn't going to be in another situation like the one he and Di had been in when they had to drive critically ill Sarah to the hospital themselves, and they couldn't even call for help if they needed it.

Only days later, Sarah peered from her window seat and watched the Sydney skyline fade into the distance. It was Sarah's first flight. Just after takeoff, the plane's floor had shuddered as the pilot retracted the landing gear.

'What was that?' she demanded.

Mark gave her a reassuring look from his isle seat. 'It's only the wheels – they go up while we're flying'.

After that, Sarah leaned back to enjoy the ride, pretending to be on the Big Dipper at the Easter show. 'This is awesome!' she squealed over the engine noise.

After the plane reached cruising altitude, the flight attendant gave Sarah a colouring book with crayons and a children's lunch pack.

Sarah yelled loud enough for the other passengers to hear. 'Dad! When will we be in Melbourne? I hope not ever. I want to stay here!'

Passengers across the isle leant forward and smiled.

Mark looked at his watch, 'We'll be there in about an hour, Jogue. Try not to wear yourself out before we get there'.

On seeing Sarah so happy, Di relaxed her grip on the armrest. Her palms had become wet during takeoff and she searched her bag for a tissue. 'I'm not even sure what's happening. I've been so busy with the kids', she confessed to Mark while drying her hands.

Mark smiled and patiently explained their plans again. 'I found an integrative medical team in Melbourne. They combine conventional treatments with other things like diet and supplements. They work with an oncologist, who can give us an independent second opinion'.

'That's right, I remember now', recalled Di. 'Did you tell Dr Kotz?'

Mark looked thoughtful 'Yes I did. I called him just before he left on his overseas trip. I asked him to send Sarah's test results to the clinic in Melbourne, but he wasn't a happy camper'.

Di felt irritated just remembering their last meeting with the doctor. 'Aren't we entitled to a second opinion? It's a free country isn't it?'

Mark looked grim. 'Last time I checked'. Suddenly he could have kicked himself for having been so up-front. He gave Kotz the names and address of the doctors they were scheduled to see, but at least he had not revealed their phone numbers.

Di gave an involuntary shiver. 'I don't trust him, Mark. After threatening us like that, there's no telling...'

Mark agreed but said nothing. He stayed thoughtful for the rest of the flight. When Di dozed off, he put his seat back and ran through a mental checklist. He'd read on the internet that the purpose of a second opinion was to confirm or deny the diagnosis of the first doctor, and to offer other available treatment options. He learnt that an independent second opinion should come from a second doctor's review of the tests and scans and not from discussions with the first doctor. In fact, the two doctors should not discuss the matter at all. The second opinion was purely to help the patient choose which advice and treatment they preferred. Mark read that patients commonly wanted more information before deciding on a course of treatment. To his surprise, he found out that in a large number of cases the second opinion proved the original diagnosis or prognosis to be incorrect.[6] Besides, no doctor was infallible and two opinions did – after all – seem better than one. Mark thought that a good doctor would not mind if another doctor looked at his handiwork.

The only problem Mark could anticipate was that, despite his requests, Dr Kotz had not yet sent Sarah's test results and medical history to the Melbourne doctors. However, he hoped the paperwork would be there when they arrived. Mark didn't realise at the time that according to the AMA (Australian Medical Association) Code of Ethics, doctors are ethically required – on the patient's request – to make available to another doctor a report of the patient's test results and treatments for the purpose of a second opinion.

Many more thoughts occurred to Mark. Like Di, he was also disturbed by the doctor's statement that things 'could get very messy'. At the time, he was not aware that the ethical informed-consent procedure requires doctors to answer the patient's (or parents') questions and provide them with enough information to make an informed decision. Doctors are also required to disclose to patients the benefits and risks of the proposed treatments and discuss any alternative treatment choices that may exist. Ethically, consent cannot be legally obtained under duress – it must always be a voluntary decision.

During the trip, Mark also worried about the family finances. He didn't know how much more time off work he could get or how long this trip would be, but for now, his boss was on side.

Before too long Mark's ears were popping. Di gripped the armrest again and Sarah whooped as she did on the show-rides. When the plane banked on the approach to Tullamarine airport, Mark caught glimpses of Melbourne from the window opposite. It was their only hope right now.

The family caught a tram into the city. Unlike the brassy nouveau riche of Sydney, Melbourne was elegant, with its English Victorian architecture lovingly preserved under a netting of tram wires. In Melbourne, people discussed issues of cultural merit in coffee houses over lattes and Viennese pastry. Di loved the old trams. It reminded her of her own childhood, when she had lived in

---

[6] Rose 2000, Clauson 2002 .

Melbourne and caught a tram to school every morning. She also loved seeing Sarah so excited. With her nose pressed against the window, Sarah took in the sights: the brasseries and tall oaks that lined the streets.

They found the Melbourne integrative health clinic just a short walk from the tram-stop. The building was old but friendly looking, with an awning over the entrance.

In the waiting room Dr David Milne, a tall, bearish man, greeted them enthusiastically. He enjoyed patting his patients on the back and giving them the high-five. Although he was not a physician, Milne was an allied health professional with experience in complementary treatments, who collaborated with Dr Tim Sales, a holistic GP.

Milne invited the family into his cluttered but cosy office and offered them a seat, with Dr Sales soon joining them. Sales had an irregular face with enormous eyes. He was more reserved than Milne was, but they worked well together as a team.

After introductions all round, Dr Milne opened a jar of liquorice and offered some to Sarah. She took a handful and popped a few in her mouth.

'Hello Sarah', said Dr Sales. 'It's nice to see you looking so well. Do you know why you're here today?'

Sarah shrugged her shoulders.

'Your parents have brought you here so we can talk about which combination of treatments might help you best. In a few days, you will be seeing another oncologist and after that, we will combine his suggestions with ours and come up with a plan to help you feel better. Is that okay with you?' asked Sales.

Sarah nodded, her cheeks still bulging with liquorice.

Mark and Di smiled. The lollies were definitely an icebreaker.

'Did you get any test results from Dr Kotz?' asked Mark. 'I asked him twice to send them to you'.

Dr Milne searched through Sarah's thin file. 'No. There's nothing here. But don't worry. With your permission, we will ask Dr Kotz ourselves. Meanwhile, Dr Sales will take some blood to check the tumour markers. Your appointment with the oncologist here is in a few days. Once you've seen him, we can integrate his suggestions with some of our complementary treatments here '.

The parents both nodded. It made sense that there must be more than just one way to help Sarah.

'What kind of options can you offer us in the meantime?' Mark asked.

Dr Milne was quick to answer. 'Much depends on what we discover when we get Sarah's file from her NSW oncologist. But for now, we can recommend an anticancer diet that is supported by several clinical studies. It consists of a plant-based diet containing various fresh fruits and vegetables, such as broccoli, known for their anticancer properties. You might want to substitute red meat with white meats such as fish and organic chicken. That means also cutting out junk foods, artificial colouring, preservatives and excessive sugar'.

Mark nodded. 'I read about that on the internet – why don't cancer doctors know about it?'

Milne smiled. 'That's what we'd like to know'.

Sales added; 'The other evidence-based complementary treatment we can offer you at this stage is nutritional supplementation, which helps repair the body and strengthens the immune system, which is responsible for killing cancer cells. We can show you the clinical studies,' he offered. 'We refer to "complementary" as treatment often given in combination with other cancer treatments like chemo or radiotherapy'.

'Yes, we really want the best of both worlds for Sarah', said Mark. 'My wife and I have already seen research on the diet and nutritional therapies and we're here to find out what proven treatment the oncologist can offer us as well'.

Di had a good feeling about this discussion. The doctors were helpful and she felt confident and hopeful for the first time since Sarah's operation.

Both Sales and Milne went on to describe other complementary treatments, such as oxygen saunas, for which less clinical evidence exists but which are entirely harmless. Treatment with these saunas, they said, is based on the known beneficial effect that oxygen has on the body, and most patients find them both invigorating and relaxing. Later, after Dr Sales had finished examining Sarah, he allowed her to try it. She sat in a tent that came to the level of her neck, with warm oxygen inside. Sarah quickly lapsed into a deeply relaxed state, in which she remained during the entire 45-minute treatment.

That evening the family traveled to their relatives' home at Yarra Junction, a semi-rural area just outside the city. There, Di's brother and sister-in-law were happy to put them up, even though they were busy with their own small children. The extended family was closely knit, with an unspoken agreement that each family member could go to the other for help or shelter if needed.

At the dinner table that night Mark and Di shared enthusiastically about the healing treatments they thought could help Sarah, and about their plans to return to the clinic daily for treatments over the next three days until they could see the Melbourne oncologist. For the first time since Sarah's diagnosis, the parents felt they were making headway. Finally, somebody was sitting down and talking to them.

Over the next few days, Sarah returned each evening to Yarra Junction glowing and hungry. After three helpings at dinner, she played games with her cousins until bedtime.

On the fourth day of Sarah's treatments at the clinic, Dr Sales rushed out of his office to exuberantly announce that Sarah's tumour markers were dropping even over the short time they'd been there. It was a good sign.

That afternoon the family had their appointment with the Melbourne on-cologist. Sales gave Mark a copy of the blood results to take to the specialist. It was all they had. There was still no response from Dr Kotz and they had no previous scans or blood test results to go on. Worse still, no tumour histology results were available, so crucial to determining a prognosis or treatment. At that stage, no one but the NSW oncologist knew exactly what type of germ cell tumour Sarah had, how virulent it was, and to which stage it had progressed. Cancer treatment options vary considerably depending on these factors. Patients with late stage ovarian germ cell cancers have poor prognoses and are eligible for less toxic treatments with fewer side effects than chemotherapy, to preserve their quality of life. These patients are also given palliative treatment options and the freedom to choose the treatment that best suits their needs.

The next day at 2 pm, the family caught a cab to the Melbourne oncologist's surgery. The family enjoyed the trip to his rooms, which were located in a leafy, affluent part of Melbourne. The cab let them out in front of an elegant and well-kept Edwardian-style office building. Once inside the foyer, the parents searched the directory and found Dr George Billings listed on the third floor.

Mark chose to go up the stairs rather than take the old-fashioned lift. 'I wonder what he can do without any test results', he reflected on his way up.

Sarah scooted up the stairs behind her father.

Di came last. A pain had started in her left leg and it slowed her down. 'Maybe he'll order his own tests', she replied.

Mark stopped to let her catch up and made a mental note to take the family down in the lift on the way out.

'You might be right', Mark agreed. 'And maybe you should see somebody about that leg'.

Inside Dr Billing's office, the phone rang. His receptionist answered it and switched it through to the doctor's room. Billings sat at his desk with a fruit juice and a half-eaten sandwich. He'd had a busy morning and this was his last appointment, before taking the afternoon off.

When his phone rang, he answered it impatiently. 'I thought I told you to hold my calls until after my last appointment', he told his receptionist.

The receptionist interrupted, 'I think you'll want this one – an oncologist from New South Wales'.

'All right then', he snapped as he took the call. For the next few minutes, Billings nodded his head while listening silently to the caller.

After fifteen minutes, the switchboard's light stopped flashing, and the receptionist saw the doctor had finished the call. Mark, Di and Sarah sat in the outer office looking at the coloured pictures of melanomas on the wall.

'What's that?' asked Sarah, pointing to the image of the black cancerous growth.

Mark didn't have the heart to talk to her unnecessarily about cancer. 'It's just a mole, Jogue'.

'Well, it sure is a yucky one!' she replied exuberantly.

The receptionist stifled a smile and announced that Dr Billings would see them now.

The doctor opened his office door and ushered them in. He seemed outwardly friendly, but a little tense from the start. To the parents he appeared a dignified, silver-haired man in conservative clothes with framed pictures of his wife and grown children on his desk. He brought another chair in for Sarah.

Mark started: 'I'm sorry we haven't been able to bring any previous records, except the tests Dr Sales did; and those show the tumour markers have dropped'.

Dr Billings put up his hand as if to stop Mark. 'Don't worry about it. It's unnecessary'.

Mark glanced at Billing's desk. A slim folder contained a single sheet of paper. The doctor then took a brief history and made a cursory examination of Sarah – not as thoroughly as might have been expected for someone intending to treat a patient. Di then helped Sarah down from the examination table and readjusted her top and skirt.

Mark volunteered to solve the problem of the missing records. 'We would be happy to pay for any scans or tests you might need for a second opinion', he offered.

The oncologist held his hands up again. 'No, no, don't worry. I suggest you go back to New South Wales and take the chemo'.

Di looked puzzled, while Mark struggled to stay unruffled. 'We'd be happy to choose the chemo, if someone could just give us some evidence it would work on Sarah's problem. That's why we're here!' Mark said, sounding frustrated.

The doctor shrugged. 'That's my advice'. He made no effort to supply them with information they wanted. 'Maybe your doctor there can help you'.

Mark shook his head in disbelief. 'At least, could you tell us if there are any other treatment options for Sarah?'

The oncologist admitted there were other options, but would not elaborate. He seemed hesitant about discussing Sarah's problem at all. Only later did Mark discover that the doctor had already spoken with Dr Kotz, and that specialists tend to be reluctant to contradict each other.

Mark asked the doctor's opinion about continuing with the complementary treatment until they could find more information about the chemo.

The oncologist considered his reply carefully. 'That would be all right in the end stage of cancer treatment, but Sarah's case is at the diagnostic stage'.

Mark asked, 'If the treatment is so good at the end stage, then wouldn't it be even better at this early stage?'

The oncologist made no reply to this and seemed eager to end the consultation.

Mark felt there was much information the doctor was withholding but they had no choice but to leave when the consultation was over. Feeling vaguely troubled, the parents went to the outer office to pay the doctor's bill. They left the doctor's surgery with the mistaken impression that their daughter was in the early stages of cancer.

After the family left his office, the Melbourne oncologist dictated a letter – not to Dr Sales, who had referred the family to him, as was the usual doctors' etiquette, but to Dr Kotz. The letter reassured Kotz that he had directed the family back to him, with Billings adding that he had no more appointments scheduled with them. The letter was in the mail to New South Wales the following day.

On the way back to Yarra Junction, the parents were troubled. They had come for an independent diagnosis, prognosis and treatment suggestion, and had expected the Melbourne specialist oncologist to review their daughter's case on its merits. If the doctor had no paperwork, then how did he make his decision?

The day after seeing the Melbourne oncologist, Mark received a surprising call on his brand new mobile phone. It was Dr Kotz wanting to know when they were coming back to New South Wales for his treatment. Mark was shocked to hear from him and reminded him that he had not yet seen any studies on the chemo. He told the oncologist about the complementary treatment which they intended to continue at home, given that Sarah's tumour markers were down. During that conversation, both agreed that the tumour markers would need to be closely monitored, and if they rose significantly, a new treatment plan would have to be made. However, they did not discuss what that treatment should consist of. Meanwhile, Mark assured the oncologist he would take Sarah to the family GP each month for tumour marker blood tests and a check-up. (The lab automatically sent the GP and the oncologist a copy of each test result, with which they could monitor Sarah's condition.) Finally, Mark told Dr Kotz they were returning home the next day and assured him they would see him on their next scheduled appointment early in the New Year.

The doctor did not sound happy by the end of their discussion. Later he made a short note in the clinical records, confirming their agreement to monitor the markers. He added that Sarah was 'off having alternative therapy'. He had also written Dr Sales' name in the notes, with the doctor's phone number, which he had looked up himself. He planned to contact each doctor who had anything to do with Sarah.

The next day the family had packed to leave on the afternoon flight to Sydney. They dropped into the clinic on the way to the airport, for their last consultation. Mark told Dr Milne about the fruitless oncology consultation they'd had the day before. Milne told him he would look into it and stay in touch by phone. When Sarah popped her head around the corner, Milne gave her a high five and allowed her to raid the liquorice jar. Meanwhile Di stocked up on supplements from the clinic's dispensary while Mark learnt how to use the portable oxygen sauna that folded up like a tent for transport. When Dr Milne left the room to get a fitting for the sauna, the family caught sight of Dr Sales as he left his consulting room.

Mark was in a good mood and approached Sales. 'I want to thank you for everything you've done for us', he said, shaking the doctor's hand.

Sales looked flustered and embarrassed. Mark noticed something had changed since yesterday.

The doctor sounded nervous. 'Thanks. But, if your situation goes legal, I'll have to do whatever it takes to protect myself'.

In an instant, the parents' smiles disappeared. What was illegal about getting a second opinion, they wondered. And what had happened to Sales since last they saw him, when he was so pleased about Sarah's progress?

Sales left just as Milne returned. He saw Mark was shocked and asked him about it. Mark told him about the doctor's sudden change of heart.

'Don't worry about it', said Milne. 'There's a health war going on behind the scenes. These days it is an act of bravery just to give cancer sufferers choices – and it's not without professional risk. Some doctors get spooked. But I'm still here for you', he patted Mark on the back effusively.

Mark left it there. Their friends had just arrived to give them a lift to the airport. But he wondered what kind of war this was that made patients the meat in the sandwich.

Within the hour, the family had passed through the checkout at Virgin Blue airlines. They sat in the airline's departure lobby on a row of seats directly facing the tarmac where a huge aircraft stood with its nose facing them. In the cockpit sat the pilots carrying out their pre-flight checks. Sarah pressed her face against the floor-to-ceiling window and waved to them.

Moments later Sarah was beside herself with excitement. 'Look Mum, they're waving back!'

Di laughed when she saw the pilots waving again at Sarah. She found herself imitating Sarah's exuberance and joined in. When the pilots smiled and waved back at Di, she buried her face in her hands and blushed.

Now it was Mark's turn to be amused. 'Thanks fellas!' he said, as he gave them the thumbs up. 'We need all the friends we can get right now'.

When the pilots returned to their work, Sarah continued to watch the ground crew prepare the aircraft they would soon be boarding. It gave Mark and Di a moment to talk in private.

'What did you think about the Melbourne oncologist's second opinion?' asked Di.

Mark shook his head. 'That was no second opinion'.

'What was it then?'

Mark thought about what Dr Milne had said. 'I'm starting to think people with cancer are like a commodity that oncologists don't want to share with other doctors'.

'Why won't anyone tell us whether that chemo will work on Sarah – it seems a pretty simple question', asked Di.

'You're not wrong', agreed Mark. 'I've never seen doctors so cagey as when we ask that. To be honest, I'm getting tired of asking it and they must be getting tired of dodging it. But I reckon it's time to find out more'. Mark reached into his pocket and removed his wallet while Di looked on curiously. After searching around his billfold, he pulled out the crumpled piece of paper Dr Kotz had given them with the names of the three chemo drugs scribbled on it. 'I'll have to do some research into these and get us some answers', he said.

Di tried to decipher the odd names on the creased paper. She soon gave up and checked on Sarah, who was now inspecting the fake presents under the tinsel Christmas tree in the airline lobby. It reminded her that Christmas was only a week away and she hadn't done any shopping yet. Mark had been off work for so many days, she wasn't even sure there was any money to shop with.

Christmas morning of 2002 came all too soon. Mark had brought home a week's pay from his job at the mine on Christmas Eve and with it, he and Di went on a last minute shopping expedition. That night they stayed up well past midnight wrapping presents and realised they'd gone through Mark's entire pay packet. It was all worth it the next morning when the kids woke up to a sea of twinkling lights with presents under the tree. All six were up at dawn and 15-year-old Laura tried her best, as the eldest, to make them wait until Mark and Di were up. Christmas that year took a different tone. The kids were confused about Sarah's illness and the parents could not explain it to them since the doctors hadn't told them much either. It would take Di weeks to settle the children again after the weeks she and Mark had been away with Sarah.

After a boisterous morning, the family went to Ruth and Jim's for a Christmas lunch that included Mark's siblings and their families. When they returned, they were astonished to find that representatives from local community organisations had left Christmas presents for the kids at the door, while Mark's union had passed the hat around. Mark and Di appreciated the community spirited gesture enormously and the proceeds got them through the Christmas – New Year break.

With some of the pressure now off, Mark used the break to catch up on work around the farm. He even managed to finish digging the dam with the dozer. With some lucky rain, they would have plenty of feed and water for the cattle in the coming year.

On New Year's Eve, Mark retreated to his study and closed the door. Finally, he was in the mood to tackle some research. Mark opened his wallet and removed the folded paper the oncologist had given him with the three intravenous chemo drugs scribbled on it. They were the ones the doctor wanted to give Sarah, and next to the drug's names, he had written the doses he wanted to give her. In a few days, they were due to see Kotz again and they needed some answers.

When Mark typed the first drug's name into the search engine, to his horror he found its side effects listed as kidney failure, baldness, rash, and a risk of developing other cancers years later. He discovered this drug was so toxic in its high dose intravenous form that it even killed a small percentage of patients outright. On the other hand, he was surprised to read that its oral form was only a fraction of the dose and had almost no side effects. He found a number of clinical studies that supported the low dose approach for many cancers, including ovarian cancer.[7]

Mark was starting to become very concerned about the serious, toxicity-related side effects of the high doses of intravenous chemotherapy that the doctor was proposing to give Sarah. He wondered if Kotz could give her this drug in smaller, more frequent doses instead and he made a note to ask the oncologist that.

Mark then typed in the second chemo drug and discovered it caused hearing loss or deafness in almost 80 per cent of children receiving it. In addition, the drug's listed side effects were kidney failure, vomiting, skin rashes, temporary or permanent blindness, bone marrow failure (complete immune system collapse) and even death from its toxicity.

When he keyed in the third drug, he read that it too could cause kidney failure and also lung damage, as well as nausea, vomiting and rashes, and again death from toxicity. In addition, he read the manufacturer's warning not to use these drugs on children. If these three chemo drugs were as toxic as described by their own manufacturers, Mark wondered how they would affect Sarah when given in the maximum tolerated doses that the oncologist wanted to use on her.

After reading this information, Mark printed it out. He felt suddenly angry at having these deadly drugs pushed on his daughter without anyone answering their questions first. What was going on, he wondered. Why didn't doctors show them any studies about the effects of this chemo, or whether it had even been proven to work for a problem like Sarah's? And why had no one told them about the safer low-dose option?

When the printer issued the last sheet, Mark switched off the computer. He felt sick as he clutched the information and returned to the living room. It was

---

[7] Zhang 1995.

11 pm. In an hour, it would be 2003 and he wondered just what the next year would bring.

Di was lying on the couch reading a book. Mark had not seen her so relaxed for a while. When he gave her the pages, he immediately regretted shattering her peace of mind the way his had been shaken in the past hour.

'This is maybe why they won't tell us much', Mark said cynically. 'I'm sorry. It's a heck of a way to ring in the New Year'.

In the first days of January 2003, Dr Kotz was already at his hospital desk writing a letter to the family's GP about Sarah. In it, he claimed an 85 per cent chance of curing Sarah. He made no mention that Sarah was at an advanced stage of her cancer – that despite the tumour having been removed, it was of a type that would recur despite chemotherapy and that she had a poor prognosis. Likewise, the doctor mentioned nothing of the family's dissatisfaction with their treatment and their desperate search for a second opinion in Melbourne. Instead, he alleged, 'the family live somewhat of an alternative lifestyle'. He ended the letter by stating his intention to involve the child protection authorities if the parents did not consent to chemotherapy.

The GP received the oncologist's letter not long after. Unfortunately, the GP did not contact the family for their side of the story.

A few days later, on a hot January day, Mark and Di had a battle of wills with Sarah. For the first time she had balked at going to a doctor's appointment.

'I don't want to see Dr Kotz', she complained. 'I want to swim in the river'.

Mark knew how she felt – he was not looking forward to having another standoff with the doctor either. But he said nothing. At this stage, there seemed no other options.

Di packed drinks into the esky for the trip while Mark's job was to convince Sarah. He put his arm around her and let her whine until she got it out of her system. After all, she'd been through more than the average kid in the past two months. After a while, she quietly climbed in the car and spent the next two hours in the back seat with her arms crossed.

From where the oncologist sat, it was clear Sarah had recovered very well from the major surgery. She looked bored, but far from ill. He aimed a weak smile at her, which she largely ignored.

Mark had several questions for the doctor that day. 'Could you perhaps give us a copy of the biopsy results?' he asked. 'We don't even know the name of Sarah's condition'.

The doctor gave a frustrated sigh as he wrote the type of tumour Sarah had on a piece of paper and handed it to Mark, along with a consent form he wanted him to sign.

Mark ignored the form and took the piece of paper, carefully folding it before putting it in his pocket. 'About the chemotherapy you recommend – are there any less toxic alternatives?' Mark asked.

The doctor appeared frustrated again.

Mark continued. 'I learnt some of those drugs could be taken in smaller doses by mouth with almost no side effects'.

'I told you before – absolutely not', the doctor interrupted.

Mark sensed they were heading toward another standoff. He gave the doctor a chance to offer them some information but when nothing was forthcoming, he thought it was the right time to let the doctor know where he stood. 'Given the success we are having with the tumour markers falling and Sarah's very apparent vitality, we would not at this stage consider intravenous chemotherapy', said Mark.

The oncologist looked unhappy.

With that, Mark reminded the doctor of the agreement they'd both made to monitor Sarah's tumour markers and to discuss another plan if their levels rose. He added that he and Di had not discounted the oncologist's treatment, but that they still knew nothing about it as it related to Sarah's illness and wanted to continue the immune-supportive treatments for the time being until they could decide on the next step.

The doctor balked and shook his head.

Mark continued. 'We certainly want our daughter under the care of a specialist. Would you continue to see Sarah and monitor her tests and scans while we continue with the present therapy – unless things change and she needs another treatment plan?'

'No, no, absolutely not', replied the doctor adamantly.

It seemed the lines had been drawn, but the parents were not sure whether the doctor had just told them he wouldn't do the scans or whether he'd given them the sack.

'As I've said before,' repeated Mark, 'we will continue to take Sarah to our GP for monitoring'. With that, he stood up, and Di followed. Sarah was only too happy to leave.

On the way home, Sarah was impatient. 'Will it still be light enough for swimming when we get home?'

Mark glanced at the clock on the car dashboard. It was nearly 4 pm. 'You might just get a quick dip in before dinner, Jogue', he said.

Di looked at Mark. 'What are we going to do now?'

'We'll have to find another specialist', answered Mark. 'Somebody a little more – flexible and communicative'.

Di looked discouraged. 'I'm beginning to wonder where we can find an oncologist like that'.

'There must be a lot of good oncologists and plenty of excellent hospitals around. We'll just have to find them', Mark replied hopefully.

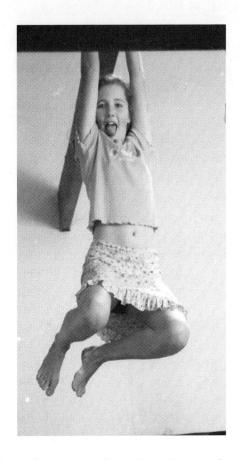

Eleven-year-old Sarah swinging from the rafters not long after her first operation, December 2002

GETTING VERY MESSY

**Respect your patient's right to choose their doctor freely,
To accept or reject advice, and to make their own
Decisions about treatment or procedures.**

AMA Doctors' Code of Ethics

From month to month all eyes were on Sarah's tumour markers, while she remained oblivious and spent the summer months having fun with her siblings. Her sister, Hannah, writes of that time:

Sarah used to play schools with us. She was the teacher, I was the teacher's aid and Leah and Josh were the students. Sarah organised assignments for Leah and Josh to do.

Sarah wanted to turn the old dairy into a granny flat with bedrooms, toilet, and a lounge room for us to sleep in. She also wanted to have a fete in the backyard where she could do activities with children and teach them how to paint.

Meanwhile we used to go over to the quarry together and bring a half a big blue drum that Sarah called a canoe and then go canoeing in it at the quarry. Seems there was heaps of slime in the water, which Sarah didn't mind, especially on hot days. Sarah also carved her name on the rocks in the quarry.

We used to go canoeing in the big dam that Dad made; and from the clay in the bottom of it, she would mould pots and clay balls for us and teach us how to do it.

Sarah and I used to catch wild ducks and get sticky tape and put a tag on their leg with a made up name on it. We also used to catch yellow, black and white striped grubs from up at Grandmas'. When she put them in a yoghurt box, they'd hatch out and fly away as butterflies. Sarah loved catching tadpoles and watching them grow into nice green frogs.

One day we went to a fair down at Newcastle where Sarah bought two hermit crabs and I bought one. On the way out of the big gates, we heard Sarah screaming in the back seat. To our surprise, she had a hermit crab latched onto her lips and it wouldn't let go. Dad stopped on the side of the road, jumped out of the car and flew around to Sarah's side. He finally unlatched the crab from her lip and drove home. Sarah had a dent in her lip and from then on Dad called the hermit crabs 'Lipstick' and the other one 'Smacker'.

In February of 2003, the Westley children started the new school year. Since Sarah had been keeping relatively well, Mark and Di did not want to risk her health by insisting she attend a full school day in addition to two long bus rides each day. They discussed it with the deputy headmaster and after that, teachers sent Sarah's schoolwork home with her younger siblings each day. She was now officially in Year 6.

When she was not busy with schoolwork, Sarah often wandered up to her favourite place. From 'Sarah's Hill', she looked toward the peaks of the Barrington Tops. There she watched monarch butterflies swarming around milkweed patches. She loved the way their luminous orange markings glowed in the sun. Sarah had learnt that monarchs drink the milky sap from the milkweed plant for a special substance that repels predators. The creatures showed no fear, as if they knew no one would harm them. Sitting up on her favourite hill, Sarah felt as free as those butterflies.

After a few months on her supplements and oxygen therapy, her parents noticed how well Sarah was looking, and made the decision to continue to allow Sarah to do her schoolwork at home for a while longer. Di had managed Sarah's care without outside help until Ruth offered to take over Sarah's school lessons and treatments. For the first time in weeks, Di had more time to devote to the other children. She could finally catch up with the housework and slip into town for food shopping, as long as she was back before 4 pm. Each afternoon when the school bus came to drop off Sarah's siblings, Ruth dropped Sarah back home. Once every few weeks, the parents took Sarah to the GP and her tumour markers remained at reasonable levels for a few months.

Ruth wrote in her diary of that time:

> *Sarah responded very well and was able to walk around the cattle with me, sometimes a journey of over 3 km, over steep hilly country. She helped with the household chores, gardening, and feeding the sheep and poultry, and I gave her maths, English and spelling lessons.*

The lessons were hard going at times. Lately Sarah had less taste for dry facts than before. 'Why would I have to know that?' she asked her grandmother about a math theory she thought had no relevance to her life.

Sarah found her English and spelling lessons less interesting than running across the pastures in her bare feet, the smell of the earth, the cows, and freshly cut firewood.

Sarah's quality of life was almost as good as it had been before her operation four months previously. She was full of vitamins, minerals, anti-oxidants and as much organic food as she could eat. She grew a centimeter taller over that time and weighed a healthy 43 kg. However, her sporty red cheeks belied her grim prognosis.

April and May brought the usual mild autumn and a cool winter. From her upstairs window, Sarah watched the Jacaranda leaves turn yellow on their fern like stems before drifting to the ground. The sunflowers her father had sown that summer on the river flats had gone to seed and attracted flocks of white cockatoos. In the veggie garden were strewn dozens of butternut pumpkins in the dense tangle of vines, plumping up for winter when her mother would make them into delicious soups and stews.

In early May, the farm cat had her last litter for the year. The days grew shorter and the nights brought a light frost. After school, the kids collected firewood and Di lit the iron stove before nightfall when it got cold. The Monarch butterflies had long since headed for the coast.

Each month Sarah's parents took her to the GP for a blood test, and by late April, Mark was spending more time in his study. Tests showed that Sarah's tumour markers were rising again, even though she remained active and vital. Since Mark and Dr Kotz had struck an agreement that another treatment plan would be necessary if the markers rose, Mark wanted to be ready for the next step. Over the past two weeks, he had devoted all his spare time to finding another medical team that included an integrative oncologist who combined conventional treatments with nutritional supplements. During Mark's internet search, he was pleasantly surprised to find that most of the well-known major US cancer hospitals in New York, Boston, Texas and Los Angeles offered integrative or complementary approaches as well as standard chemo and radiotherapy. It was a good start, but he was particularly looking for fully equipped cancer hospitals offering complementary treatments, along with a choice of non-toxic treatments or low-dose chemo options. Online he discovered a number of integrative oncology clinics and hospitals that offered this, in the UK, USA, Germany, France, Thailand, Singapore and Switzerland. One hospital's website stated:

> *Because we love our patients as ourselves and are bound by oath to do them no harm, we only offer therapies that have the potential to improve the patient's health without compromising the quality of his/her life. If we believe that a conventional therapy is necessary, we will make it available, but it will be administered in a way that will not cause the negative side effects generally associated with conventional therapies.*

Despite a lengthy search, Mark found no Australian hospital that offered these options, but a local man told him about the Integrative Health Clinic[8], located about two hours from where they lived. While considering overseas options, Mark made an appointment at the clinic to explore Sarah's treatment choices in Australia.

As it happened, the Integrative Health Clinic Mark had discovered was the medical clinic I had co-founded with a medical partner in 2001. I had been working in the public hospital system as a health professional for 30 years[9], including ten years in neurosurgical intensive care. In more recent times, I had developed a greater interest in natural medicine and returned to university to earn a science degree and qualifications in nutritional and complementary medicine. I also earned a diploma in journalism and have regularly written investigative articles as a freelancer.

At the clinic, we offered standard medical services, along with evidence - based complementary medicine. From the day we opened its doors, the clinic

---

[8] A pseudonym for the clinic existing at the time; it is no longer in operation. Also referred to herein as 'the clinic'.
[9] As an RN.

was immediately popular with patients who wanted treatment choices tailored to their needs. Our patients were usually independent types who didn't want doctors telling them what to do, think and feel. They wanted to collaborate with their health care providers and if necessary discuss information they had found on the internet or other places without having doctors becoming angry about it. They also wanted a comprehensive range of novel complementary treatments, and since I had extensive experience in hospital intensive care units, I set up and ran the clinic's intravenous program, which included IV vitamin C and a range of intravenous vitamin and antioxidant therapies.

In May, Mark and Di brought Sarah to the clinic for an appointment. Sarah pranced around the consultation room, making it difficult to conduct an examination. From the beginning, I noticed something special about Sarah. Despite her serious cancer, she seemed the happiest little girl I had ever seen. Everyone at the clinic sensed her joy and exuberance and it lifted our spirits just being around her.

Sarah's mother was shy and dignified while Mark was a man of few words. Together, they considered the hard evidence before making decisions and it was clear they had common sense and excellent critical reasoning skills.

Even more obvious was their love and concern for Sarah. They were discerning about the information they exposed her to and spoke to her in an age-appropriate way, while respecting her wishes and views.

Sarah was clearly well cared for. A quick stint on the scales showed that, despite her illness, she was in a healthy 68th percentile for her age in weight; while in height she was considerably taller than the average eleven-year-old. She had long limbs, clear eyes, red cheeks, and shiny hair that hung in loose curls past her shoulders. She did not complain of pain or discomfort and moved her body freely while performing her mischievous antics.

Mark had managed to obtain Sarah's blood test results from the family's GP, who had initially refused him copies but later allowed him the results over the phone, which Mark had written down and filed in his own folder. These results showed gradually rising tumour markers. The only other information Mark had, concerned Sarah's tumour type. On his last visit, Mark had asked the oncologist for the biopsy results which he had refused to hand over. Instead, the doctor wrote the type of tumour on a piece of paper, which Mark now took from his folder and showed to us. Otherwise, the parents had no paperwork relevant to their daughter's illness – an unusual situation, since most parents came armed with scans, blood results, and histology.[10] Without these, no prognosis or treatment plan is possible.

Like the Melbourne doctors, we were out of the information loop and did not know which stage of cancer Sarah was in or what her prognostic indicators were. This information was crucially important and we could do almost nothing without it.

Oncologists determine a cancer patient's prognosis – their chances of survival – by calculating several prognostic indicators after surgery or biopsy. This depends on the patient's type of cancer; its size, position, and whether it has metastasized or spread to other organs (Rosai 79).

The first step is usually 'staging' the cancer, which is the process of determining the degree to which the cancer has spread. Oncologists allocate a Roman numeral between I and IV, denoting the extent of spread. Stage IV indicates a late stage terminal cancer with a poor prognosis that has spread to the liver, spleen or other distant organs. Stage I, on the other hand, denotes the cancer has not spread. This carries the best prognosis for the sufferer with high chances of a five-year survival or even a long-term cure, depending on the cancer type. Within the stages are sub-stages: for example IA, IB, and IC. Stage IIIC cancer is considered advanced, while stage IV is late stage or terminal and has no sub-stages. Both of these stages usually carry poor prognoses (Rosai 79).

The next prognostic indicator that oncologists use is the grade of cancer, indicating its virulence or tendency to spread. Low grade or grade 1 cancers are not generally aggressive and are not prone to spread. They carry the best prognosis, especially if diagnosed early in stages I or II, before metastasising to more distant sites. On the other hand, grade 3 cancers are the most aggressive and prone to spread and recur, even with chemotherapy or other treatment. A grade 3 cancer diagnosed in stage III, when it has already spread, generally carries a poor prognosis (Rosai 79).

The next prognostic factor depends on the type of cancer. This was the only information Mark was able to elicit from the oncologist – but only a scribble on a paper and not a histology report.

Germ cell tumours (GCT) are a family of uncommon tumours. They arise from the immature reproductive cells of the testes and ovaries and manifest as

---

[10] According to *Good Medical Practice: A Code of Conduct for Doctors in Australia,* doctors are ethically required to give patients all information they request and keep them informed of all information including examination and test results, giving patients adequate opportunity to question or refuse intervention and treatment.

various types of ovarian and testicular cancers in children, and less commonly in adults. Of the many different subtypes of germ cell tumours, some are benign (non-malignant) and carry an excellent prognosis while others are highly malignant cancers that are lethal regardless of the treatment. Some are relatively more common, while a few are extremely rare. A long-term retrospective study found the survival rate of benign germ cell tumours in both girls and boys to be 96 per cent, and for malignant tumours, only 42 per cent survived for five years (Malogolowkin 90). However, these types of studies can easily be misinterpreted since both girls and boys are included in the groups, yet testicular germ cell tumours carry a better prognosis overall than ovarian germ cell tumours. For example, young males diagnosed in Stage I with low grade or benign tumours have five-year survival rates close to 100 per cent (Pectasides 06). In girls, on the other hand, ovarian germ cell tumours, even in the early stages, carry a worse prognosis, while some girls diagnosed with high grade late stage malignancies who relapse after chemotherapy typically have less than a 10 per cent chance of still being alive five years later (Murugaesu 06).

Along with several confounding factors surrounding germ cell tumours, such as gender, stage, and grade, the greatest confusion can stem from still another factor – their individual sub-types. Firstly, germ cell tumours themselves are a family of tumours so uncommon that relatively few studies exist of their individual sub-types. As stated earlier, most existing studies mix in testicular with ovarian germ cell tumours, even though testicular tumours have significantly better prognoses. Many studies also mix in several different germ cell tumour types, including both benign and malignant tumours, which tends to give false five-year survival rates. These general germ cell tumour studies do not necessarily apply to specific germ cell tumour sub-types, the worst of which cannot be compared with an entire group of germ cell tumours. Simply put, this would be akin to comparing a crate of mixed fruits to a pineapple. These germ cell tumour studies with both benign and highly malignant tumours mixed in can mislead even experienced clinicians when researching prognostic data about specific germ cell tumour types. For a clinician who has never treated a rare sub-group of germ cell cancer, the confusing data can be a minefield, and ethically the clinician is required to request the parents' permission to consult more experienced colleagues who have treated these rare germ cell tumours [11].

In Sarah's case, she had developed three malignant types of ovarian germ cell tumours. The first was dysgerminoma, the lesser in severity of the three,

---

[11] AMA Code of Ethics

which carried a 70–80 per cent five-year survival rate, even in its more advanced stages. This tumour spreads through the lymphatic system and gives off the telltale βHCG – the tumour marker discovered at the second hospital where Sarah was misdiagnosed as being pregnant[12].

Sarah's second ovarian cancer type was a rare and malignant variety called yolk sac tumour otherwise known as endodermal sinus tumour. It typically produces alfa-fetoprotein (AFP), the tumour marker the oncologist discovered in Sarah's blood at the regional hospital. This tumour typically spreads through the blood as well as seeding cancer cells throughout the abdominal region. From a review of the medical literature that specifically deals with yolk sac ovarian tumours, one prominent study cites the prognosis for patients in stages III and IV as being 30–25 per cent respectively (Nawa 01). This means that three quarters of patients with this cancer who are in stage IV die in the first five years, despite chemotherapy and other treatments. Another study corroborates these findings, stating that survival rates in the later stages were 'abysmal' (Ayhan 05). In a recent study, Swiss researchers support these findings, showing that any positive outcome occurs only when patients with this tumour are diagnosed early, in stage I, when 5-year survival rates are upward of 87 per cent (Dällenbach 06). However, in the advanced stages, the researchers claim, patients with yolk sac ovarian tumour have the same poor prognosis as women with late stage ovarian epithelial cancer (where only 10–15 out of every 100 patients are still alive at the five-year mark) (Dällenbach 06).

The prognosis after relapsing from this tumour is even grimmer. One recent study, which included girls as young as eight years old, showed that all who relapsed from this tumour after chemotherapy died of progressive disease (Ayhan 2005). Another study that included girls as young as five years old concluded, that even with up-to-date chemotherapy, the five-year survival rate for girls with stage IV yolk sac ovarian tumours is only 25 per cent, and of the ones who relapsed after chemotherapy there were no survivors in the studied group (Tong 08).

Sarah's third cancer type was the extremely rare and lethal ovarian embryonal carcinoma. This aggressive cancer produces both AFP as well as βHCG tumour markers. As one researcher put it, embryonal carcinoma is more frequently found in testicular germ cell tumours, and is 'vanishingly rare' in the form of ovarian germ cell cancer in girls. It was virtually unknown until researchers R. Kurman and H. Norris first described it in histological detail in

---

[12] Rice, 1999 and John Hopkins Pathology, 2001 .

1976, after finding that girls and young female patients with it rarely survived (Meriwether 71). In 1990, Japanese researchers reported a six-year survival in a young patient with stage II embryonal carcinoma, but stated that the prognoses in the latter stages are not as optimistic (Ueda 90).

With all three tumour components, Sarah's cancer was classified as a 'mixed germ cell tumour'. The prognosis of mixed tumours depends entirely on the characteristics of its individual components and the stage of the tumour. For Sarah it was a worse case scenario – she had two of the worst possible cancer types, of the highest virulence, at the latest stages, with a near certainty the cancers would recur despite any form of treatment. According to the available research specific to her tumour types, Sarah had, at the time of her diagnosis, a less than a 30 per cent chance of surviving five years, despite surgery or the gold standard chemotherapy. Her high grade, late stage tumours carried an almost certain chance of recurrence no matter what treatment was used, after which time she had an almost zero chance of survival.[13] Therefore, her treatment options should have been flexible and included measures to preserve the quality of life she had left.

Usually oncologists propose treatment options to patients according to the risk versus benefit principle – taking into account the patient's individual preferences, the likelihood of a cure, the seriousness of the side effects and risks of treatment, and the willingness of the patient to tolerate the risks and discomforts. Ethically, the decision should be made in honest discussions and in partnership with the patient and/or family.[14] In treating children with cancer, best clinical practice means considering the child's point of view (Shield 94). Treatment options normally encompass a reasonable compromise between preserving the patient's quality of life versus the likely benefits, harms, and emotional and physical costs to the patient and family (Reuben 04). There is no reason why any poor prognosis late stage cancer patient should be forced into any treatment against their wishes and, in particular, into one with few if any likely benefits.

Sarah's case qualified her for some of the newer cancer treatments with fewer side effects aimed at preserving quality of life. She was also permitted palliative treatments, which should be offered to all children with ultimately

---

[13] Kawai 2006, Nawa 2001, Ayhan 2005, Dällenbach 2006, Tong 08, Fujita 93, Ueda 90.
[14] Informed Consent, Parental Permission, and Assent in Pediatric Practice. Committee on Bioethics PEDIATRICS, Volume 95 Number 2, pp. 314–317, February 1995.

terminal conditions.[15] Her late stage cancer also entitled her to supportive treatments, including the complementary treatments she was already receiving.

Cancer patients, and particularly those in the last stages, require accurate information about their condition in order to make appropriate decisions. Doctors are ethically required to be honest about the diagnosis and prognosis, especially when their patients are facing an ultimately terminal condition and wish to know the details of their illness, as in Sarah's case. The AMA Code of Ethics requires doctors to:

> *Recognise the need for physical, psychological, emotional, and spiritual support for the patient, the family and other carers, not only during the life of the patient, but also after their death.*

When the parents brought Sarah to our clinic, they saw themselves as being in an impossible situation and wanted the best care possible for their daughter. We knew about hospitals overseas that offered integrative cancer treatments, but were unaware of any in Australia. This included metronomic chemotherapy, a form of low dose chemo, conveniently taken in tablet form.[16]

Clinicians in the US, Europe and Asia have used metronomic chemotherapy for the past 35 years on a variety of adult and paediatric cancers, and it is well tolerated by children (Kamen 00). In daily low doses, the drug(s) attack the tumour's blood supply and in many cases keep the cancer from spreading. Instead of maximum tolerated dose (MTD) intravenous chemotherapy, many oncologists prefer metronomic chemo as first line treatment for solid tumours, as well as maintenance therapy for children with blood cancers. The treatment is increasingly used as salvage chemotherapy[17] on patients with solid tumours who have relapsed after standard chemotherapy (Kerbel & Kamen 04, Andre 08).

Coincidentally, while Sarah's parents were searching out this option, Lisa,[18] a young Italian woman with ovarian cancer, was being admitted to Dr Riccardo Samaritani's unit at San Carlo Sanità Hospital in Rome. She had

---

[15] Academy of Paediatrics 2002.
[16] Metronomic chemotherapy (MC) is the administration of chemotherapy at doses below the maximal tolerated dose on a frequent schedule of administration, with no prolonged drug-free breaks.
[17] Salvage therapy is a form of cancer treatment given after the cancer does not respond to standard treatments.
[18] A pseudonym

relapsed after having had standard intravenous chemotherapy treatment. When her oncologist prescribed a further round of the high dose intravenous chemotherapy, Lisa's cancer grew out of control, even while she was receiving the treatment. The new tumour growth obstructed her bowel and she required a colostomy. The oncologist expected Lisa to die and, as a last resort, he prescribed metronomic chemotherapy. The treatment immediately stopped the growth of the already advanced tumour, while Lisa experienced no side effects from it. (Samaritani 01, Gasparini 01).

In view of the innovative cancer treatments available internationally, Mark and Di's requests for information about overseas cancer hospitals were entirely reasonable and under their present circumstances, it seemed a good idea to take Sarah to a major cancer centre with experience in her rare cancers, while she was still well enough to travel.

The parents said they would take some time to consider their options. Meanwhile I detailed a full, nutrient-dense nutritional protocol for Sarah to maintain her general health and stamina.[19] I then gave the parents written information about a number of overseas cancer hospitals that offered specialist care, imaging, surgical facilities, complementary medicine and metronomic chemotherapy, as well as standard chemo and radiation.

The parents left the clinic with Sarah late that afternoon. On their way home, Mark stopped at a suburban village shopping centre for some cold drinks. When leaving the supermarket, he passed a post office and had an idea.

'Do you have passport application forms?' Mark asked the woman behind the counter.

The postmistress smiled. 'We sure do, just for yourself?' she asked.

'I'd like three please'.

The woman was happy to oblige and handed over the paperwork.

Mark returned to the car with the drinks.

'What took you so long, Dad?' asked Sarah, as she grabbed one of the orange juice drink boxes her father was juggling.

Di looked at the passport application forms. 'What's that?'

Mark looked from Di to Sarah. 'What would you say if we found a hospital that offered us more choices?'

'Do I have to see that doctor again?' whined Sarah from the back seat.

---

[19] Known as nutritional loading.

'Which one, Jogue?' asked Mark.

Sarah pulled a face. 'You know. The one at the hospital who gets in a bad mood'.

Mark grinned and shook his head. 'No Sarah, this hospital is overseas where you'd be seeing a different oncologist and a whole team of people who could help you'. He unfolded one of the pamphlets and started reading.

'What kind of people?' persisted Sarah.

Mark chuckled. 'Well let's see, it says here that the hospital has some special doctors who can work together to get you better. You could probably keep taking your supplements and oxygen treatment along with the cancer medicine they prescribe for you. A special dietician can make you organic food and juices just like your Mum does for you, and there's a counselor, a massage therapist, and a surgeon on staff'. Mark lowered the pamphlet and looked directly at Sarah. 'But we'll have to travel overseas to America', he added.

Sarah's eyes widened. 'Could we go on the plane?'

Mark laughed. 'Yes. But I'm warning you, that trip would take a lot longer than the one to Melbourne'.

Sarah looked wildly excited. 'Yea, Dad. Let's go now!' she squealed.

Mark turned to Di. 'What do you think?

Di had been thinking about their predicament. 'You'll get no argument from me. But can we afford it and would your folks be willing to look after the other kids?'

Mark had an idea. He did a mental calculation of how much he could raise from selling half his cattle herd and he was almost certain his parents would be willing to look after the kids. 'It would take a bit of organising. But I think it's our best bet for now', he said.

Di took the passport applications from Mark and stowed them in her hand-bag. She would have to start on them as soon as they got home.

It was the first time Mark and Di had been in total agreement so quickly on such a hefty issue.

On the way home, Sarah lay across the back seat with her seatbelt awkwardly attached and watched the sun flickering through the trees as they drove. Her parents were in a good mood and chatted all the way home.

Over the next few days, Mark and Di gathered the necessary documentation for their passport applications. Di searched for Sarah's mislaid birth certificate, while Mark established a folder dedicated to the travel arrangements and hospital information. He costed airfares and learnt more about the cancer hospital they intended taking Sarah to in the US. The process of completing travel arrangements would take a few weeks and he kept the ever-expanding file open next to his computer.

When they had gathered all their documents together, the parents planned to drive to the larger township of Taree, 150 km away, to have them processed. Then they would be free to travel. The main hold-up came when Mark's birth certificate was also misplaced. Meanwhile, Sarah had another appointment coming up with the GP, for the May tumour markers.

On the morning of 2 May, Caitlin Grimes, the social worker at the regional hospital, left Dr Kotz's office after a meeting. Over the months, they'd had regular meetings about the Westley family, including one with the head of the paediatric department.

Grimes knew a lot about the family. She had met them when they had first arrived with Sarah at the regional hospital. She had profiled them as being the types who were apt to be difficult and instructed the nurses to watch the family closely. The family had asked a lot of questions about Sarah's treatment and wanted proof. But today, there would be no more questions. The oncologist had authorised her to take action. The social worker did not think other cancer treatments existed, apart from the one the oncologist wanted, and by all accounts she felt justified in the drastic action she was about to take. She had dealt with the child protection department (DoCS) before when other parents had baulked about their child having chemo. The problem was more common now that people looked on the internet.

After reviewing her notes one final time, the social worker called the Department of Community Services (DoCS) Hotline, a special phone line dedicated to reporting child abuse. When a child protection caseworker took her call, the social worker alleged that Sarah was a child medically neglected by her parents, and that they had not arranged urgent medical care for Sarah. The child protection caseworker made an official record of this complaint.

Grimes then further alleged that 'The parents are affiliated with a religion which prohibits them from allowing Sarah to have chemotherapy'. The caseworker at the other end noted this false statement. Grimes went on to claim that the parents were preventing Dr Kotz from giving their daughter lifesaving chemotherapy. The social worker did not mention that Sarah was in the advanced stages of cancer, and that the matter was not a medical emergency, but more a matter for honest discussion about treatment options between the doctor and the parents. Likewise, the social worker did not mention that the oncologist and Mark had made an agreement to monitor the tumour markers for the time being, and then formulate another course of action if they rose significantly. Now was that time, but the doctor had chosen to report the parents to the authorities rather than have those planned discussions with them. The social worker also failed to inform the department of the family's desperate attempt to seek a second oncologist's opinion and how they had been stopped from receiving that independent opinion. Finally, there was no mention that the family GP was monitoring Sarah every few weeks. Instead, the social worker's report sounded as though the family had done nothing about Sarah's illness.

On hearing the complaint, the child protection caseworker told the social worker that, because of her status as a health professional, she would class her child abuse complaint as 'urgent'. In turn, she asked Grimes for a letter from Dr Kotz confirming the complaint. The department required his expert opinion as to Sarah's prognosis with treatment. The department would action the complaint as soon as the caseworker received the doctor's letter. Unfortunately, this was not the first unfounded report that hospital personnel had made to the child protection department about Sarah. This report now resided in the department's case file alongside the previous, outlandish report alleging that Sarah was 14 weeks' pregnant.

Three days later, on 8 May, the oncologist wrote his letter to the department. In it, he withheld the same relevant information the social worker had. He claimed that the family had not returned to him since they had been to see 'a couple of people in Melbourne who dabbled in alternative therapy' – by which he presumably meant the Melbourne GP and specialist oncologist the family had visited for a second opinion and supportive treatment. He did not mention that the family had seen him in January after they had returned from Melbourne, when all parties had agreed to monitor the tumour markers month by month – an agreement the doctor recorded in Sarah's clinical records. Finally, he maintained to the department that his treatment had an 87 per cent chance of a permanent cure, and without it, Sarah would not survive.

On receiving the oncologist's letter, the department began an immediate investigation. Caseworkers issued urgent requests for information under Section 248 of the NSW Children and Young Persons (Care and Protection) Act 1998. They contacted those who'd had contact with the family, including; Sarah's school principal, Dr Milne, Dr Sales, the family GP and others. The letter's tone made it clear to the recipients that they were compelled to answer all the department's questions under threat of legal consequences. Following the letters, caseworkers contacted the recipients personally. They interviewed them by phone and transcribed their answers into legal affidavits.

Soon the department's aggressive investigational methods hit pay dirt. When a department caseworker contacted Dr Sales in Melbourne, the doctor behaved as he had warned Mark he would do, should the case 'go legal', and agreed to make out an affidavit against the family. The document seemed to be Sales' attempt to distance himself from the family to avoid any unpleasant professional consequences, and it proved useful to the department.

Without delay, the primary school principal returned the questionnaire in writing, replying: 'Sarah is always well groomed and cared for. She is a well mannered and co-operative student'.

Dr Milne, however, declined to answer the letter and would not be interviewed by caseworkers, believing that there is no law broken when people choose second opinions or other treatments.

Finally, the department interviewed the family GP. Unfortunately for the family, the doctor repeated the incorrect speculations originating from his discussions the previous November with Dr Little, the hospital registrar who had alleged Sarah was pregnant and that the family was part of a religious sect that did not believe in modern medicine. To make matters worse, the GP had also been primed in January when Dr Kotz wrote him a letter reiterating Sarah's likely cure with his treatment and telling him of his intention to contact the child protection department should the parents not agree or co-operate with him. The GP, who had seen the family on a regular basis, still sought no other side to the story. He now repeated this incorrect information to the caseworker, who recorded him on 13 May as having said about the family: '...they are misguided by their religious beliefs ... belong to a sect ... and have an alternative lifestyle and beliefs'.

This doctor's contribution added more fuel to a fire already well out of control.

Meanwhile, the family remained unaware that the doctors and the Department of Community Services were building a case against them.

While DoCS investigators were digging deep to make their case, Mark and Di completed their passport applications and were ready to finalise their travel arrangements to take Sarah to the US cancer hospital. Mark's next day off work was 15 May, when they'd planned to travel to Taree to put their passport applications in for processing and to organise tickets from a travel agent. Within 14 days, they would be on a flight with Sarah to a state-of-the-art cancer hospital that offered metronomic low toxicity chemotherapy as well as her usual complementary treatments. The US hospital was fully equipped with operating theatres, CT and MRI scanners, surgeons, oncologists, nurses, counselors, integrative doctors, naturopaths, dieticians, a chef, and cancer support personnel.

By mid-May, the growing DoCS file on the family was transferred from head office to the department's regional branch office. Like the family, the case file would also travel to the coastal town of Taree, located in the Manning river basin. The town was named after the 'tareebit', an Aboriginal word meaning the 'tree by the river'. The name refers to the sandpaper fig, a species of tree that grows prolifically along the rivers and creeks and nourishes the caterpillars of Sarah's favourite ethereal purple moonbeam butterflies that swarm around the river lands after hatching.

The DoCS office in Taree backs on to the Manning River. Gary Boggs headed the branch in charge of child protection for the greater region, including Gloucester.

Ironically, the department is overshadowed from the north by the Three Brothers Mountains, the site of the Dream Time legend of a witch who stole the fabled Aboriginal children from their family. For Indigenous Australians the legends still live today and in the future. For the child protection personnel, if they know it at all, the legend is probably nothing but folklore. Over the last fortnight, that team of caseworkers from the Taree office had worked tirelessly to 'protect' Sarah from 'parental neglect'.

On 14 May, a caseworker from Taree DoCS phoned the Westley home. Di took the call and was shocked to hear from the child protection department, since she had no children in need of protection from abuse or neglect. When the caseworker wanted to come to the house that afternoon Di asked her instead to come the following day, on Mark's day off. True to her country traditions, Di spent the rest of the afternoon baking scones for official guests the next morning.

After the kids went to bed, Di stayed up until Mark had finished his late shift in the early hours of the morning. After telling him the news, both were intrigued by the scheduled visit, and thought perhaps the child welfare people had found out about Sarah and were coming to help families like theirs with a sick child to look after. They thought it was awfully nice of them.

The next morning, on 15 May, Mark phoned an acquaintance who'd recently been to the house and had commented on how well Sarah looked despite her serious illness. The man had worked in the police force before retiring and was familiar with the child protection department's way of doing things. He was shocked to hear of the caseworkers' planned visit that morning. Mark asked him whether they might be coming instead to help them or assist them with the cost of Sarah's illness.

The man gave a bitter laugh. 'Perhaps, once upon a time. But these days they're more like the GESTAPO'.

When Mark asked advice on how to handle the interview; the man warned him not give them any extra information.

'Why not?' asked Mark. 'Wouldn't it be easier just to have a chat with them?'

The man let out a howl. 'No! These people don't chat, they write out affidavits. Everything you say can be and will be used to incriminate you'.

'Incriminate us in what?' demanded Mark. 'We haven't done anything wrong'.

'They'll do whatever they want. You shouldn't even let them into your house', Mark's friend replied.

Mark couldn't help a cynical chuckle. It all seemed too unbelievable 'That's a bit much', he retorted. 'They're supposed to help us. That's what they're there for'.

The man was adamant. 'Their system is coercive, not charitable. They have police powers, and do not mind using them. Nobody tells them what to do, not even parliament. Here's hoping you're never tangled up with them. Once you are, they'll never let you go. Like I said, do not let them into your house. Call a lawyer instead'.

Mark could hardly believe the man's advice. It went against his deepest-held beliefs. He'd always strongly felt that people everywhere, even in government departments, were reasonable if given half a chance.

'And one more thing', said the retired officer. 'Don't, whatever you do, tell them you want to take Sarah overseas, or they'll make sure you'll never step outside your front door again without them knowing about it. These people are not averse to using dirty tricks either. So be careful'.

An hour later, it was nearly lunchtime, but nobody was hungry. Sarah's aunt and baby cousin were visiting the house, while Sarah was over at Ruth's having her treatments and school lessons. Just on noon, two caseworkers from the Taree office drove up the drive in a white compact car. They knocked on the door and for a few moments, Mark and Di were frozen to the spot. Maybe the friend had been right after all and they shouldn't let them in, they thought.

While they deliberated, Sarah's aunt scuttled into another room, protectively clutching her baby.

Mark opened the door to two caseworkers wearing business suits. Gillian introduced herself first. She was the younger and did most of the talking while Judy was a quieter, middle-aged woman. Mark invited them in while Di offered them a seat at the table she'd already set for morning tea. Di went to the kitchen to fix the pot of tea and retrieve the scones. As usual, she was more than happy to let Mark do the talking.

From their seats at the table, the women scanned around the house. They peered into the kitchen and living room, and even down the hallway towards the study. Just as Mark was starting to feel scrutinised, Gillian spoke to him in an official tone, using frequent psychological terms. She said the department had received a report that Sarah was not receiving appropriate treatment for her condition, and that her tumour markers had risen. Di was just pouring boiling water into the teapot and was shocked to hear the woman claim they had not taken care of Sarah. She immediately returned to the dining room. Like Mark, Di thought that if the women only knew the truth they would see that they were doing everything possible to help Sarah. She joined Mark in listing their numerous efforts to get Sarah the best possible treatment. For the time being, however, they followed their friend's advice and withheld the information about their plans to take her to the overseas hospital.

Feeling somewhat shaken, Di served morning tea while the women questioned Mark closely about Sarah's complementary treatment. He painstakingly explained the basic premise for the treatment; that the oxygen was detrimental to cancer cells and the supplements helped Sarah's energy and vitality. Judy asked him what medical supervision Sarah was having. Mark replied that the Melbourne team and the local GP were monitoring Sarah's tests and that several months previously they had consulted another oncologist for a second opinion. He explained that he had recently found another specialist, but again stopped short of mentioning the overseas hospital. When the caseworkers wanted to know who it was, Mark told them he and Di were currently discussing it with staff at the Integrative Health Clinic. The caseworkers wanted the details of the clinic, which Mark told them he would provide later.

Mark and Di expected that this information would reassure the caseworkers that Sarah was indeed getting regular and continuous medical care, but the women seemed to find this of little interest. They were more interested in what the parents' view of chemotherapy was. Mark explained that he was not against it but that he and Di wanted to see evidence it would work, especially in the high doses the oncologist had in mind that were known to kill the patients on occasion. He added that despite many requests they had never received this evidence from the oncologist. He explained that they did not know why the doctor withheld this from them; perhaps because he had not encountered Sarah's type of cancer before. Perhaps evidence was difficult to find, he speculated.

The caseworker asked whether this was why they had not gone back to see the oncologist. Mark explained that they had in fact gone to him in January, that since then they had been watching the tumour markers and that now it was time for another treatment plan. He repeated that the main barrier between the family and the oncologist was the oncologist's refusal to provide them with information. This had made it difficult to make decisions and they felt they had to go to another doctor. Mark stressed again that this was the most serious decision they'd ever had to make and they needed all the information they could get to make the right one.

Mark noticed the bland expressions on both caseworkers and wondered what they might have done if it were their child. He began to sense that the caseworkers were not hearing him and that the more he talked, the deeper he was digging a hole for himself. Both caseworkers had taken out their notepads and were writing prolifically.

When Judy asked whether their decisions were influenced by their religious beliefs, Mark was stunned. He explained that he and Di were non-denominational, not allied with any organised religion or sect, and that neither of them consulted anyone but medical practitioners on medical matters. He added that he and Di had made every decision so far based solely on the medical information at hand, and when the oncologist had with held information, they had been forced to find it themselves among clinical studies or by asking other doctors.

When Gillian asked what their current plan was, Mark replied that in light of the latest blood test they now planned to see new doctors for the next step in Sarah's care. He noticed the discussion was now becoming circular – he had already told them there was a new plan now the markers had risen. Were they trying to catch him out, he wondered.

When not busy writing, both caseworkers peered through the archways leading to other rooms looking for the missing Sarah. Mark wondered whether they thought a critically ill and pitifully neglected child lay somewhere behind those closed doors. When the caseworkers finally asked where Sarah was, Di told them she was at her grandmother's house having school lessons. When the women insisted on seeing her, Sarah's aunt came out from an adjoining room and volunteered to fetch Sarah from Ruth's.

Judy waited until Sarah's aunt was gone. 'We will have to serve a legal notice on Sarah', she announced.

The parents were disturbed to hear this and Mark wondered how anyone could rightfully serve a legal document on an 11-year-old child. As far as they'd been led to believe, the visit was meant as a simple discussion. This now felt more like a betrayal and maybe even a trap. Perhaps they should have consulted a lawyer first and not let them in, Mark thought.

Just as Mark and Di were about to question the caseworkers further, Gillian searched in her briefcase and produced a document for Mark. She then handed him a legal notice stating that under Section 173 of the Children and Young Persons (Care and Protection) Act 1998, he and Di were forced to take Sarah to Dr Kotz at a specified time the following week.

Mark was alarmed when he realised this could interfere with their trip to the overseas hospital. 'Couldn't we take Sarah to another doctor?' he asked. 'An oncologist *we* had in mind?'

Gillian seemed troubled at first but quickly regained her footing. 'It's really important that you agree to at least take the first step with us and get this complete assessment done on Sarah', she said in an official tone.

Mark understood the embedded refusal in the dry language, but he stood his ground. 'Look, we were about to take Sarah to another specialist anyway, but we do not want to return to Dr. Kotz'.

The caseworkers looked uncertain for a moment.

Mark was tense about having their plans ruined. He looked at Di and saw she'd chewed her thumbnail ragged.

The women gazed at each other as though communicating non-verbally.

'Perhaps we can accommodate you somewhat on that', said Judy with a faint smile.

'Yes', agreed Gillian as she rose up from her seat at the table. "I'll be happy to make arrangements for you to see another oncologist of the department's choice – if you don't mind letting me use your phone'.

Mark was caught by surprise and showed her to his study, without first having had time to put away his open files. Gillian went to Mark's desk and hesitated before picking up the phone as though expecting him to leave. He returned to the dining room pale with nerves. What he had thought would be a sensible discussion now felt like a legal investigation. At the table, Di sat uncomfortably while Judy continued scrutinising their home.

Mark's talk with the retired police friend now ran unchecked through his mind and he wished he had taken his advice. He read the summons again and wondered what kind of powers these people had and what they were trained to do. Mark had always been up front with people because he and Di had never done anything wrong. He had always believed they had choices, yet this summons compelled them to take Sarah to a doctor they had never met.

While Gillian was out of the room making phone calls to doctors, Sarah arrived from her grandmother's house. She burst in through the front door looking bemused, wondering who wanted her in the middle of her school lesson.

Judy stared at Sarah. 'Who is this?' she demanded.

Sarah came around the table to sit on her mother's lap. 'It's Sarah', said Di. The caseworker looked confused and took a moment to consult her paperwork. From Caitlin Grime's complaint and Dr Kotz's letter, she had expected to see a child whose medical treatment was neglected. She looked from the paperwork to Sarah and back several times. The strangeness of it lingered for a moment, as the child with red cheeks and shiny long hair did not accord with the department's paperwork.

Sarah sat waiting to hear what the woman wanted. Finally, Judy asked her to come outside with her. Sarah reluctantly went as far as the doorway.

The caseworker used a well-rehearsed monotone: 'Hi Sarah, we're from the Department of Community Services, have you heard about us?'

Sarah tried not to giggle at the woman's rehearsed formality. 'No', she replied.

The woman handed Sarah a piece of paper. It was a summons. Sarah took it, uncertain about what to do with it. She did not know that some pieces of paper could cause problems.

The caseworker told Sarah: 'My job is to work with families and make sure that children are being cared for properly. The reason I am here today is that we have received some information that you are not well. I understand that you had an operation in November and we just need to check and see how everything is going. Is that okay?'

'Yeah', said Sarah, bewildered.

The caseworker continued: 'I have spoken to Mum and Dad and given them this piece of paper, which is basically asking them to take you to a doctor for a complete up-to-date assessment. Because you are 11, you are old enough to understand and be included in these discussions. So this piece of paper here is the same as what I have given Mum and Dad and it is asking them to take you to see a doctor next week. Do you understand?'

Sarah was silent, unsure about why this woman wanted her to go to another doctor. (Later, the caseworker noted in her report: 'Sarah did not say very much at all'.) As far as Sarah was concerned, she had been seen by no less than 10 doctors and had undergone dozens of examinations including an operation over the previous six months. Only three days previously, she had been to the family GP for a blood test. She went to him once a month. She was having daily oxygen treatments, and felt quite well at present. She also knew her father had made further appointments and plans for her to see other doctors in just a few days. And in a few weeks she would be in an aeroplane bound for a large American cancer hospital for further treatment. Sarah would have found it incomprehensible that someone would come to her home with a piece of paper to say that she must go to a doctor, when she thought that she was already seeing plenty of doctors.

Gillian, who had previously left the room to make the phone call, now reappeared after 20 minutes. When she saw Sarah, she looked confused. 'Did you find Sarah?' she asked.

'She's right there', said Mark as he pointed to his red-cheeked daughter, who was clutching the summons.

Gillian stared in disbelief at Sarah and watched her carefully as she went to sit on her father's lap.

'Did you find another oncologist?' asked Judy, trying to return her colleague's attention.

Gillian was still bewildered. 'Yes, I did', she answered distractedly, before snapping back into her official manner. 'I've made an appointment on 20 May for you to take Sarah to an oncologist in a Sydney-based hospital, and you must take her there – by law', she warned. 'Here are the details'.

Mark took the sheet of paper and the caseworkers left soon after.

With the women gone, Sarah's aunt emerged from the room she had retreated to. Sarah shrugged her shoulders and left the summons on the kitchen table before going outside to search for caterpillars. Mark picked up the paper and wondered whether anyone had the right to issue an eleven-year-old with a summons.

With Sarah out of the room, Di got up to wash the dishes. 'She was in your study for a long time', she said.

Mark returned a worried look and headed off to check his papers. It was the first time he'd ever felt violated in his own home.

The caseworkers returned to their Taree office almost two hours later. Judy stayed back late to write up her report. In it, she stated:

The child arrived with her aunty and her baby cousin. I observed the child to be tall, slender; she had rosy cheeks, good skin tone, bright eyes, and no visible signs of being ill, bouncy, active and apparently not incapacitated due to her illness.

However, these notations, along with the parents' ongoing efforts to have Sarah's medical needs properly attended to, did not stop the department's investigation – if anything, it was accelerated. The director of Taree office, Gary Boggs, consulted with internal legal advisors at the Sydney office the following day. Caseworkers from head office were already involved after receiving the oncologist's letter. Doctors' letters were taken seriously and always carried more weight than a complaint from an ordinary person, whose motives the department sometimes scrutinised. Doctors suffered no such scrutiny and the matter now had captured the interest of some people in high places within the department. The Director-General himself would become involved soon.

Mark and Di lay in bed that night, both unable to sleep. The alarm on the dresser showed 1 am. In the sky hung a half moon that softly lit the tall eucalypts outside their bedroom window.

'Are you still awake?' asked Di.

'Looks like I'm not the only one', quipped Mark.

'Do you think we can still take Sarah overseas?'

Mark had been mulling over that question himself. 'Not right now. You saw those legal summonses. If we put our passport applications in, there's no telling what they'd do to stop us. We're forced to see that doctor in Sydney, before we can do anything else'.

'What are we going to do if we can't get Sarah to that American hospital?' asked Di.

'I don't know', said Mark. 'Maybe the DoCS oncologist has some answers for us. Meanwhile, nobody can stop us going to the Integrative Health Clinic and then on a quick trip to Melbourne. What do you think?'

Di thought for a while. 'Sounds like that's all we *can* do right now'.

'After we do what they want, let's hope they leave us alone, so we can get Sarah out of here for proper treatment', added Mark.

Di already knew the answer before asking the next question. 'Is this what the oncologist meant when he said things would get very messy?'

THE WHOLE BOX OF
FROGS

Treat your patient with compassion and respect.

AMA Doctor's Code of Ethics

Not long after the caseworker's visit came the day Mark and Di were legally required to take Sarah to the Sydney oncologist. The family had arranged appointments with their other health practitioners on the same trip, which made the department's demands to drive the 660 km round trip to Sydney slightly more tolerable.

The night before the trip, temperatures dropped to freezing, leaving a lace of frost on the pastures the next morning. Early on 19 May, Mark packed the family's mini-van for their road trip, first to see us at the Integrative Health Clinic and then on to Sydney where they planned to stay the night with family friends in the west Sydney suburb of Ryde. The next morning, from Ryde they had only a quick trip to the city hospital to see Dr Roger Capewell, the oncologist the child protection department had demanded they see. After their appointment with him, they planned to set off on the 900 km trip to Melbourne by car to consult with the Melbourne integrative health team there.

While Mark checked the oil and tyres on the van, Di prepared the other five children for school. At 8 am sharp each day the school bus stopped at the mailbox. The driver was not one to wait for kids who were even a minute late, so for the next 10 days, while the parents were away with Sarah, they had a schedule worked out. Their other kids would stay with Ruth and Jim; Ruth would drive them to the bus stop, and Laura would get them to the bus on time and shepherd them back home in the afternoon. The children would spend a few hours at home to feed the animals and do their homework, before Ruth picked them up and took them home with her for the night.

The kids hugged Sarah goodbye before they ran for the bus. She liked to languish under the warm covers until just before her mother headed upstairs. The floor was cold in winter, except when her father stacked the downstairs combustion stove with hardwood and left it burning all night. Then it left a warm patch on her bedroom floor just above the stove.

An hour later, Di locked the door and they set out, heavily packed, for the long trip. Mark had recently bought the mini-bus to make travel with the large family more comfortable. With plenty of room in the back, Sarah made a cubby across the rear seat with quilts and pillows. As Mark steered down the drive, she glanced back through the rear window. The homestead was covered in frost and looked like a Christmas postcard from England. She would miss the farm while she was away, but it was all right this time of year – there were no more caterpillars or butterflies until spring.

In an affluent suburb of Sydney, Dr Capewell prepared to leave for work. As usual, he had an impossibly busy schedule. Not only was he an oncologist in a major city hospital, but also a research scientist involved with several cancer research organisations.

Capewell arrived at the hospital at 9 am. His secretary had a latte ready on his desk; without speaking to her, he closed his office door. He enjoyed reading oncology journals for a few minutes each morning. Cancer research was a competitive industry. Each year Capewell had to apply for millions in grants to keep his research going, and it paid to find out what others were doing in the field, just to get an edge on the funding.

The phone rang and he reluctantly picked it up. It was his personal assistant. 'Will you take a call from DoCS about your appointment tomorrow with the Westley family?'

'If you insist', he said as he finished his coffee.

It was the child protection caseworker from the Taree office. 'Just touching base to make sure you understand what the department is requiring of you in the Westley case...'

'Yes' interrupted Capewell. 'A full, thorough medical assessment. I have worked with DoCS before and undertaken section 173 assessments'.

'Then you would know we require a written letter or report from you as soon as possible after that', the caseworker reminded him.

'Just a minute', said Capewell. He put the phone down and searched his in-tray for a file on the Westley girl, but found nothing. In the six days since the department had legally appointed him, no one had sent him any records. At least Dr Kotz from the regional hospital had briefed him last Friday.

'Could you get the parents to bring down any scans, test results and any information they have?' he asked.

'I'll contact the parents and request they take these documents with them to their appointment', answered the caseworker.

After the call, the caseworker tried for most of the day to contact Mark and Di at the farm, but the phone rang out each time. By chance, in the late afternoon Laura answered the phone. She and the kids had just come off the school bus. The younger ones were outside feeding the animals while Laura was at the computer doing her homework. Their grandmother was due to pick them up any minute.

Laura told the caseworker that her parents had already gone to Sydney and would be staying with friends at Ryde overnight before their hospital appointment the next day. The caseworker wanted the friend's number, but Laura didn't have it handy. It would have made little difference – Mark and Di simply did not have any scans or tumour histology results. That had been their problem from the beginning – the oncologist had refused them that information and kept them in the dark about Sarah's true prognosis.

The following day was 20 May. The family had enjoyed spending time with their friends in Ryde. Just after lunch, dressed in their Sunday best, they left for the city. Mark negotiated the busy city streets and one-way lanes only to find the hospital car park was full. The hospital was a massive concrete structure jammed between other inner city buildings without a park or a patch of grass in sight. Once inside the front lobby, Sarah giggled at the clown statue as they walked past.

The family arrived in the upstairs cancer ward on time for their 2.30 pm appointment with Dr Capewell. When they knocked on the oncologist's office door, he opened it promptly. The doctor was stylishly dressed with a multicoloured tie that was obviously meant to cheer up his paediatric patients. Just inside his office stood his desk and a small examination cubicle butted up against the opposite wall. In the corner sat the oncology social worker who was already busy taking notes before the family had said anything. The oncologist introduced first himself and then the social worker. The parents sat down in front of the doctor's desk while Sarah sat on Mark's knee.

'Do you know why you're here?' opened the oncologist after everyone was seated.

'We had no choice in the matter', answered Mark.

The doctor paused and smiled faintly. 'Did you bring any scans or test results?'

'No, we've never been given any', said Mark.

'Is that so?' asked the doctor somewhat surprised. 'Then what do you know about your daughter's illness?'

Mark wondered why the doctor was asking him this. Didn't he have Sarah's medical records? Nevertheless, he related what little he had been told of Sarah's illness.

The doctor listened carefully and made notes in the file. 'Perhaps I should have a feel of her tummy. If you'd like to come with me?' he said, pointing to the examination bed in the corner.

Di took Sarah's hand and helped her up on the bed. Sarah co-operated and let the doctor feel her abdomen.

'Hum, that feels pretty normal', he said to himself before taking her pulse. When he'd finished, he washed his hands and returned to his desk to make notations in Sarah's file. After that, he ordered a pathology test.

Di returned to her seat with Sarah and waited for the doctor to speak.

When he put his pen down, the oncologist addressed Mark and Di with his verdict. 'Though I can feel no abnormality at the moment, your daughter's tumour markers are rising and she will have to have chemotherapy'.

'Do you mean the kind of chemo with the serious side effects? asked Mark.

'Yes, of course this chemo has side effects', said the doctor, matter-of-factly. 'That includes hair-loss, vomiting, bleeding, and even a three-per cent risk of death. But we are very hopeful for a cure for Sarah'.

Sarah heard this and gripped her father's arm. The doctor was talking about her as if she weren't there. Di was horrified and seized Sarah's hand. She hoped she hadn't understood what the doctor said about her.

'Isn't there another type of chemo that isn't as toxic?' asked Mark.

'This is the only treatment for your daughter', said the doctor.

Mark and Di could almost hear each other's thoughts. They had been at this point before.

'Do you think we could see some studies that show your treatment would work on Sarah's tumour?' asked Mark.

The doctor aimed an uncertain glance towards the social worker. 'Well, I don't have any here right now, but when you come next time, we can provide some papers for you'.

The social worker promptly made a note to find some of these studies.

'Meanwhile', said the oncologist, 'I want to order a blood test, a bone scan, and CT scan for Sarah. The earliest I can book the CT scanner is next week on May 26. Do you agree to bring her back then?'

Mark and Di both agreed.

The doctor continued. 'At this stage I won't order any other treatment. But it would be helpful if you would consent to the chemotherapy today'.

The parents reconsidered briefly but they knew no more than before. At least this doctor had promised to provide the information they wanted next time they came.

'No', said Mark, 'we will wait until your test results come through and until we see the information you will give us about the treatment. Then we can let you know. We'll be back next week. Meanwhile we're traveling to Melbourne to have the oxygen sauna checked, and we will be seeking other advice about what you have told us'.

Capewell found the idea of other advisors disagreeable but could do nothing to stop them. There, he ended the session.

After the conference, Mark wanted to be out of Sydney before rush hour. Both parents were worried about the confronting things Sarah had heard the doctor say. All was quiet while Mark dodged the traffic. An hour later they traveled south west on the Hume highway towards Melbourne. The trip would take about 12 hours. Near Goulburn, the temperature suddenly dropped from the cold winds off the snowfields. Mark stopped at a picnic rest stop for a hot cup of tea from the thermos. Di produced some fruit and a few rice crackers with cheese from the esky. Sarah looked distracted and wouldn't eat.

'Aren't you hungry?' asked Di.

'What does 'toxic' mean?' Sarah asked.

'It's a poison', answered Mark.

'Is that what that doctor wants to give me?'

Di gave Mark a desperate sideways glance before covering her face.

Mark tried to soften the shock for Sarah. 'Well, not exactly. We're still discussing the best choice for you'.

'No Dad, I heard what he said – hair falling out, vomiting and bleeding. He even said I was gonna die!'

Mark folded his arms around Sarah while Di looked away to hide her tears.

'Now you listen to me, there's nobody going to do anything without your permission and ours. Right now we're trying to find the best treatment for you and there have been no decisions made yet'.

Sarah began to cry. 'But Dad, you told me we're going on a plane to a hospital to get me better'.

'I did Sarah. I did'.

'When are we going then?' she demanded.

Mark held her tighter. 'We can't go right now. Maybe in a little while'.

'Why can't we?' Sarah wailed.

Mark hesitated. 'Because those ladies who came to our house want us to take you to Dr Capewell. We should give him a chance to help you', he said softly.

'Well, I don't care about them and I don't want to see him again', howled Sarah.

Mark patted her soothingly. 'It's all right. Your Mum and I are here. It's going to be all right, Sarah'. Mark struggled to hold back his own tears, while Di retreated to the mini-van for a tissue.

For the rest of the trip, Sarah was unusually quiet – as though something inside her had changed.

The next day was 21 May. In the morning, Dr Capewell's oncology social worker phoned the DoCS caseworker to brief her about their previous day's conference.

'We met with the parents yesterday and found them to be quite strange', said the social worker.

'In what way?' the caseworker asked.

'They were passive and difficult to engage', complained the social worker. 'They would not enter into any scenarios that were posed to them by Dr Capewell and myself until the test results were known. The natural mother was very quiet and did not speak. The parents indicated to us that they plan to go to Melbourne to see their therapist and agreed to return next Tuesday, May 27, for a CT scan and a full blood count'.

The child protection caseworker asked how long the tests would take.

'It will take just a day or two and then Dr Capewell will determine what treatment plan to suggest', explained the hospital social worker.

'Were you able to provide the parents with any written information?' enquired the caseworker, '...as this was important to them'.

'No, not yet', admitted the social worker. 'The parents requested articles on chemo, but were not given anything. I am organising for the information to be provided to them when they return', she explained.

After finishing his rounds at 4.30 pm, Roger Capewell phoned the DoCS caseworker from his office. His impressions of the conference were more optimistic.

'The interview went well', he told the caseworker, not realising what effect his mention of death from the treatment had on Sarah. 'And I feel the parents are willing to consider chemotherapy. They needed to see all the information, and facts and figures. I explained all this to them', he said confidently.

'Did you provide them with any written information?' asked the caseworker.

'No', he admitted. 'But the hospital social worker will organise this when they return'.

'How did you find the parents' presentation?'

The doctor became irritated. 'The parents sounded weird about being part of a large organisation ... I don't feel it's only the family's decision, but perhaps the church or influences from grandparents and extended family members', he speculated.

Since the parents had not discussed these issues in the conference, it was clear the previous psychosocial profiling was at work again.

When the caseworker pressed the doctor for more information, he added, 'The parents' behaviour and decision-making about basics shows significant departure from normal behaviour in our society'.

The caseworker made a note of this for an affidavit. 'If they agree to [maximum tolerated] chemotherapy, will you be able to treat Sarah?' she asked.

'Although I am reluctant to take on any difficult patients I would be happy to take on the case on the condition that the parents comply and follow instructions', replied Capewell sternly.

Before the phone call ended, the caseworker assured the doctor of her complete support. She understood the doctor's requirements, and would ensure the department used whatever means it had to carry out his treatment plans – even if that meant acting immediately, before the doctor had received the results of the most recent tests and scans, and before any studies had been supplied to the parents. During the next few days the caseworker sought advice from the department's legal section about how medical treatments could be forced on Sarah. Unfortunately, no one – not the social worker, caseworker or the doctor – enquired how Sarah had fared during the meeting, or how she felt hearing for the first time that she could die from the treatment.

Once they arrived in Melbourne, the family met with Dr Milne to discuss Sarah's progress and the oxygen machine. On having it routinely tested, Milne discovered the machine needed repairs. Meanwhile a new one had to be ordered, but this would take several days, which would cause the family a slight delay in getting back to New South Wales.

While at the clinic, the family also encountered Dr Sales. They exchanged a few awkward words. The doctor did not mention his talks with Dr Kotz or that the department had persuaded him to prepare a legal affidavit about them. With a sheepish look, Sales disappeared as soon as he could get away.

While in Melbourne Sarah became unwell with what Di thought was a mild stomach bug, but she improved after a few days on clear fluids and bland food. Before the department's visit to their farm, Sarah had been relaxed, able to cope with her illness and maintain an active lifestyle. Now the stresses of the past week took a new toll on her. She had been upset and withdrawn since the conference with the oncologist. Another conference was scheduled in a few days' time, during which Sarah's scan results would be discussed. The parents hoped the doctor's discussions would be honest, but not as brutal as they had been before.

After being delayed a few extra days in Melbourne while the oxygen machine was repaired, the family headed back to Sydney. Mark had phoned Dr Capewell with news of their delay and asked to reschedule their appointment for three days later.

Capewell agreed, but became alarmed about this change and immediately phoned a caseworker from the department. 'I received a message from Mr Westley saying that he could not make the appointment for the CT scan on Monday, but would like to reschedule for Thursday. He also agreed to attend at 1.00 pm on Friday for the results and a discussion with me. I told him this was okay, but I am concerned he may not show up', explained the oncologist.

The caseworker took his concerns seriously. For this important meeting on Friday, DoCS had scheduled several caseworkers to be present while the oncologist discussed his plans with the family.

'Would a teleconference be okay instead of having staff attend in Sydney for the meeting on Friday?' asked the caseworker.

The oncologist agreed to a teleconference, but now both were concerned the meeting would not go according to plan. The caseworker hung up from the doctor's call and immediately phoned the department's internal legal advisor. It was now a matter of determining what forces could be brought to bear against the family at a moment's notice if they didn't show up.

True to their word, on 30 May, the family headed towards the hospital for Sarah's rescheduled appointment for CT scans – unaware of the goings-on behind the scenes. They had left Melbourne the previous day and spent the night in the country town of Gundagai, which they'd left early that morning. Now they were stuck in the Sydney traffic battling the lunchtime crowds. They were running an hour late for the scans – a fact that made Capewell tense when he found out, even though their appointment with him was for the following day. However, once the family was at the hospital, the radiology department staff was kind to Sarah. It was not long before they had inserted an intravenous catheter to inject the contrast dye that would help show up any abnormal lumps on Sarah's scan. A few hours later, Sarah had finished the bone scan, blood tests and CT scan. She returned to Ryde with her parents to stay overnight with their family friends. They would return the next day for the appointment with Dr Capewell.

By evening, Mark and Di were exhausted, but Sarah had a hearty appetite and cleaned up two large bowls of vegetable soup and toast. She stayed up playing a few rounds of board games until 10 pm, after which she went to bed and slept soundly all night. Mark and Di were worried about the next conference with the oncologist. Sarah had been depressed after the previous one, and the trip had served as a distraction that lifted her spirits again. Now they were unsure about how she would be able to handle the next onslaught.

The family arrived at the hospital by lunchtime the next day, in ample time. While in the waiting room, Sarah met another girl her own age and the two happily clowned around in the hospital corridor.

Behind the scenes, a teleconference was set up to allow several child protection caseworkers to hear the discussions. This time Dr Capewell seemed far more interested in Sarah's rare cancer and ushered the family into a larger conference room on another floor. When the parents entered the room with Sarah, it was already crowded with three junior doctors and the social worker – the same young woman who had told the caseworker that the family was 'strange' because the parents would 'not enter into any scenarios' before they had read the studies and before the test results had come through.

Three empty chairs were set out for the family, but only two were close to each other, forcing Sarah to sit away from her parents. She chose instead to sit on her father's knee so that she had both parents close by. The meeting was patched in by teleconference to include five child protection caseworkers. It started at 1.20 pm, with eight people present and five at the end of the phone line.

After a round of obligatory social greetings, Dr Capewell professorially addressed the room. Unlike at the first appointment, he was now fully versed in the details of Sarah's tumour, and seemed intensely interested in it. 'We have the results', said the oncologist. 'The X-rays are abnormal and show a large tumour in the spleen and another small growth quite close to the surface of the skin in the groin. The large one is in the base of the spleen. It also has a type of cystic mass which could be a haematoma...'

Sarah knew what a tumour was and suddenly turned pale. Di reached for Sarah's hand and Mark closed his arm protectively around her.

The oncologist continued to address his registrars and announced his treatment plan for the tumour. 'For this recurring germ cell tumour, the current therapy is [maximum tolerated dose] intravenous chemotherapy for three to four cycles – that should shrink the tumour and then she will have surgery to remove the tumour. I need to consult with a surgeon about removal of the spleen but will make a decision regarding this after chemo'.

After a short pause, he addressed the family directly. 'With the chemotherapy we give her a very good prognosis [20] – but without it she will die. But again, there are some side effects we have to make you aware of. This chemo can cause hair-loss, nausea, vomiting, bleeding, infection, peripheral neuropathy [nerve damage], and secondary cancer in another location, lung fibrosis and anaphylaxis [allergic shock]. And', the doctor added, 'up to 3 per cent of children die from the chemotherapy'.

The other three doctors appeared fascinated and took down notes, while over the intercom the caseworkers recorded the conversation.

Mark felt Sarah trembling. As if she were not there, the people in this room were talking about opening her up, taking out her organs, and injecting her with drugs that killed as many as three children out of a hundred from the treatment alone, and crippled many more from the side effects. During her previous bout of cancer, the surgeon had talked to her gently. Now these people were casually discussing her life and death without taking any real interest in how she felt or what she thought about it.

Those in the room fell silent and waited for the parents' reply. Only the social worker continued taking notes and the department personnel remained silently listening through the speaker on the table.

'What about the studies?' asked Mark.

---

[20] When tumours of the type Sarah had, recur and spread, they attract a prognosis of an almost zero per cent 5 year survival.

'Oh, yes of course. We have it for you here and I'm sure you'll find it supports what I've just said'. Capewell located a French scientific study he had put aside and handed it over to Mark. For a while, he waited for Mark to flip through it. Mark scanned it briefly until he came to a few statistics that troubled him, and raised a number of questions about them. For a while, the two discussed issues around the paper. Capewell was adamant the study supported his treatment plan and became impatient to move on. He wanted the parents to sign the consent form and then he wanted another blood sample from Sarah.

Mark saw that Sarah was upset by what had been said about her during the conference. 'I think my daughter has had had enough', he said. 'She needs to go home now for a rest, and we will think about what you have said'. Mark stood up.

The oncologist looked at Sarah closely for the first time. 'Your daughter does not look very well. I want to take some blood from her now'.

Mark moved protectively in front of Sarah, 'I don't think so. The poor kid has had enough. We'll go to our local GP tomorrow for the blood test, if that's all right with you'.

The oncologist approached Sarah, wanting to examine her, but she shied away from him.

The doctor turned to Mark instead. 'What are your plans then? We need to start chemotherapy'.

Mark agreed there had to be a plan. 'Sarah needs to be back with her siblings to relax and calm down for a day or two. I'll make a decision in a few days, by June 4th, and let you know – after I've read the material you gave me'. Mark gathered his family to leave. Both parents realised Sarah was in shock after what she had heard and they needed to get her home as soon as possible.

The doctor was not happy, but agreed to let them go. This ended the conference.

After the meeting, the oncologist phoned one of the child protection caseworkers who had been listening in via the conference call. He told her he thought the parents would eventually agree with his treatment plans. According to the transcripts obtained some time later, Sarah's emotional welfare did not arise during this discussion either. The caseworker was focused on how the doctor's treatment could be enforced if the parents did not agree, and made no enquiries about Sarah's emotional distress on hearing the doctors discussing the possibility of her death, in front of her.

Shortly after the conference, Dr Capewell wrote a letter to the child protection department. In his letter, dated 30 May, the oncologist stated that he agreed with his colleague Dr Kotz that with the administration of chemotherapy, Sarah's chance of a cure was '...of the order of 70–80%. Cure means that she will grow into a normal healthy adult'.

The oncologist did not mention that with the cancer's recurrence and the spleen now involved, Sarah had almost no chance of surviving. The doctor's claims for a cure to the child protection department, would prove devastating to the family and seal Sarah's fate.

Dr Capewell's views and his support of Dr Kotz now galvanised the caseworker into action. Once again, she phoned the department's internal legal advisor. Normally the Children's Court heard these matters; however, for reasons that have remained unclear, the department explored the idea of taking the case to the Supreme Court if the parents did not consent to the oncologist's plan. The department was now seeking a way to haul in a terminal cancer patient by force – an almost unheard of scenario.

Mark drove his family home in shocked silence. The four hour trip seemed endless. Just past the Newcastle turnoff the rain started, first lightly and then in sheets. Mark turned the wipers on full. Sarah sat mute in the back seat until the dark weather set in, when she started quietly sobbing. Di motioned Mark to stop and he immediately pulled onto the narrow roadside shoulder. There the family van stood in the rain with its hazard lights blinking. For a long time cars sped by oblivious while the parents were in the back of the van trying to comfort their daughter.

'Promise you won't ever take me there again', sobbed Sarah.

Mark lowered his head, not knowing what to say, while Di rummaged in her bag for more tissues.

'Promise!' demanded Sarah.

'I can't do that right now', said Mark gently.

'Why not?' she wailed.

Mark struggled but managed to keep a veneer of composure. 'From what they told us today, what you have is very serious, Sarah', he said. 'But I promise that your mother and I will be with you every step of the way. I have to read some information the doctor gave me when we get home. After that, we will all have to make some decisions'.

Sarah glanced desperately from one parent to the other. Mark cupped Sarah's face in his hands. 'Listen to me', he said. 'We all need to settle down for a while at home, and when your mother and I have read this new information we'll have a chat about what is the best option. Okay?'

Sarah nodded and relaxed slightly. Di cleaned Sarah's face with a tissue and held her tight, while Mark went outside to compose himself. The rain did not matter to him anymore. He hardly noticed it.

For the rest of the trip Sarah burrowed into the bed quilt and pulled its corner over her head. In the last few hours of the trip, darkness came, and she fell sound asleep.

When nearly at the front gate, Di checked to see if Sarah was asleep before turning to Mark. 'First they tell us nothing and then they do our head in. That treatment they want to give her sounds extreme, with all those kids dying and being maimed by it'.

Mark was weary from the last 10 days' travel. The emotional day had drained him completely. 'So far they've only told us what to think. This study is the first independent information they have ever given us. Let's see if it says the higher dose chemo works first before we can decide if it's worth taking the risk of her dying from the treatment', he answered.

Di was getting sweaty palms just thinking about the terrible options they were facing.

'Crikey, you're right though', Mark added. 'They sure laid it on us today. The whole box of frogs'.

STORM WARNING

A weather front is a boundary between two masses
Of different densities. The storm develops
When they both collide.

Wikipedia

While the parents had been away in Melbourne and Sydney with Sarah, the farmhouse had grown cold to its bones. When Mark finally turned into the driveway he just wanted to crawl into a warm bed, but his first job at home was to find dry firewood and light the combustion stove. Di's leg was aching and she yearned to put it up for a rest, but she had to start dinner instead. While Di cooked, Mark hauled several loads of luggage into the house. Sarah disappeared upstairs into her room. Outside, everything seemed in order. Muttley and Pooch were well looked after and happy to see them. The chooks were in their roost with the door closed. Sarah's siblings had dutifully fed the animals each day after school before Ruth collected them for the night.

While Di took a light supper tray upstairs to Sarah, Mark drove over the hill to his parents' house to collect the kids. When they saw Mark's car lights, they ran out into the rain to greet him and piled into the van, eager to see their sister again. Ruth and Jim waved goodbye from their doorway. In the rush, Mark forgot some of their belongings and went inside the house to gather them. On his way out, Ruth saw her son's face up close.

'You look tired', she said.

Mark didn't stop. 'You could say that', he answered.

Jim gave his son an encouraging pat on the back as Mark rushed past. 'Take care, Son', said the old man.

At home, Di had an expedient supper of soup and toast waiting on the table. The children were happy to see their parents but had wondered what was up with Sarah when she'd gone to bed early. While Di and Clara attended to the younger kids' baths and bedtime, Mark and Laura washed up the dinner dishes. Di fell exhausted into bed not long after the children.

By 11 pm, the house was still cold. Mark put on a few extra logs and thought of turning in. Instead, he went to his study and fished around his briefcase for the clinical research Dr Capewell had given him (Culine 1997). In his cramped home office, he adjusted the reading lamp and sat down at the desk to look at the research paper. It was written in technical jargon that would not be easy to decipher. For a few minutes, he stared at it uncomprehendingly. The house was quiet. He had forgotten how still it is in the bush. Their friends' house at Ryde was always surrounded by Sydney traffic. At home, only the living room clock chimed on the half hour.

Mark bore down on the document, making a determined effort to understand each word. It was well past midnight before he had finished the first two pages. The study was of 54 girls with various malignant ovarian germ cell tumours, of which a small number were types resembling Sarah's. All the girls had had surgery to remove the tumours, followed by the type of chemotherapy the oncologist wanted to give Sarah. The chemo was used either as a first line treatment or, in a few advanced and recurrent cases, as a last ditch salvage treatment. Mark got a lucky break when he discovered the third page, where a concise table listed three groups with different types of germ cell tumours at various stages, including their responses to the chemotherapy.

Since Mark now assumed from the scan results that Sarah was in the more advanced stages of cancer, he searched the advanced disease column where a few girls were listed with tumour types similar to Sarah's (including many with tumours much less virulent). There he discovered that even with chemotherapy only half of the girls had survived to the end of the study. One girl had died of liver failure from the chemotherapy. He wondered how many of those girls were alive today, since the study had started in 1980 and ended in 1992. He did not realise at the time that the study included many with tumours less risky than Sarah's and that other studies focusing only on Sarah's types were far less optimistic. Nevertheless, Mark started to get an idea of the seriousness of Sarah's situation when he read the bottom row. For a moment, he was confused. Hadn't the oncologist told them Sarah's tumour was recurrent? Did this mean that her cancer had advanced even further and her chances were even worse? This would put her into the bottom group with those who had recurrent tumours. In that row, a girl with a tumour like Sarah's was listed. To Mark's horror, he noticed that she was now dead. Even with the treatment the oncologist proposed, in the recurrent tumour section of the study, there were no survivors.

Suddenly Mark felt ill. Why would Dr Capewell give him this study to support his treatment when the kids were dead, and then make claims of a cure? Was this some kind of a terrible joke? Mark felt his stomach about to heave and just in time, he made it outside into the fresh air. It had started to rain again, but at least the water felt clean on his face.

Four hours later light flooded the home office. Mark awoke groggily with his arms stiff from sleeping on them. He'd had terrible dreams. They had come for Sarah – they had come to steal his daughter. His desk was in disarray, and he felt like a truck had backed over him. He rubbed his eyes as last night's appalling discovery assaulted his mind again. In the rest of the house, he heard the children. They were already up, but he could only sit there among the jumble of papers, still in shock.

Di came to the study door, herself bleary eyed. She surveyed the scene, shook her head, and left for the kitchen to start breakfast.

Di sent the five other children off to catch the school bus, but left Sarah sound asleep upstairs. When the kids were gone, Mark emerged from the study for a cup of hot tea. Outside, the rain had set in to a constant drizzle. For the first time, he noticed that the southerly wind seemed to seep through cracks in the house he never knew were there. Di had the kitchen wood stove burning and hot water was on tap.

'You look terrible', said Di as she poured tea into two mugs.

Not as terrible as I feel on the inside', answered Mark.

Di surveyed Mark's crumpled face. 'Any good news?'

Mark took a hot sip and waited for it to warm his stomach. 'Not at all. Seems those kids with the type of recurrent tumour Sarah has, didn't fare too well on that treatment they want to give Sarah. They're...' Mark paused. 'No longer alive'.

Di fumbled her mug and spilled the tea over the tablecloth. 'What? What's going on Mark?' she demanded as she fetched a cloth from the kitchen.

Mark's hair still stood on end from his night in the study. He raked his fingers through it. 'That's what I'd like to know'.

Di wiped up the spill and limped back to the sink. 'What are we going to do?' she asked fearfully.

Mark rubbed his face until some colour returned to it. 'I don't know who we can trust right now. We already know the child protection people are not listening. Not to us anyway. If we could just buy some time, get them off our backs and get her overseas into safe hands for treatment'.

'I'm really worried about her', said Di. 'Did you see her yesterday when the doctor told her she would die without his chemo and then straightaway told her she could die of the chemo too? What do they expect the poor kid to think?'

'Yes. I saw her being gutted right there in that room', agreed Mark. 'Since those last two trips to Sydney she's been going downhill fast', he added bitterly.

'What if they force us to sign for that chemo?' asked Di.

Mark slammed down his cup. 'How can we? Knowing those other kids are dead from it, or despite it?'

It was Di's turn to be angry. 'Then why do they tell us they're going to cure her with it?'

'I don't know. I don't know', Mark said irately. 'But one thing I do know. Either it's a barefaced lie or they don't know what they're doing. Either way doesn't make me real happy'. Mark got up and put on his coat and old bush hat.

'Where are you going?' asked Di.

'I'm checking the cows'.

'It's wet'.

'I don't much care', he muttered. 'And you'd best have that leg seen to'.

'I will – when I get a minute', answered Di.

They both heard Sarah stirring upstairs before she came down. This time she took the steps instead of sliding down the handrail. She looked tired, but brightened up when she saw Mark in his raincoat.

'Hey Dad! Wait for me'.

Mark drove the utility around the cattle with Sarah. He hadn't checked them for the ten days they were away. He'd already sold a few dozen to raise money for Sarah's overseas hospital expenses. That left some of his best cows to sell later if necessary. At least there were no calving problems this time of year. The cows had calved by April and the young ones could already fend for themselves. Most of the herd stood together in small groups with their rumps facing the wind. The southerly swept a cold drizzle through the valleys keeping the temperature down to a chilly 14° C.

Mark drove up to Sarah's favourite hill, where he stopped the utility for a while. From there, they both tried to spot the igneous cliffs of the Barrington Tops in the distance, but rain clouds shrouded the mountains. Instead, they enjoyed the view into the vale, with their cosy homestead nestled into the valley below, its chimney smoking with burning iron bark.

Sarah caught sight of a huge bird gliding overhead. 'Dad. Look!' It was a hawk with a massive wingspan.

'What's he doing out today when the mice are all inside!' cried Sarah excitedly.

The bird's grace fascinated Mark. 'Look again', he said.

They both watched the bird wheeling around the sky, around an invisible bubble of air, on motionless wings, in perfect freedom.

'Dad', said Sarah finally.

'Yes Jogue'.

'I know I could die of cancer. If we can't go on that trip you promised, I just want to spend the time I have left right here with you and Mum and the kids'.

Mark looked away to hide his thoughts from her. He'd promised himself he would never tell Sarah what he'd found out last night. Instead, to be scrupulously fair, he wanted to ask her which treatment she wanted, solely based on what the oncologists had told her. 'What about that chemo the doctor told you about yesterday? Do you want to try it?' Mark asked.

Sarah shook her head. 'No way Dad', she said firmly. 'That doctor said I was going to die without it and die with it too. So what's the point? I saw a kid who had it and died anyway. I want to die happy and be free'. Sarah paused and searched the sky for the hawk again, 'like that bird up there', she said.

The hawk was still riding the same thermal. It had not flapped its wings once.

Mark wondered what Sarah had seen or heard while in the children's cancer ward last November that gave her that idea. He was fighting back his own tears now.

'What do you think of the supplements and the oxygen treatment?' he asked.

'They're okay', said Sarah. 'I'm pretty sure they make me feel better'.

Mark steadied himself. 'Sarah, you're going to need some more treatment soon. I'm just not sure yet what kind or where'.

Sarah brightened. 'Does that mean we can go on the trip?'

'There might still be a chance. We'll just have to see. Meanwhile your mother wants to talk to you separately about what treatment you want. You need to be honest with her too'. Mark wanted Di to know exactly what Sarah's wishes were. There was no telling what the future held and Di had to know every inch of what was going on in case, for some reason, he was out of the picture.

Mark had to conceal his troubled thoughts again from Sarah. If it were not for the child protection department, they would already be safely overseas with Sarah instead of the chilling position they were now in.

Recalling the clinical study he had read just hours ago made him shudder. He would need a trustworthy qualified professional to go over it as soon as possible, to see if he had read it correctly. Mark had promised to phone the oncologist the day after tomorrow with his decision – he would ask him about the study then. Meanwhile, in the next few days Sarah desperately needed some rest, while he and Di made a plan.

Respite on the farm lasted barely a day. There was no time to make a plan or to seek advice. The next day was 3 June. The rain had stopped and the sun raised the temperature to 15° C. The family was just beginning to unwind from the mind-numbing stresses of the past two weeks when a child protection case-worker phoned the Westley house at 9.05 am to set up an appointment for later that day. Two hours later, Judy and Gillian, the same two DoCS caseworkers, turned up. The pair had been involved from the beginning. Unbeknownst to the parents, they were among several other department staff who had listened in during the conference with Dr Capewell. The parents invited them in and told them Sarah was at her grandparents' house for her treatment and home schooling.

'We want to speak with you first anyway', said Gillian.

'Yes. Tell us about the treatments Sarah is having', said Judy.

For the second time Mark later regretted speaking with the caseworkers rather than seeking legal advice. At that time, however, he still believed open-ness would resolve all issues, so he went on to tell the caseworkers about the oxygen treatments and supplements. He also included information on a few other complementary treatments Dr Milne had told him about in Melbourne.

'Does Sarah know that chemotherapy is available to her?' asked Gillian.

'Yes,' he answered. 'Dr Capewell explained it all to her day before yester-day'.

'Have you had a chance to ask her about it since?' asked Judy.

'Yes', answered Mark, 'and she told me what she thought of it'.

'And what did she say?' asked Judy eagerly.

Mark took a slow breath to gather his thoughts. 'Sarah told me that after hearing what the doctor had said, she would rather die and be happy than go through it all and die anyway'.

'Really?' asked Gillian disbelievingly.

'Yes, and she came to this conclusion herself', added Mark.

The caseworkers looked astonished.

Both women turned to Di for confirmation.

'Did you speak with your daughter about this, Mrs Westley?' asked Judy.

Di nodded.

'And what did she say to you?' asked the other caseworker.

Di answered without her usual hesitation. 'I asked Sarah: "If that chemo was the only chance you had, would you have it?"'

'What did she say?' asked both caseworkers at once.

'She told me: "No way, I would rather die happy"', said Di.

The caseworkers murmured to each other for a few moments.

Finally, Gillian assumed the leadership role and announced, 'We are going to have to interview Sarah separately about her wishes'.

Mark had been completely unprepared for the department's visit. He now tried to decide whether to tell the caseworkers about his shocking discovery in the clinical study or take it up with the oncologist, since he had promised to phone him anyway with his decision. For the time being, he chose to remain quiet, since the child protection people seemed to take no notice of what he was saying in any case, and he was not sure what powers they had or how they planned to use them. Meanwhile, the caseworkers were eager to visit Sarah over at Ruth and Jim's house and urged Mark and Di to come with them.

The caseworkers knew the way to Ruth and Jim's without directions, and Mark and Di followed close behind them in the family van. Once there, the party interrupted the school lesson Sarah was having with Ruth. The women roamed around the house and closely inspected the oxygen sauna and the vitamin pills. They asked so many probing questions that Mark hoped they would ask the oncologist just as much about his treatment. Perhaps then, the whole mess could be cleared up before it got out of hand.

When they had thoroughly inspected the house, the caseworkers took Sarah out into the backyard, away from the family, to interview her.

'What did you find out in Melbourne?' asked Gillian.

'Erm, I don't know', answered Sarah warily.

'What do you know about chemo?' asked Judy.

'I know I don't want it'.

'Why?'

'I would rather stay home'.

The women then asked her what she thought chemotherapy was.

Sarah answered: 'It kills cells. You lose your hair and everything'.

'Has anyone ever asked you if you want the treatment?' asked Judy.

This seemed a relevant question since no doctor had ever asked her that.

'Yes, and I don't ever want it', said Sarah adamantly.

Gillian asked her what she would do if the 'treatment' did not work – without specifying which treatment she was referring to.

Sarah answered: 'I don't know. I'll probably get sick again'.

'Will they be able to fix you?' asked the women.

It was a question that she could not possibly answer. 'I don't know', answered Sarah, bemused.

Sarah was certain about what she wanted and why, but the caseworkers weren't accepting her wishes. They gave her a handwritten questionnaire to fill out before going inside to speak with the parents again. Before Sarah could complete the questionnaire, the caseworkers wanted the parents' immediate consent to chemotherapy on Sarah's behalf.

'I can't do that', said Mark adamantly.

'Why not?' asked the caseworkers.

'Because there is absolutely no evidence the treatment will work in Sarah's case', answered Mark. 'And you heard her say yourself that she doesn't want the treatment or the side effects that come with it'.

The caseworkers were not happy and conferred among themselves.

'We will need your decision by the end of tomorrow', said Gillian.

Sarah had already made her decision, but Mark suspected it was not the decision the department expected of her.

After farewells to the adults and a syrupy goodbye to Sarah, the caseworkers left the grandparents' farm. Two hours later, they were back at the Taree office. One caseworker transcribed the conversations into legal affidavits while the other obtained more legal advice from head office about the next step.

After the caseworkers had gone, the parents and grandparents stood speechless in the living room.

Sarah broke the silence. 'Why do those ladies come to our house all the time?'

Jim gave a bitter chuckle. 'That's what we'd like to know'.

Ruth and Di ushered Sarah into the kitchen where they would put the kettle on for a cup of tea and find some biscuits Ruth had hidden in her cupboard for a special occasion, while Jim stayed in the living room with Mark.

The old man looked confused. He lifted his thick glasses to wipe his watering eyes. 'Son, what's going on here?' he asked.

Mark had tried to spare his father the details because of his poor health. 'At best it's a terrible misunderstanding', explained Mark.

'At worst?' asked Jim, searching Mark's face for a clue.

Mark lowered his voice to a whisper. 'At worst? They want her. For what reason, I don't know'.

'Let's hope it's the former', said Jim as he sat down heavily on the couch. 'Our family has been here since the wild colonial days. We've come through droughts, fires, floods and two World Wars. Son, I know you're man enough to sort things out and protect your family. What are your plans after this visit?'

His father's support strengthened Mark's resolve. 'I'm going to call the oncologist at the hospital. It's time for a talk', he said.

An hour later, Mark returned home to place the first of several calls to the hospital in Sydney. It was time to tell Dr Capewell about their decision and he desperately wanted to tackle him about the study. However, each time he phoned, the switchboard operator told him the doctor was unavailable. Once, Mark was transferred directly to the doctor's personal assistant. She told him that Capewell was in Coffs Harbour.

Mark did not know it yet, but behind the scenes, decisions had already been made. By then the oncologist was leaving the heavy lifting to the child protection department.

The next day, Wednesday 4 June, started out like any other. An overnight frost melted into a sunny winter's day. Sarah's five siblings went to school at the usual time and Mark took Sarah to Ruth's for her schooling and treatments. Mark planned to do some chores around the farm, but first, he had to phone his boss to let him know he needed a few more days off to handle the gathering storm with DoCS.

Meanwhile, Di tried to rest her leg, but found things soon got too busy. The caseworker from Taree DoCS phoned twice before lunch to ask if they had made a decision to consent to the chemo yet. Both times Di had to call Mark in from the paddock.

After the first call, Mark tried phoning the hospital again on the off-chance Dr Capewell had returned from his trip, but he was told the doctor was not in. There seemed no way to resolve this issue and he felt trapped. After the department's second call, the caseworker issued an ultimatum – they would have to make a 'decision' to consent immediately.

The family was put under unbearable strain. After lunch, Mark brought Sarah home from Ruth and Jim's to have another talk with her. The department had forced them into quizzing Sarah again about her wishes, asking the same impossible questions.

At home, Mark asked Sarah whether she had any questions about what the oncologist had said in Sydney.

Sarah exploded. 'Yes I heard what he said. Okay? I've already told you. I don't want the stuff that can kill me and then die anyway. I just want to be here with you, and do the stuff we've been doing and be happy'.

'Okay, okay. We've got it', said Mark as he looked at Di. 'But now we have to tell the caseworkers what you want, and what we think is right for you'.

'Well, tell them then', griped Sarah.

'Maybe you could help by filling out that questionnaire they left the other day', said Di.

'I don't want to!' cried Sarah. 'I want to go outside and see the ducks'.

'Your mother's right', said Mark. 'Off you go, up to your room and fill it out. We're not allowed to help you with it. And when you're finished, we'll go feed the ducks together and see how many eggs there are today'.

Sarah inched up the stairs protesting all the way. After a half-hour, she brought down the filled-out questionnaire. Her answers left no doubt that she was informed about the doctor's proposed treatment and didn't want it.

As a stress reliever, Mark took Sarah with him in the utility to check the fences after lunch. They stayed close to the house in case Di needed them.

While the family felt unbearable pressure bearing down on them, the atmosphere in the Taree regional office was tensing up as well. The regional director and several caseworkers were teleconferencing with head office in Sydney to discuss an application to the Supreme Court. They wanted to seek an order to administer the treatment by force.

At 1.20 pm, the child protection caseworker phoned the Westley house again. 'Have you made a decision?' she demanded.

Mark tried to explain again. 'Sarah has been fully informed by the oncologist of the treatment he proposes and the side effects, and is adamant that she does not want that kind of chemotherapy. She wants to keep using what we have been using and look at different options. As far as I can see, there is no evidence the treatment will work on Sarah and Di does not want it – full stop. Personally, I can't change Sarah or Di's mind. That particular chemo is the last option'.

That was the wrong decision as far as the department was concerned. The caseworker answered tersely: 'Given what you have told us about your decision then I need to advise you that I will consult with a legal representative and this may mean that the Supreme Court will become involved'.

Did Mark hear right? Did she say the Supreme Court – just for wanting a different treatment option for their daughter? This was starting to feel surreal.

The department officials had not listened to them or Sarah,[21] and the whole thing was on a collision course.

For Sarah's sake, Mark tried one last time. 'Please understand that we have looked into it and believe there are better options than the one being proposed. We're concerned about the known toxicity of the treatment and the fact that no one can tell us how successful this would be'.

Mark tried to explain that the treatment was not known to work in Sarah's case, but the caseworker, he knew was not listening.

Finally, he told the caseworker: 'I have spoken with Sarah. She is aware of the risks both ways ... that's our final decision and my wife and I have made it with Sarah'.

The caseworker repeated: 'You realise then that the department may need to have some of these decisions made by the Supreme Court'.

'Then so be it', said Mark.

When he hung up, he saw the questionnaire with Sarah's answers lying on the table. No one had asked them for it because it seemed that no one cared what Sarah wanted or what he and Di felt was best for her. Their views were not the department's and now they were threatening them with court.

Di stood in the kitchen. She had only heard one side of the conversation, but saw in Mark's face that it hadn't gone well. Di's voice was tinged with fear. 'What are we going to do?'

'We have to get Sarah overseas for treatment. This is our last chance', said Mark grimly. 'Tomorrow we're going to Taree. Let's get those travel papers together and put them in for processing. And while we're at it, we'll do some food shopping'.

Di sank slowly into a chair at the dining room table. She was too shaky to stay upright.

Mark looked through the French door windows to check on Sarah. She was the only one strangely at peace, collecting eggs from the duck pen, with Muttley close on her heels.

---

[21] The United Nations *Convention on the Rights of the Child* to which Australia is a signatory states in 1.23 Article 12(1): 'Parties shall assure to the child who is capable of forming his or her own views the right to express those views freely in all matters affecting the child...'

DARK NIGHTS

Protect the right of doctors to prescribe, and any patient to receive,
any new treatment, the demonstrated safety and
Efficacy of which offer hope of saving life,
Re-establishing health or
Alleviating suffering.

AMA Code of Medical Ethics

On the morning of June 5, the child welfare department launched legal proceedings against Mark and Di in the New South Wales Supreme Court in Sydney. The parents were at home and easily contactable, but the department chose not to inform them of the hearing. Instead, caseworkers scheduled the hearing ex parte – to be conducted without the parents' knowledge.

In court, DoCS barristers referred to Mark and Di as 'defendants', while the department was the plaintiff seeking orders to place Sarah into the care and custody of the State.

The department's evidence included letters from both oncologists, Drs Kotz and Capewell. The latter claimed in his letter to the court that Sarah had an 80 per cent chance of a cure with his chemotherapy, stating: 'Cure means that she will grow up to be a normal healthy adult'.

However, neither oncologist mentioned that Sarah was in the final stage IV of cancer although Dr Capewell had recently confirmed this by his own tests. The judge was unaware that Sarah's end-stage ovarian cancer was reasonably expected to have a fatal outcome, even with treatment, making a cure improbable. No one informed the court that, as a result, Sarah had different needs from a cancer sufferer in the early stages. In accordance with the paediatric medical practice guidelines[22], Sarah was entitled – from the time of her diagnosis – to palliative and supportive care and quality of life options. This means that the

---

[22] WHO 1995a: 'Palliative care begins when a child's life threatening illness is diagnosed and continues regardless of whether the child receives any kind of treatment, including curative treatments'.

parents and child were entitled to seek out options with fewer side effects, just as they were attempting to do.

Had the judge known of Sarah's poor prognosis, granting emergency powers to the department would have been an unlikely outcome. However, without this crucial evidence, and without the parents there to defend themselves, the court granted the department all its requests, including an additional order compelling Sarah to report to a hospital or police station within two hours. From there, the parents were to surrender their daughter into the custody of department caseworkers. In effect, Mark and Di's parental rights were being severed.

While the court was issuing a summons against them, Mark and Di were busy planning a trip to Taree to make the necessary travel arrangements to take Sarah to the US cancer hospital.

The morning of 6 June was overcast with drizzly showers. Still unaware of any court action against them, the parents saw their other children off to the school bus. It was Friday and they hoped to get the urgent passport applications through and perhaps travel as early as the following week. They planned to start packing for their trip after returning home from Taree that day. Mark also made a mental note to remind himself that he still had to sell off a few more head of cattle next week to ensure sufficient funds for the hospital fees.

At 10 am, Mark locked the doors, put Muttley on the chain, and headed down the drive towards Taree with Di and Sarah. The family was using Ruth's car while their mini-van was being serviced. Mark glanced in the rear mirror. Sarah looked relaxed in the back seat.

Not far from home, Mark crossed carefully over a ford through fast-flowing water. The river was up from the recent rains, and he reminded himself to take the long way around coming home in case the river rose even higher while they were away. Once across the waterway, Mark turned onto the road to Taree that ran along the river. For several kilometres, the gravel road was edged by a steep embankment, forcing Mark to drive slowly to stay on the narrow road while dodging the rain-filled potholes. Just after a tight bend, Mark noticed a hefty boulder had fallen onto the middle of the road on a section edged by a steep river bank. He braked and looked for oncoming traffic. From the other direction, he saw a light-coloured, compact car approaching with two passengers inside. Since he was closer to the boulder, he swerved around it and drove past the other car, which had to steer to the edge of the embankment to let him pass. Mark and Di could make out two women passengers in the car, before the vehicle was out of sight. Mark shot a brief glance at Di and she shrugged her shoulders. They both preferred to dismiss the incident.

An hour later the family arrived at Taree, but Sarah said she was hungry and wanted lunch before they made any other stops. It was lunchtime by then and the parents felt peckish themselves. Mark parked the car in the shopping centre car park and, after a quick round of the supermarket; they stopped at the food court for lunch. While eating their sandwiches Mark caught sight of his sister-in-law, and called out to her.

Di's sister was surprised to see Mark and Di, and rushed over to their table.

'What are you doing here?' she demanded. 'I've tried to call you all morning'.

Mark chuckled. 'What do you mean?'

Di's sister looked around nervously. 'I got a call this morning from a friend who works at the hospital. There's a police alert out for you. Anybody who sees you should take Sarah to the nearest hospital or police station'.

Mark sprang to his feet and motioned his sister-in-law to the far corner to prevent Sarah overhearing. 'What the devil are you talking about?' he whispered.

'Seriously, whatever this is about, you should get out of here right now', she insisted. 'You can stay with us for a while until you get this sorted or I can take you to a solicitor's office. We know somebody here in town. Just let's go and we can talk somewhere else'.

The compact car on the narrow gravel road that morning had contained two DoCS caseworkers. They carried a document they intended to serve on Mark and Di, demanding they surrender their daughter to them. When they found no one at home, except Muttley the dog straining on his chain and barking furiously, the caseworkers hurried to the grandparents' house.

A few minutes later, Ruth opened her door to two caseworkers dressed in suits with a document they were determined she should accept on behalf of Mark and Di. Ruth looked at the official-looking stamped papers and refused to take them on her son's behalf. Jim was splitting firewood in the bottom paddock and she wanted to discuss it with him first.

The caseworkers were dismayed at Ruth's refusal and demanded to know Mark and Di's whereabouts. Ruth truthfully told them that she wasn't sure exactly where they'd gone – either to Taree or Raymond Terrace – before suggesting they put it in Mark and Di's mailbox.

With this, the women grudgingly left. On their way back to the Taree office, the caseworkers returned via Mark and Di's house. At the bottom of their drive stood an upended steel drum mailbox that served the family and other house-holders for mail deliveries. The caseworkers left the documents there in plain sight, and weighed them down with a rock. The papers were loose and without an envelope.

Some time later Ruth had second thoughts and drove down the road to Mark's house. In the communal mailbox, she found the open document, its pages whipped around by the wind. Ruth was unfamiliar with legal documents, but felt this was so serious she started trembling. She rushed home to show the papers to Jim, who despite his thick prescription glasses could not decipher the document either. They both assumed it had something to do with Sarah.

Moments later, Mark rang from a public phone in Taree and Ruth blurted out the news. He asked his mother to read the document to him over the phone, but she could hardly speak.

Never mind Mum', said Mark. 'I think we've got the kind of trouble that needs a lawyer. Could you do us a favour and pick the kids up from the bus stop when they get home from school, and I'll call you when I know what's going on'.

'Of course I will', said Ruth. 'And be careful, Son'.

Ruth looked at her watch after the phone call and realised she and Jim had only a few hours left before they had to collect the kids from the bus stop. She placed the papers behind the glass cabinet in the kitchen before she and Jim headed out to the bottom paddock to shift the cattle and split the rest of the firewood. They were gone for at least two hours. When they returned, Ruth smelled a faint trace of cigarette smoke in the house. She noticed the dog was agitated, and she followed the animal to the kitchen. There, she looked at the glass cabinet where she had placed the summons only two hours previously, only to find that it was gone. After that, Ruth and Jim never left their doors unlocked again. [23]

---

[23] At the time of this publication, Mark discovered in an FOI document that the caseworkers had evidently realized their failure to properly serve the summons on Mark and Di, and returned to retrieve it a few hours later from where they'd left it in Mark's mailbox. However, Ruth had meanwhile retrieved it, taken it home, and placed it behind the glass kitchen cabinet. When the caseworkers found it missing from the mailbox, they went to Ruth and Jim's house to take it back and found no one at home. Mark believes that the document was taken from his parent's home at that time.

By early afternoon, a party of four agitated people walked into the legal office of a country lawyer. Mark tried to explain his problem to the receptionist, who surveyed the worried group with a child in tow. A lot of desperate people came into their law firm for help, but this family looked very decent and well mannered.

'Just a minute', said the receptionist as she got up from the desk. 'I think we've got just the man for you'.

After a few minutes, a big, rough-hewn man came out and escorted Mark, Di, Sarah and Di's sister into his office. Two hours later, Mark had explained only part of how they'd tried to help their daughter and the obstacles they'd had in getting information from the doctors.

Something about Mark's story made the lawyer take the case. Unfortunately, there was little to go on, since no paperwork was available at that moment and no documents had been served on Mark and Di. On the other hand, the medical history alone – or at least the details known to Mark – took several hours to relay and record. Without the documents, the lawyer knew nothing of the orders issued the previous day. It was now after office hours on Friday evening. This weekend was a public holiday – the Queen's Birthday – and nothing more could be done until the next working day on Tuesday, when the lawyer assured Mark he would contact the department for a briefing. Meanwhile, the lawyer advised Mark to write down all the details he could recall into a notebook and bring it back with him for their next meeting on Tuesday. The lawyer then cautioned the family to be careful until he could make the necessary enquiries and ensure their rights were represented. Mark told him he would make plans to lay low for a few days until the lawyer could find out what was going on.

It was the middle of winter and outside it had already grown dark. The parties shook hands before Di's sister brought her car to the rear entrance to take Di and Sarah home with her. On the way, she would drop Mark off at the shopping centre car park where his mother's car still stood. From there, Mark would drive it to his brother's house at Gloucester. If they had to lay low, they would need a fresh change of clothes and Sarah's supplements.

Mark left the shopping centre car park after 6 pm for the trip back to Gloucester. It was a moonless night, made even darker by thick cloud cover, and the car's high beams barely lit the road.

After an hours' drive, Mark spotted his brother's house and turned into his driveway. His brother had been waiting for him and stood with the shed door open for Mark to drive straight in, after which he closed the door immediately behind him. Mark sat in the car for a moment with his heart pounding. He had never felt hunted before. Next to him was parked his brother's utility, fully packed for them with their clothes and Sarah's supplies.

Mark wasted no time. He gave his brother a thank-you wave, swapped vehicles, and drove out with his brother's utility straight away, leaving his mother's car in the shed. Mark sped back down the drive and swerved onto the road to Taree.

On the lonely back highway connecting Gloucester with Taree, Mark encountered a white government car on the road in front of him. In his rush, he passed it and caught a glimpse of official looking occupants inside. Not knowing what else to do, he throttled the utility and left the car behind at speed.

It was already after 8 pm when Mark arrived back at his sister-in-law's house. Di's sister and her husband had taken good care of Di and Sarah, but they all looked anxious.

'Get your things together. We're going', said Mark.

'Where to?' asked Di.

Mark wanted no one else to know where they would be. 'Just trust me on this one'.

After saying their goodbyes, the family bundled up in warm clothes and piled into the utility. The temperature had dropped to a chilly 6° C and the icy drizzle made conditions even colder. Inside the utility's cabin, Mark turned the heater on. The three sat in front, with no lights but the dashboard's eerie glow. Sarah snuggled up to her mother. Di was worried about her. Sarah wore the same hunted look as they all did and she wondered what kind of lasting impression this would make on her daughter's young mind. None of them had ever felt this kind of fear before. They headed north on the Pacific Highway, like fugitives in the night. Their destination was almost halfway up the NSW coast and it would take at least four hours to get there. It was a long and painfully quiet trip, with no one knowing what to say.

They arrived in South West Rocks in the middle of the night – terrified, confused, and exhausted.

At almost the same instant that Mark and Di arrived at their secret location, a police officer knocked on Ruth and Jim's door. Ruth was terrified to see a constable in the middle of the night, but he seemed respectful and she invited him in. The portly country cop had lived in the district a long time and he knew the family. The summons he carried gave him the power to enter Ruth and Jim's home and seize their property. He asked where Mark and Di were, but Ruth and Jim truthfully knew nothing of their whereabouts. In a sympathetic tone, the officer then asked questions about Sarah's illness. Ruth put the kettle on and made him a cup of tea, while Jim filled him in on the details he knew about. After a long chat, the officer reassured them all would be well soon enough. He was a seasoned cop, and well aware of the wide powers the court order gave him, but he used his own discretion and treaded softly. This was a small town and he knew the family to be responsible and law abiding – in fact, one of the pillars of the community. As far as he was concerned, the matter would all work out in the end. Two hours later, at 1 am, fortified by strong tea, the officer squeezed behind the wheel of his cruiser and disappeared into the frosty night.

After the officer left, Ruth and Jim had little rest that night. In the other rooms lay sleeping the five other Westley children. The grandparents wondered what on earth they could tell them in the morning, when they didn't even know themselves what was going on.

Saturday 7 June dawned a few hours later. The family slept fitfully in the flat a friend had lent them at South West Rocks. Mark woke up in the holiday house bedroom, only to be assaulted again by memories of the day before. He knew somebody wanted Sarah but he wasn't sure why. He would do whatever necessary to protect his family, but constant vigilance came at a price. He'd only been able to catch a few hours' sleep.

Di stirred next to him. She too looked worried, even in her sleep. This weekend, Mark decided, he had to gather his thoughts and write down details of all that had happened since Sarah got sick.

Meanwhile Sarah was in the second bedroom sound asleep. When she woke up, they would tell her that this was just a short holiday, but Mark suspected this would be futile; after yesterday, Sarah knew someone was hunting them. They would just have to make it a pleasant day for Sarah, but he would stay alert. From the bed, Mark peered outside through the half closed Venetians to check for any unusual activity. He wondered how their other children were faring, but couldn't take the risk of phoning his parents. A chilling thought kept intruding into his mind: Would DoCS go to his parents and take the other children if they couldn't find Sarah?

Ruth and Jim's morning was dismal. The children woke up and wanted to know where their parents and Sarah had gone. They'd been worried ever since Sarah had told them that two ladies had visited on two different occasions and taken her outside to ask her questions about whether she was being properly taken care of. Laura especially wanted to know why the police had come in the middle of the night. Ruth and Jim hardly knew what to say. They were sick with worry and felt a heavy responsibility to protect their other five grandchildren. They began to wonder whether the department had the power to take both Sarah and the other children.

'Your parents are just on a bit of a trip with Sarah. They'll be back soon', said Ruth as reassuringly as possible. 'Just the same, I want to show you something'.

Ruth gathered up the five kids and led them outside. Together they walked up to the orchard. It was overgrown with tall grass high enough to hide an old cubby house that had once been a playroom for children of generations past.

Ruth opened its creaky door. 'Let's see if you can all fit in here'.

Laura understood what her grandmother was doing and made it into a game for the four younger ones. Soon Clara caught on and helped Laura shepherd the youngest two into the cubby. The oldest girls squeezed in last of all and closed the door from the inside.

'Good!' exclaimed Ruth, as she fought back tears. 'Now you can do this if ever a stranger comes to the house'.

The smaller children burst from the cubby giggling while Ruth dried her eyes with her apron. 'Now let's go up and have breakfast', she said.

Back in the kitchen, Jim boiled the jug. Despite his poor vision, he saw Ruth's red-rimmed eyes. 'What's the matter?' he asked.

Ruth stared at him for a long time. 'Hiding those kids is something I never thought I'd have to do'.

On the same Saturday morning, the child protection department called in emergency staff to arrange another Supreme Court hearing. The caseworkers had been thoroughly frustrated by their bungled attempt to serve a summons on Mark and Di and remove Sarah from her home. A senior department official contacted a Supreme Court Justice on Saturday morning June 7, and asked the judge for an urgent court hearing that day. This is a move usually reserved for the most heinous situations and is not normally used against people who simply want to decide on a treatment for their illness. The justice was led to believe the matter was an extreme emergency, rather than one concerning a late-stage cancer patient, and he granted the department its emergency hearing. He was also not told that the department itself had bungled the service of the summons. At that stage, it was made to appear that the parents were evading the summons and the grandparents were shielding Mark and Di from its service, necessitating stronger court orders. The caseworkers stated in an affidavit, that they had returned to retrieve the summons from Mark's mailbox some hours later, (presumably after returning to the Taree office and then realizing they had wrongly served the summons), and after finding it missing they had returned to Ruth and Jim's house. They then wrongly claimed Ruth had handed it to them, while making no mention that there was no one at the house when they'd returned. Worse still, caseworkers withheld from the court how the summons had been removed from the house while Ruth and Jim were not at home.[24]

A few hours later, in the special Supreme Court session, the department's barrister sought stronger orders than before, requesting that parental rights be revoked and Sarah be made a ward of court. In effect, DoCS's caseworkers would be Sarah's new parents. To achieve this, the department requested even wider powers – including extra force – to haul Sarah in.

The hearing occurred without the parents' knowledge and without giving them an opportunity to defend themselves or refute the claims in the caseworker's affidavits. Though the family had engaged legal counsel the previous evening, it was now Saturday, and the lawyer knew nothing of it either. Since no summons had been served, not even a seasoned lawyer could realistically imagine a special Saturday session would be called in the Supreme Court, merely because a patient wanted a treatment other than the one a doctor had ordered.

With no new testimony other than the oncologist's original letters, the court granted the department's harsh demands, and also took the unusual step of authorising police and department personnel to use force to enter any premises or stop any vehicle or vessel suspected of transporting Sarah in order to take her into custody. The department was now legally Sarah's parent. She could be apprehended by the SWAT team and without search warrants. Within the hour, police and hospitals received a new alert: 11-year-old Sarah was to be taken into the department's immediate custody, by any force necessary.

---

[24] Mark was not privy to that court hearing and not aware of the caseworker's claims. The department withheld the caseworker's affidavit and other court records of the ex-parte hearing from Mark for the next 7 years until an FOI request recently turned it up in December 2009.

By midmorning, another cruiser was dispatched to the Westley grandparents. On seeing the vehicle, Laura and Clara hurried up to the orchard with the three little ones and hid.

The same police officer knocked on their door and made another round of enquiries about Sarah's and her parents' whereabouts. Ruth and Jim still did not know where they were. The new orders authorised the officer to use maximum force on the family but instead he remained respectful and left the grandparents alone. They were relieved when the officer did not ask about the other children. [25]

Later that day, Ruth got a phone call from a retired police officer who wished the family well. 'Just keep your car in the garage and out of sight for a while', he advised, 'if you know what I mean'.

Clear and sunny weather followed the recent rains in the small seaside town of South West Rocks. Sarah was enjoying the beach and the surf was up after the high winds. Seagulls wheeled around overhead, diving down for small fish. Sarah frolicked on the sand, looking for seashells and bright pebbles. Later the family sat down to a feast of fish and chips, calamari, and prawns. Sarah ate twice the amount her parents could manage.

Mark had started jotting down all the details he could remember about the past seven months. Once he started writing in the diary, streams of painful events escaped from his pen, making their nightmare all too real.

Sarah and Di returned to the beach after lunch without Mark. The ocean glistened in the wintry afternoon sun. They built sandcastles together until the tide came in and swept the sand sculptures away.

None could have imagined what had happened in court that morning.

Monday, 9 June was the Queen's Birthday public holiday. Mark could wait no longer for news of his other children and called his parents from a public phone. Jim answered and was relieved to hear they were all right.

On impulse, Mark laid a trap to see if their phones had been bugged. As a boy, he had read his share of detective magazines but never thought he would

---

[25] In 2004, the department drafted a new amendment to its NSW *Children and Young Persons (Care and Protection) Act 1998,* empowering caseworkers to remove other siblings in the family without being required to state any reasons for doing so. Had that amendment, passed by Parliament in 2005, been in force in 2003, Sarah's siblings could have been taken away.

use the information in his life. At the end of the call, he told his father he was leaving New South Wales and heading up to Queensland with Sarah. He intended no such thing, but his father took him at his word. Mark later discovered through friends in the police force that a police alert had gone out to watch for vehicles with a child on-board heading north towards the state border. He knew then that his family's telephones were being illegally monitored – a problem that would plague them for a long time to come.

On Tuesday, 10 June, Mark left early for the four-hour drive to Taree in his brother's white utility for an appointment with his solicitor. Before Mark's arrival, the lawyer had phoned the department to let them know he was the family's legal representative. He then asked the department for an up-to-date brief about its activities in relation to the family. This started a volley of phone calls and a complex round of negotiations. Meanwhile, with the lawyer now identified, the department would soon know Mark's whereabouts. It was only a matter of time before Mark would show up at the legal office.

By 10 am, Mark drove into the lawyer's office car park, where he immediately noticed a man and a woman in two separate cars watching the parking lot from different positions. Mark parked in the farthest corner, and after twice making sure the utility's doors were locked, he hurried into the rear entrance of the legal office. The receptionist ushered Mark into the inner office; moments later, process servers entered the office foyer and served court documents on the receptionist.

While the receptionist signed for the documents, Mark sat in the lawyer's office receiving news of the two court hearings that had been held without his knowledge. It shocked him to the core to learn that he was forced to give up his daughter immediately – that she was a ward of court and that he and Di had lost their parental rights to decide what was best for her. This seemed incomprehensible, since they had done all in their power as parents to deal with Sarah's illness and discuss their concerns with the doctors in a reasonable manner.

After the immediate shock, Mark told his lawyer he wanted his say in court. His lawyer prepared an affidavit that included the material Mark had written down over the weekend. It set out for the court the parents' thoroughness in dealing with Sarah's health issue, the research that had been undertaken and the treatments she had received. It included the parents' doubts about the oncologist's proposed treatment and their attempts to gather other specialist opinions. When the lawyer finished drafting it, Mark swore to the document and the legal secretary prepared it for court.

Before too long the department's barrister phoned the lawyer again to storm him with fresh demands; insisting Sarah be taken to Gloucester hospital within two hours or he would charge the parents with contempt of court. In addition, the barrister threatened to charge the lawyer for contempt if Sarah did not turn up at the hospital. The lawyer put the barrister on hold and explained to Mark the department's demands. Mark replied that two hours was a physical impossibility since Sarah's current location was four hours away, but he promised to deliver Sarah to the Gloucester hospital the next morning without fail. The lawyer got the barrister on the line again and told him Mark's answer. He found the barrister's response heavy going, but managed to get an agreement after a difficult negotiation. When the lawyer hung up from the exhaustive round of talks, Mark added in private that, although his promise to bring Sarah to the hospital was rock solid, either he or Di would accompany Sarah at all times until the legal mess was sorted out, regardless of any court orders. The lawyer saw Mark's determination and realised he wasn't about to lose his parental rights without a stand-up fight.

Still feeling outraged, Mark left the legal office and headed towards his brother's utility in the rear car park. He recalled that he had carefully locked it, but as he came closer, he immediately noticed the driver's side door had been interfered with. It was unlocked and ajar, as if someone had hastily broken in and left in a hurry. Inside, he noticed the loose change he'd left on the passenger side console was still there. He quickly scanned the interior for any devices, but could find nothing immediately obvious. Feeling unsettled by the break-in, he left as quickly as possible with a terrible feeling he was now being tracked.

Mark drove back to South West Rocks while closely watching his rear vision mirror. Worse than being followed was the prospect of telling Di and Sarah that Sarah had been made a ward of court and that she had to submit to all the caseworkers' and doctors' demands – including all medical procedures – whether she wanted them or not. It occurred to him that anybody who forced Sarah into anything against her will would have their work cut out for them. At that point, Mark still did not comprehend the full implications of what had occurred that weekend. It just seemed like a nightmare from which he wanted soon to awaken.

Mark called his parents from a phone booth at Bonny Hills, to tell them the news. Jim was horrified and said he and Ruth would come to Gloucester hospital the following morning.

Two hours later, Mark was back at the South West Rocks flat to break the news. When Di and Sarah became upset at what he had to tell them, Mark decided to stay put for the night, to let them get over the shock, and leave early in the morning for Gloucester.

After Sarah went to sleep, Mark and Di leaned on the balcony railing. The new moon was bright enough to cast a cool glint on the water. The surf roared in the distance. In another time, it would have been a romantic night. Instead, it felt like an omen of terrible days ahead.

Mark noticed Di seemed fragile. 'How are you holding up?' he asked.

Di gave an ironic chuckle. 'I still have those application forms in my bag. This means we can't take Sarah for treatment, doesn't it'.

Mark had forgotten about the trip in the panic of the past few days. It now struck him as ironic that each time they tried to take Sarah to a doctor or hospital of their choice, the department totally derailed them. 'According to them', said Mark, 'we're not her parents and we don't get to choose anymore'.

Di turned and glared at Mark angrily. 'Don't you ever say that again!'

Mark put his arm protectively around her shoulders. 'Di', he started gently. 'I've got to see a barrister tomorrow'.

Di swung from his grasp and backed away. 'Not tomorrow. They're taking Sarah to Sydney and we've got to be with her'.

Mark grasped on to the railing. 'You'll have to go with her', he replied softly.

'What?' Di was beginning to sound panicky. 'I can't do that on my own'.

'We have no other options', said Mark carefully.

Di panicked and flailed her arms at him. 'I can't, Mark!' she cried as she grasped at his jumper. 'Do you hear me? I just can't!'

Mark cradled her while she softly wept on his shoulder.

'I'm only a mum', she sobbed. 'They won't take any notice of me'.

'Listen to me carefully', murmured Mark into Di's ear. 'These people mean business. They have a lot of power. They are terribly misinformed and they are serious about taking our daughter. Right now, we have to save our family. We all have to do things we don't usually do right now. You'll need to do my job sometimes and I will have to do yours. Right now, I need to prepare for court in a couple of days and hopefully undo the damage they've already done'.

Di dried her eyes with the back of her hand. She knew Mark was right; she would have to be Sarah's protector whenever he wasn't around. It meant she would have to get over her shyness. It was scary, but she had no choice.

There seemed nothing more to talk about and they were both exhausted. Before going to bed Mark checked on Sarah and made sure the doors were locked. When the lights were out, he peered through the Venetian blinds. On the road across the street, a light-coloured car was parked. He stared at it for a minute and noticed the inside light quickly flicker on and then off. There seemed no doubt a person was in the car. From his dealings with the department so far, it didn't seem too far-fetched to think they had surveillance on them. Mark mentioned nothing to Di and returned to bed. He spent a restless night, sleeping with one eye open.

The next day was 11 June. The department phoned the matron of Gloucester hospital to notify her that an emergency patient (an 11-year-old girl) was due to arrive at the hospital by lunchtime. From there, the department scheduled an ambulance to transport her to Taree airport where an emergency aircraft was waiting to fly her to Sydney.

At 11.45 am, a large group of family members arrived at the Gloucester hospital, including Sarah and her parents, Laura and Clara, Ruth and Jim, and two of Sarah's aunts. For a while, the hospital staff didn't know where to put them all. When a nurse asked where the patient was, Mark brought Sarah forward. The nurse stood disbelieving that this athletic girl with red cheeks was the sick patient needing an emergency airlift to Sydney. When she'd recovered from her surprise, she showed the family into a large recreation room where they could wait until the ambulance came to collect Sarah at 1 pm.

Unfortunately the ambulance was five hours late, and so, during the wait, Sarah and her sisters played games in the rec room. When they got bored, they played hide-and-seek on the hospital grounds and set pranks on the staff, running off giggling afterwards.

The ambulance finally arrived at 4 pm. The paramedics scanned around for the emergency patient, and were just as surprised as the nurses had been to discover it was Sarah – a tall, cheeky girl. By then, Sarah was in a playful mood. She joked with the paramedics and looked forward to what she considered a joy ride. After allowing Sarah time to say goodbye to the rest of the family, the paramedics led Di and Sarah to the waiting ambulance. Di sat next to the stretcher while Sarah bounded up on it but refused to be strapped down. The ambulance arrived at Taree airport just after 6 pm.

On the airport tarmac stood the waiting emergency air ambulance, a specially outfitted fixed-wing aircraft fully crewed by medical staff – piloted and operated by the Ambulance Service of NSW. The aircrew guided Sarah and Di up the ladder into the medically equipped aircraft. Sarah giggled with delight. She was overjoyed to travel on an aeroplane again; by now, it was her favourite pastime. This flight was different from the commercial plane she had taken with her parents to Melbourne. It had a lot of interesting equipment inside and an aircrew just for her, without any other passengers. Before takeoff, the crew tried to strap her to the stretcher. She tolerated the restraints until after takeoff, when she insisted on sitting up. For the remaining 330 km flight to Sydney, she joked with the crew.

After an hour and a half, the night flight was on its approach to Sydney airport. The crew had never encountered such a bright and lively 'emergency' patient before, and they'd thoroughly enjoyed themselves.

It was Di who was sick by then. After the stress of the previous weeks and the turbulent motion of the small aircraft, Di felt queasy by the time the flight descended through the light drizzle and landed on the runway. She was relieved to get out of the small aircraft and onto solid ground again. But she was not there for long – an ambulance stood waiting on the tarmac to rush them to Dr Capewell's ward at the city hospital.

While Sarah and Di were in the aircraft 5000 metres overhead, Mark made his way to Sydney by road. The following day he had an appointment with a Sydney barrister who would represent the family in court. It was a woman barrister, whom he hoped would work as hard to uphold the family's rights as the Taree lawyer had done so far. The two legal representatives were meant to work together – the lawyer was in charge of the paperwork while the barrister's job was to appear in court.

Mark hoped the next hearing would allow him to put his own side forward. Surely once the judge had heard all the facts, the department's run would be over. So far, the department officials had had it all their own way and had caused only havoc. They certainly knew how to wear down their opponents – he hadn't had a decent night's sleep in weeks.

Di and Sarah arrived at the city hospital late that evening and ED staff transferred them immediately to Dr Capewell's hospital ward. Sarah was tired on arrival, but as soon as night duty staff finished admitting her, they wanted to take a blood test and start chemotherapy. Sarah was terrified and refused. When they insisted, Sarah told them she wanted to wait until her father arrived. They were surprised at the girl's nerve and reluctantly left the room.

Just as Di had settled Sarah down to sleep, two night nurses and a doctor arrived, trailing two orderlies behind as backup. Without further explanation, they converged on Sarah. Four staff held her down while a fifth forcibly took blood and inserted an intravenous catheter.

With the cannula taped to her wrist, Sarah was shaking after the forceful procedure. For a few moments, Di was paralysed with shock until she recalled the promise she had made to herself and to Mark the night before.

Di leapt from her seat. 'What are you doing?' she demanded.

'We're going to start chemotherapy', answered the doctor who had taken the blood.

'You need permission to do that!'

'We already have it', said the doctor.

'You do *not* have it. My husband will be in court tomorrow. Until then you will get off my daughter and leave her alone!' Di surprised herself with her own grit. Even the doctor was startled and backed away.

Sarah glanced terrified from her mother to the staff members, who one by one retreated from the room.

'Please don't leave me alone, Mum', she begged after all the staff had gone.

Di retrieved two extra cotton blankets from Sarah's bedside cupboard. 'I'm not going anywhere', she answered. Being careful of the newly inserted cannula, Di covered Sarah with the blanket before settling into the armchair next to the bed. She intended to stay there until morning, when she would probably have to deal with the oncologist in person.

The next morning Dr Capewell arrived to examine Sarah. Di stayed close by and no one mentioned the events the night before.

On returning to his office, the oncologist wrote a letter and faxed it to the department. Later that morning the department's barrister from the Crown Solicitor's department took the letter to court with him.

Mark arrived in court with his barrister at mid-morning. The department's barrister was already there. When the court came into session, the judge who presided over the matter was not the one who had granted the department emergency powers. This judge took some time to read the previous judge's orders and expressed surprise at the unusually wide powers the department had been granted. Now he had before him the child's parent and the family's barrister and could hear the defendant's evidence.

Mark's barrister presented Mark's affidavit to the court, while the department's barrister presented Dr Capewell's letter.

Although Sarah had been emergency airlifted, the oncologist reported her condition that morning as non-urgent: '...the tests did not show any abnormality requiring urgent action. She had an uneventful night. This morning she is not in pain from the tumour mass'.

Further into his letter, the doctor stated that the mass had almost tripled in size over the past two weeks but he maintained his prognosis of around an 80 per cent chance of cure. He then added: 'If Sarah does not receive chemotherapy within the next few days she may die...' [26]

The oncologist did not mention Sarah's late stage of cancer or that she only a slim chance of survival despite any type of treatment. On this, the new judge remained tragically misinformed, just as the previous judge had been.

After reading Mark's affidavit, the judge remarked that it appeared clear that Sarah's parents had in fact been dealing with her illness with the seriousness and thoroughness it deserved. Mark also heard the judge remark that he would not consider forcing a medical treatment on a person with less than 50 per cent chance of survival. In other words, had he been accurately informed of Sarah's poor prognosis, which was considerably less than the judge's 50 per cent benchmark, the judge would have thrown the matter out. Unfortunately, however, as the oncologists had concealed this information not only from the court but also from the family, tragically Mark was unable to inform the court of Sarah's true prognosis, which would have entitled her to receive her chosen treatment.

Instead, based on the inaccurate evidence before the court, the case continued. The judge made orders allowing Mark a few days to prepare further submissions, since the family's side of the matter had not been heard. The judge ordered the chemotherapy postponed until he could consider Mark's material.

Unfortunately, while the department had had months to prepare its case, Mark had only a few days. This would prove impossible unless he could access Sarah's medical records in order to allow independent medical experts to read them and prepare medical reports to support Sarah's case. Since the oncologists had refused Mark copies of Sarah's clinical records and test results – even though he had asked for them, and was entitled to them – Mark's barrister now had to ask the judge for orders. Without hesitation, the judge ordered the doctors to release Sarah's medical records to the family and their legal representatives.

Incredibly, however, over the next days the oncologist defied the court order and still did not produce the medical records. Mark had a list of doctors to be briefed, but there was still no briefing material. Time was running out and

---

[26] Chemotherapy is not considered an emergency treatment.

most doctors on the list were increasingly unwilling to produce a report in 24–48 hours. Finally, Mark's lawyer briefed a doctor in London. In the rush, the doctor was given information on only one of Sarah's tumour types, dysgerminoma – the type which was least virulent – while he remained unaware of Sarah's two other lethal tumour types. This rendered the London doctor's report technically useless, even though it contained a number of valid treatment suggestions, including low dose chemotherapy and immunotherapy – two newer cancer treatments.

While the battle raged, Sarah waited in hospital for a week with Di staying at her side around the clock. Dr Capewell arrived each morning with several other doctors and students. He had not asked Sarah or Di whether they minded the strangers in the room each day, despite being ethically required to do so. From the door and often from inside her room, the oncologist lectured about Sarah's condition while his colleagues listened, fascinated, and asked questions.

Each day the oncologist requested a blood test for Sarah and sometimes two per day. Di noticed that none of the other children in the Sarah's section were having daily tests and asked the doctor about it. After her enquiry, the practice stopped and Sarah had tests less frequently. Di thought it strange and wondered whether Sarah's blood was being used for research.

By midweek, Sarah received an official visitor. Since Sarah was of the age where she was entitled to some input into decisions made about her, the judge had appointed an independent legal representative to seek her views and ensure her rights and wishes are upheld in court. This female lawyer asked Sarah whether she wanted chemotherapy. Sarah answered that the oncologist had explained everything about chemotherapy and the side effects to her, as well as the consequences of having it or not. She made it clear that she did not want that particular chemotherapy, but wanted another treatment and the regimen she had been having.

During the next court hearing a few days later, the judge weighed the evidence. In the end, it amounted to the two hospital oncologists' opinions versus the doctor in London. Since Dr Capewell had a 12-page curriculum vitae, he won the day. To make matters worse, Sarah's court-appointed legal counsel appeared on her behalf and told the court: 'Notwithstanding those views which Sarah has expressed, it is in the best interests of the child for chemotherapy to occur'.

This clinched the judge's decision, and he ordered Sarah to have the chemotherapy. He also allowed her to continue her complementary therapies and supplements while undergoing the treatment.

Despite the small concession, Mark was upset with the way the hearing was unfolding. Before it ended, Mark told his barrister that he wanted more time to have medical reports prepared and for that he needed the clinical records the oncologists refused to hand over. When his barrister failed to raise the issue in court, Mark had the first stirrings of doubts about his legal representative. However, after the verdict the barrister disappeared back to her chambers and was unavailable for a discussion. Instead, Mark urgently phoned his lawyer in Taree to see if anything could be done to stop the treatment until they had the necessary medical documents.

In a desperate measure to buy more time, the lawyer faxed a letter to the hospital placing the responsibility on the oncologist should Sarah die or suffer severe disability or side effects from the treatment. For the first time, the oncologist felt the heat and was infuriated. He demanded the letter be retracted before he started the chemotherapy.

The following day, the department stepped in and once again urgently applied to the court for even stronger orders. The judge agreed and, with the court barely adjourned, the parties rushed out to use their cell phones.

In the hallway, Mark phoned the ward and asked to speak with Di. While he waited for the staff to get her, he glanced at the date on his watch. It was Friday, the 13th of June – a day he would never forget.

Further down the hallway, the department barristers phoned Dr Capewell at the hospital. Minutes later, the oncologist instructed hospital staff to prepare the chemotherapy. It would be forced on Sarah, and it would commence at 6 pm that night.

SARAH'S NEW PARENTS

Make sure that you do not exploit your patient for any reason.

AMA Code of Medical Ethics

It was the evening of Friday the 13th, and Dr Capewell was preparing to leave the hospital. He looked forward to relaxing on the weekend. It had been an eventful week, and he was pleased to have scored a victory in court. So confident was he of winning, that he instructed the medical staff days ago to hook Sarah up to a saline IV to keep her vein open for chemotherapy. Capewell's oncology registrar was in charge of the ward on the weekend and would take care of everything.

The IV apparatus with its drip counter was mounted on wheels so Sarah could push it around on her walks down the hall. For Sarah it was like being on a plastic leash. During the week her father was in court, she scooted the IV around the ward so fast that a nurse put a 'Learner Driver' sign on it. But the fun was about to end. Just before 6 pm, staff converged on Sarah. Doctors and nurses wearing goggles, gloves and plastic aprons came from all directions with chemotherapy equipment.

From the hallway, Di watched the staff racing towards Sarah's room. She had moments before taken Mark's call and received the news. Mark told Di that he would have to fight the Friday night Sydney traffic and could not say how long he would be before arriving at the hospital. Di returned to Sarah's room and found it full of hospital personnel. Immediately, a nurse instructed her to put on rubber gloves and an apron when handling her daughter's bodily fluids, or when touching her skin. Another nurse in safety gear reprogrammed the IV drip machine and changed the bag from saline to an IV bag containing yellow fluid. An oncology registrar stayed in the background, ready to intervene if necessary.

'What's that?' asked Sarah.

'You're going to have chemotherapy now', said the nurse.

In a panic, Sarah moved to the other side of her bed, stretching the IV line attached to her. 'But I told you I don't want it', she cried.

The oncology registrar moved in closer and told Sarah she was going to have it whether she wanted it or not.

'But I've got rights', insisted Sarah.

'You've got no rights', replied the doctor firmly. 'You're a ward of the court'.

'What do you mean?' demanded Sarah.

'DoCS have ordered this', said the doctor, 'and there's nothing you can do about it'. He shot a warning glance over to Di.

Sarah turned to her mother hopefully. 'Mum?'

Di had never felt so powerless before. Mark had told her that any move seen as interference with the chemo would result in contempt of court charges and possible prison for either or both parents. Di realised she could no longer stop the staff doing whatever they wanted to her daughter, and wept helplessly.

Sarah searched frantically around the room for signs of her father while staff continued their preparations unfettered. They were confident now that no one had the power to stop them.

Sarah huddled miserably in bed. She suddenly realised that her parents had no more say in what happened to her. People who did not know her now made decisions for her. She found it a strange feeling to have no say over her own body. It was the first time something had been forced into her against her will. The terrifying thought occurred to her that there was nothing more to do and nowhere to hide.

The nurse programmed the buttons on the IV pump and started the infusion. Di held her breath and took Sarah's hand, ignoring the rubber gloves she was supposed to be wearing. Sarah watched as the yellow fluid displaced the clear saline in the plastic tubing and inched closer down her arm with each click of the machine. A minute later, the first drops of chemical hit her like a violent blow. She immediately felt desperately ill and retched violently. She reached out to her mother, but Di could do little more than hold the vomit bowl for her. When Sarah realised that nobody could help her, she took a sickening plunge into hopelessness and looked utterly abandoned. She tried to go inward to a safe place in her mind, but when she closed her eyes, the nausea engulfed her. Instead, she focused intensely on her mother, her only source of comfort. Di held her hand until Sarah's skin became too tender to be touched. It was only the beginning. Soon her skin became hot and her lungs felt on fire with every breath. At the same time, her teeth chattered with cold and shock.

'It feels like I'm burning and freezing at the same time', groaned Sarah. 'Please help me, Mum'.

Di filled a sponge bowl with tepid water from the basin. She wrung out a washcloth to try to cool Sarah down, but as she lifted Sarah's pajama top she gasped in horror. Red welts had suddenly developed over Sarah's body, back, and front. They were swelling up even as she watched, and when she touched them, Sarah flinched. Di was shocked at how heated her daughter's skin felt, and yet Sarah trembled with cold at the same time. Di was sure Sarah was having an adverse reaction to the drugs and she rushed out to find a nurse. Several minutes later, the nurse arrived. She looked at the welts and then made a note on Sarah's chart. 'It happens. They'll be gone in a few days', she said before leaving again.

Despite Di's efforts to think of reassuring things to say, Sarah reminded her mother that the doctor had told her that children died of the treatment she was having, and now she knew why. It really felt like she was dying, she told Di.

Each time Sarah needed the toilet; she clung on to Di and would not let her out of her sight. Di was now aware of the strong industrial smell coming from her daughter's skin and from the urine in the toilet bowl. When Di noticed her own hands burning after she washed Sarah, she tried to avoid skin contact with her and was careful to wear rubber gloves before touching her daughter in future.

Sarah had been on the chemo IV for an hour when Mark walked in. He hugged his daughter and immediately smelled chemicals on her breath and skin. Sarah could hardly acknowledge him by then; she writhed in her bed. Mark had never seen her so distressed. Her expression had changed to one of almost primal fear; as if something foreign was raging inside her. Her face was swollen, and she moaned and retched at the same time. Mark turned white. He had just spent a week in court fighting for his daughter's right to choose another treatment, and he would rather be in court for another year than see her like this.

The nurse came in to change Sarah's IV bag to another chemical. She smiled cheerfully and seemed unaffected by Sarah's distress. For a moment, the nurse sent Mark and Di out of the room.

Mark lowered his voice outside in the hallway. 'I've never seen her this bad. And she smells like a chemical factory'.

'It must be the strongest they've got', whispered Di. 'You should see her blistered skin. They didn't tell us this could happen'.

Mark covered his mouth and turned pale. 'I don't think I can stay. Give her a hug, if you can. I'll call you from Ryde. See you later'. With that, Mark strode down the hall towards the elevators.

It was nearly 9 pm, when the nurse stopped the IV. For the rest of the night, Sarah lay in bed softly moaning. Angry welts rose across her body. She complained of pain in her chest and seemed unable to catch her breath. Her supper of green jelly and ice cream stood untouched on her bedside table.

Di sat in the chair next to Sarah's bed. She'd brought her needlework but couldn't focus on it. She tried to read a story but Sarah had suddenly become hypersensitive to sound and couldn't stand the noise of someone speaking. The nurse came in to take Sarah's 10 pm observations. When she left, she switched the dim night light on.

Around 10.30, Mark phoned the ward from where he was staying at Ryde, and asked the nurse to allow him to speak with Di briefly. When Di took his call, he apologised for not staying. Firstly, he'd found it difficult to see Sarah in so much discomfort, and secondly, he thought it prudent to stay out of the way for a while. He had the impression that the department would like nothing better than to cite him for contempt for the slightest reason. He sent his love to them both and assured Di he would be back over the weekend.

After the call, Di returned to her bedside watch. She was dead tired and in desperate need of sleep, but Sarah's moans kept her awake all night.

Over Saturday and Sunday, Sarah had two more days of chemotherapy. Like a mantra, she kept repeating: 'I feel so sick'. She had not kept any food down since Friday, and was starting to lose small bunches of hair when her mother combed it. She was weak and barely able to move. She needed help into the bath, and onto the toilet, which she now negotiated like an old woman. The drugs had caused severe back pain and constant painful muscle spasms. Sarah was now curled up in bed and unable to walk.

On Monday, Mark returned to the hospital. Di showed him the welts over Sarah's torso. No one told them that, according to the to manufacturer's information, this was a listed but rare side effect of two of the chemotherapeutic agents she was given, and an indication she was sensitive to the drugs. The welts had progressed from painful raised red blisters to brown pigmented stripes. Mark retreated from the room and paced the hospital corridor for a while to cool his anger.

Later that morning Dr Capewell brought a large group of doctors and other personnel into Sarah's room and gave a lecture to them about her case. The group included the entire hospital oncology team, and their oncology fellows, registrars, residents and interns. He seemed in a good mood and hugely pleased with the treatment, even though Sarah was unable to leave her bed.

The oncologist returned later with both his registrars and announced to the parents his next plan for Sarah. 'We can use the veins in her arm for the chemotherapy, but we plan to put in a permanent chemo line into one of the vessels near her heart', said Capewell.

Mark was not ready to give up his fight in court for Sarah's right to have a less toxic treatment and didn't want Sarah to have a permanent chemotherapy line at that time.

'I don't think so', Mark said to the oncologist. 'Until we are finished putting our evidence to the court, we'd rather she didn't have another risky procedure at this stage'.

The oncologist was not happy with Mark's attitude after the court had given him free rein in Sarah's treatment. He left the room abruptly, with his registrars following behind. Mark trailed the group into the hallway and politely called out to the oncologist. The doctor stopped and turned briefly.

Mark felt the doctor had been given a blank cheque on false pretences. 'I would like to have those medical records today. The ones the judge ordered released', he said to Capewell.

The oncologist gave Mark a noncommittal reply and headed down the hallway with his registrars in tow. One of the junior doctors turned briefly and shrugged his shoulders.

For the rest of the afternoon Mark stayed with Sarah and Di, but began to feel increasingly uncomfortable about being at the hospital. By late afternoon, he felt a strong urge to leave and decided to return to his lodgings in Ryde. By 5 pm, it was nearly dark outside and he said his goodbyes to Di and Sarah. When leaving the hospital car park, the guard at the gate stopped him and asked him to wait. He took down his licence number and made a phone call in the guardhouse. While the guard was still on the phone, Mark gave him a friendly wave and drove through the checkpoint. In his rear vision mirror, he saw the guard standing on the roadway watching him.

Mark was still driving his brother's utility and he had a feeling he was being tracked back and forth from the hospital to their family friend's home at Ryde where he was staying. He wondered whether someone was setting him up for contempt charges because he was still trying to be involved as a parent with decisions concerning Sarah's treatment.

In the dark, Mark headed north-west towards Ryde. He watched his rear and side mirrors for cars behind him and took care to drive within the speed limits. Within half an hour, he arrived at his friends' home. He parked the utility under a large tree at the front of the house and locked all four doors, before hurrying inside. He was looking forward to unwinding soon from another stressful day. His friends weren't home from work yet, but a slow cooking crock-pot simmered in the kitchen with a fresh batch of minestrone soup. Mark popped a couple of slices of bread into the toaster, and helped himself to a large bowl of soup and buttered toast. After half an hour, he felt calmer and almost rested enough to read some legal documents his lawyer wanted him to check over before the next hearing. The documents were still in the utility. Mark grabbed the keys from the coffee table and went outside to retrieve them. When he went to unlock the driver's door, he was shocked to find it was already open. He glanced around and saw only the other residents' cars parked in the street and no sign of anyone lurking around. He felt sure he had locked the car doors. Briefly, he wondered if he was imagining things. Then the anger hit. He dashed into the garage to find a flashlight and returned to the utility. In the strong beam of light, Mark searched for jimmy marks on the lock, before opening the door and discovering his legal papers inside the cab were in disarray. Now he really wondered whether someone was trailing him with a GPS radiofrequency device placed somewhere on the utility. Outside of detective magazines, he'd never heard of such a thing in real life. He knelt down on the pavement and shone the flashlight underneath the car. He carefully inspected the chassis and ran his fingers along the metal skirts, but found nothing.

This was becoming too much. A few days ago, his mother had admitted to him; she and Jim had had a break-in at their farmhouse with the summons taken that she had retrieved from Mark's mailbox.

Within minutes, Mark had packed up the utility. He gunned the engine, and made a 180-degree turn outside the house. This time he headed north, towards the Pacific Highway. From there, he turned onto the F3 freeway northbound to Newcastle. He had a nagging feeling he should check out their farm and homestead, and see how their other children were faring. He had not been home for over a fortnight, ever since Sarah had been airlifted to Sydney, and he had not seen his other children over that time either.

It was nearly midnight when Mark arrived home. The farmhouse stood in darkness. He parked the utility in the shed and locked its doors. While his vision adjusted to the dark, Mark scanned the yard. Muttley and Pooch were making a racket. He found the dogs unusually agitated, when they would normally be wagging their tails when he arrived. When he let them off their chain, they circled the homestead several times sniffing the ground. Mark noticed the dogs were especially interested in the smells around the doormats.

In the dark, Mark found his way to the two French side doors under the veranda. A heavy brass lock and a deadlock secured them. Since his parents had told him of the break-in at their farmhouse, Mark had instructed everyone to keep the doors locked. He slipped the key into the lock, but before he could turn it, the door swung open. Mark stood fixed to the spot for a moment, staring through the yawning doorway into the dark living room. Maybe the kids hadn't locked the house when they dropped in after school to feed the animals. He resisted any form of unfounded suspicion and wanted to find only logical explanations to these peculiar events, but he had to admit, they really were adding up. Mark entered the house carefully. He went into each room upstairs and downstairs, turning the lights on and inspecting every corner. It was nearly 2 am before he got a decent fire going in the iron stove, and well after that before he could finally sleep.

The next day was 19 June. After a morning working around the farm and an afternoon appointment with his lawyer in Taree, Mark went up the road to his parents' house in the evening to spend some time with Ruth, Jim and his other five children. When he arrived, Laura had the kids doing their homework while Ruth was cooking dinner. The kids were excited to see Mark again and plied him with questions about Sarah. He kept his answers understated, not wanting to worry them unnecessarily. They already looked haunted when he asked them about school. Laura explained that she was keeping an eye on the younger ones, making sure they were all on the bus, that they didn't talk to strangers and never went anywhere with anyone they didn't know.

Mark looked at his parents and back to the kids. 'That's probably wise', he said. 'Good job Laura'.

When the family sat down for a meal, Mark noticed how much disruption they had suffered. His children worried about being kidnapped, his eldest daughter had to act as a security guard for her siblings, his parents were spooked when a stranger came into their home, and everyone was worried sick about Sarah.

'When is Sarah coming home?' asked Jim.

Mark took a moment to enjoy his mother's home-cooked meal. 'Di was telling me Sarah might get out on Monday. She's been there nearly two weeks', he answered.

'How's Di holding up?' Ruth asked.

Mark recalled Sarah's torment and the awful chemical smell from the drugs. 'Sarah's better off with her mother right now', he said.

Hannah was impatient to see her sister. 'Can we go with you Dad?' she begged. 'It's creepy at the house'.

Mark looked from Hannah to Laura. 'What do you mean?' he asked.

Laura was about to rebuke her sister for raising the issue, since she didn't want to worry her father. But, on consideration, she thought it might be time to be up-front about what was happening to them. 'I think she means, when we go to our house after school, sometimes things are in different places than they were when we left them. And some things go missing', explained Laura.

Mark put his fork down. He deliberately had not mentioned the peculiar things that had happened to him. 'What kind of things go missing?' he asked.

Laura looked around the table. Almost everyone had stopped to hear what she would say. 'Sometimes, your desk in the study gets messed up, Dad. And, one thing I know for sure. I'm writing to my friend about what we're all going through, and I hide the letters she writes back in a special place. The other day I noticed they were gone'.

Mark looked around the table at the other children. Their knowing expressions told him that Laura was right about their belongings at home being disturbed.

Ruth got up and cleared away the dishes to make way for the trifle she had made for dessert. She knew all too well that something strange had happened in her house too. For a moment, the whole family was reminded of the pervasive feeling that came with having their lives invaded by an unseen enemy.

Mark thought about giving his parents a rest. 'Why don't I take the kids for the weekend and maybe you could collect them from the bus again on Monday afternoon while I'm in Sydney picking up Di and Sarah'.

'That's fine with us, Son', said Jim.

Ruth nodded.

Mark then arranged to borrow Ruth's car to drive Sarah home, while he returned his brother's utility. Ruth meanwhile kept Mark's mini-van to transport the other children.

'I don't know what we would have done without you', said Mark to his parents. 'Di and I are very grateful'.

Ruth brushed it aside in embarrassment. 'That's what families are for'.

June 23 was a Monday. At morning rounds, Dr Capewell visited Sarah with his junior and senior oncology registrars and a group of seven others. Sarah's blood test that morning showed she was anaemic from the chemotherapy. It had depressed her bone marrow, which was now unable to produce enough red or white blood cells or blood-clotting cells. Despite the tests, Capewell was pleased with the chemo, and further to that, he examined Sarah and claimed her spleen had become smaller. Di sat at Sarah's bedside and noticed that the others in the room also seemed happy to see the oncologist pleased. Di was happy only about one thing: today the oncologist would discharge Sarah home. However, he did so with strict instructions to return to the hospital every 21 days for another three days of chemotherapy. Next time she came, he also wanted her to have vaccinations for meningococcal disease, influenza and pneumococcus. He also warned that, from now on, Sarah could not have therapeutic levels of oxygen under any circumstances, since the chemotherapy had caused changes in her lungs that would interact badly with oxygen and cause lung fibrosis. The oncologist left Di with strict instructions to take Sarah to the local GP or to the local hospital if she spiked a fever or had any bleeding, and to bring her back for the next chemo round in three weeks.

After his rounds, Dr Capewell dictated a letter to the family GP, and to the department and eight others, stating:

> ...I am also reporting to you that Sarah is a ward of the state. The manager at Taree DoCS is the person that I have been communicating with since the Supreme Court ruled on the 13th of June that Sarah was to have chemotherapy. Any decisions about operative or other management the Taree office will need to be informed, and consent sought for operative procedures.

Among other things, the doctor also stated: 'She continues to be asymptomatic, although in the three days surrounding giving her chemotherapy, she had some nausea and decreased appetite'.

He did not mention the raised brown welts now permanently branded across Sarah's torso.

At around midday, Mark arrived to take Sarah and Di home from the hospital. After her serious side effects from the chemotherapy, Sarah was far from asymptomatic (symptom free). She was bent over and unable to walk. She was in significant pain in her back and kidney region, which was visibly swollen. When the parents mentioned it to the staff, they were not concerned about it and offered Sarah no pain relief before discharging her from hospital. The oncologist had warned against using paracetamol in case it masked any fever or pain. He had also gone back on his promise to allow Sarah her supplements in the hospital even though the judge had permitted it. She now had to endure significant pain without any remedies or comforts.

While the parents packed Sarah's belongings, staff came in and out of the room beaming at her. When Sarah complained of feeling terrible, the nurse told her that everything would be all right.

Mark and Di went out into the hallway to search for a wheelchair since it was obvious Sarah would not be able to walk to the car. 'Where is the ambulance when you really need it?' asked Di.

'They're looking at her like a prize ewe', answered Mark. 'Compared to her healthy looks two weeks ago, she's so sick now she could, without a doubt, use an airlift home'.

The 300-kilometre trek home took well over five hours. Mark had made a comfortable makeshift bed in the back of Ruth's family sedan, but Sarah found the slightest movement agonising. Her skin burned, her muscles contracted into painful spasms, and her back ached. She also had the first of the severe, blinding headaches that would plague her each time she had another round of chemotherapy.

They arrived home with Sarah about the time her siblings stepped off the school bus. The kids wanted to see their sister straightaway, but Sarah stared empty-eyed and disinterested around the house. She asked her father to carry her straight to bed where she curled up in the foetal position, refusing much food and drink. Although it was a sunny winter's afternoon, Sarah had no energy to go outside, lying instead under her favourite lilac cover in her top-floor bedroom. Brutus stood waiting at the gate for Sarah, and Muttley stood below her window howling for her, but Sarah showed no interest in her favourite animals.

Everyone who saw Sarah was shocked by her appearance, especially since she had looked so well only two weeks previously. Sarah's older siblings tried to hide their feelings from her, but her youngest sister Leah and little brother Joshua cried pitifully after seeing their big sister again.

The next day Hannah rushed up the drive from the school bus and ran upstairs with two pumpkins to ask Sarah which one she liked best. Sarah picked one at random just to be left alone, but three hours later Di had made her favourite pumpkin soup out of it. Hannah brought the soup up on a tray and fed it to her sister. It had a dollop of cream floating in the centre to fatten her up.

The following day was 25 June, and Mark had taken an extra day off in case they had to rush Sarah to the hospital. He worked outside in the yard mending the house fence. At 18 ° C, it was an unusually warm and clear winter's day, with a wispy, high cloud cover. Mark was just cutting a piece of fencing wire when he noticed the sound of a helicopter overhead. It surprised him. He had seen few in that outlying area before and they were far from any airport flight path. The helicopter came from the south and flew a slow, deliberate circle around the house. He watched it for several minutes before it disappeared again in the southerly direction from which it came.

Mark was so determined to find the underlying cause of these strange goings on that he devised a test. That night when everyone was in bed, he personally tied the dogs to their chain and locked the doors before going to bed. He made sure the French doors were deadlocked from the inside where no one could open them without using the key. Since it was hardly ever used, only one key to the deadlock existed, and it was on his key ring. After making sure all the doors and windows were locked, Mark went to bed and put his keys under his pillow.

At around 2 am, the dogs made such a racket it woke Mark up. He got up without turning on any lights, and peered through the living room and bedroom windows for any signs of cars. Outside, all was dark around their homestead and on the road to a neighbour's property. When the dogs settled down, Mark went back to bed.

The next day Di got up early before the others. She wanted to drive the kids to school that morning and then stock up on spinach and other green leafy vegetables from the greengrocer. She thought Sarah looked anaemic and needed lots of iron-rich vegetables. Di went outside to get some clothes from the line that she wanted to dry by the fire. When Mark woke up, he headed towards the kitchen looking for breakfast, and saw both French doors swung wide open with Di in the yard heading back to the house with a bundle of washing.

'How did you get through those doors? asked Mark.

'They were unlocked', answered Di with an innocent smile.

Mark scratched his head and returned to the bedroom. He lifted his pillow and was surprised to find the keys still there. He returned to check the locks and found no signs of forced entry. Whoever opened those doors had done so with some kind of key. He figured anything was possible when a house stands empty for weeks on end. Meanwhile, he didn't want make a fuss and alarm Di. Of one thing, he was certain: from now on, he would stay alert and do whatever was necessary to protect his family and his property.

For the next three weeks friends and relatives dropped by to visit Sarah. They usually brought her favourite foods and board games, but she had little interest in either. Ruth dropped in to tempt Sarah with a homegrown chicken for dinner, baked in its own juices. Di roasted veggies and steamed spinach, and turned it all into a tasty meal of rice soup followed by roast chook, potatoes, and veg. Sarah picked at her dinner in bed from a tray while the family feasted in the dining room. Sarah did not eat her normal amounts. She had developed abdominal cramps and diarrhoea since the chemo, but with small, home-cooked meals every two hours, she managed to gain back, over the next three weeks, the kilogram she had lost in the hospital.

As soon as Sarah ventured out of bed for longer periods, she came down with a chest cold and a nasty cough. Next came the nosebleeds. The first one lasted for hours, despite Di's best efforts to staunch the flow. Then the bleeds came every day in streams and long clots. Sarah's blood clotting mechanism was impaired and she was pale from the chemo and blood loss. After one marathon bleed, Di rushed Sarah to the local hospital. The female doctor treated her in the Emergency Department. After several hours of packing Sarah's nose with long ribbons of gauze, the doctor managed to stop the bleeding. However, she told Di she was at a loss to stop future bleeds; she could only monitor Sarah's blood loss and then order a transfusion if necessary. The doctor asked why Sarah was stooped over and in pain. Di explained she had been in that condition since the chemo. The doctor looked at her sympathetically, but was unable to do more to help. She prescribed Sarah some antibiotics and sent her home.

When Sarah's problems persisted over the next two weeks, Mark and Di brought her to us at the Integrative Health Clinic. They were concerned that, even while Sarah was still sick from the last chemo, soon they would have to bring her back to the hospital for another three-day cycle. They did not think she was up to it in her present condition.

We had last seen Sarah at the Integrative Health Clinic at the end of May, only three weeks before the chemo. Now she was barely recognisable: anaemic and ghostly white, hunched over and in obvious pain from her back and flank region. Her abdomen was abnormal, and painful spasms bent her limbs. Her chest was also congested: she was breathless and wheezy and her left lower lung lobe was devoid of air entry. She still complained of loose bowel motions since the chemo and antibiotics. We recommended some medications to give her a measure of relief and pro-biotics to restore her normal gut flora and settle her diarrhoea.

The parents told us that the oncologist wanted to give Sarah several vaccinations. They wondered how she would fare without a normal immune system. It was a good question. We had nothing against chemo or vaccinations provided an assessment was made between risk and benefit. However, many vaccinations contain live organisms and are contraindicated for immune-compromised persons after chemotherapy. This was clearly the case with Sarah, and she also had several serious health issues and complications that required more urgent attention. The problem in her chest was alarming, and it seemed to us that it would be more prudent to investigate her problems further, treat them appropriately, and wait until they had cleared somewhat before imposing more risky procedures. It was obvious that Sarah had experienced severe side effects from the first three rounds of chemotherapy. Under these circumstances, the clinic issued a letter stating the reasons Sarah did not appear fit to undergo another cycle of chemotherapy until the current issues were resolved.

Mark and Di took the letter with them to the hospital a few days later, hoping the doctors would realise that their daughter was suffering serious side effects from the treatment and would agree to postpone the next round.

Long time family friends wrote about Sarah:

30th June 2003

I must say I was greatly saddened to see the vast change in Sarah Westley's condition and appearance since having chemotherapy treatment. The sight of a crippled child in constant pain, bloated and hardly able to eat was quite a shock to my wife and myself.

We have seen just how happy, active and full of energy she was until taken to Sydney on 11th June, 2003 for treatment. Sarah had been walking, running, playing games and eating as much as any other healthy child of her age.

Laura's letter after Sarah's first chemo:

When Sarah returned from Sydney she could barely walk, and when she did she was virtually hunch-backed. The last time we had seen Sarah, she looked vibrant. Now she looked as though she was suffering from anorexia and bodily restrictions would not allow her to stomach food for several days. She was literally an invalid and used a wheelchair which she barely had the strength to operate. Her abdomen was covered in purple strips like skin disfigurations and she was also extremely sensitive to touch and light.

She experienced excruciating muscle cramps and severe nosebleeds. On one occasion, Mum took her to the hospital because her nose had been bleeding heavily for at least two hours and had been passing clots over 10 cm. which set us into a state of panic.

Also Sarah, during her stay in Sydney, had developed a chronic cough due to the chemo drugs. When she coughed her whole body was tortured with deep pain and she had to use a cushion against her stomach to relieve the pain.

After the first lot of chemo, Sarah's personality had changed enormously. She was no longer the bright bubbly girl we knew. Before, she had been chirpy and never stayed down for long. She was very daring and had experienced many close shaves. We thought of her as a cat with nine lives. Sarah was always the one to do the silly things and often played pranks on not only us, but friends and family as well. We all took it in good spirit, playing along with each cheeky act. The chemo had changed all this dramatically. She now didn't even have the energy to talk to us. This was saddening and rather depressing to us, as we knew what she was normally like, and we grew to miss her mischievous tricks.

Laura Westley

THE DEPARTMENT WANTS YOUR SPLEEN

The Lie can only be maintained by violence

Aleksandr Solzhenitsyn

On 3 July, Mark and Di drove Sarah to Sydney for her hospital appointment. Today the oncology registrar was scheduled to give her a medical check-up, before the next round of chemo tomorrow.

While driving the long distance from Gloucester to Sydney, Mark thought deeply about the events of the past three weeks. He recalled all the break-ins they'd had lately, during which nothing had gone missing except legal paperwork. They'd never experienced such strange events before DoCS had entered their lives. He wondered why the documents had gone missing and why the doctors weren't giving out the court-ordered documents about Sarah. Most of all, he wondered why his barrister wasn't insisting on it, since without the medical records Mark could not protect his family's rights. Now it fell on him to get whatever documents he could from the doctors, and even this was proving difficult, since the oncologist for some reason was refusing to carry out court orders. On 1 July, Mark had phoned Dr Capewell and insisted on receiving Sarah's medical records before they brought Sarah in for any more treatment. In response, the oncologist had promised to hand over copies of some lab tests and scans, and today Mark would ask for them. This represented only a minute fraction of the total clinical records, but something was better than nothing.

As they entered the city limits, Mark prepared himself for a tense atmosphere at the hospital. When the concrete building came into view, Mark felt his stomach churning. He steered into the hospital car park and they all fell into thoughtful silence.

'Dad, I can't walk too far', said Sarah from the back seat. 'My back is too sore'.

Di turned to look at her daughter. Sarah had not needed a rest stop for the entire four-hour trip. 'It seems like your tummy is a bit better now', she remarked.

Sarah confirmed she'd had no more loose stools after the pro-biotics, and her stomach cramps had gone. She could also now stand and walk for short spurts, but Mark would still have to carry her over longer distances.

Inside the hospital, the familiar smell of alcohol swabs and stale French fries brought back dark memories for Sarah.

Once in the ward, a nurse led the family to a treatment room in the day unit, where Mark placed Sarah on the bed. In a few minutes, Dr Capewell's oncology registrar arrived and greeted them somewhat nervously. He examined Sarah and found her spleen still enlarged despite the chemo.

Mark was now confused. It had been weeks since the department had sought court orders to force treatments on the grounds that Sarah's problem was an 'emergency'. From the court documents, he learned that in some letters the doctor had told the court that Sarah's spleen was cancerous, while in others he claimed it was enlarged and bleeding. If so, why did the oncologist give her chemotherapy for a bleeding organ? Now, a month later, not only was Sarah's spleen evidently as big as before, but in addition to this, she was now suffering from the severe side effects of the chemotherapy. When Mark asked these questions, the doctor told him to wait for the answers until the test results were in.

The registrar filled out several pathology forms and instructed the parents to take Sarah to another department for the blood tests. An hour later, the results were on his desk. The doctor looked surprised. Despite the chemotherapy, Sarah still had elevated tumour markers. The July tumour markers after the chemo were roughly the same as the May levels had been when Sarah was still at home, before the chemo and the DoCS intervention. On the other hand, not only had her markers not improved, but her health was in fact considerably worse, since the chemo had impaired some of Sarah's body systems. Her blood count was down, her immunity weakened, and her kidneys were less efficient in clearing her body's waste products.

After reading the results, the doctor asked the parents a number of questions and recorded his findings in the clinical notes.

Cough on and off over last week. Significant pain with coughing so that she holds her breath to stop coughing. Abdominal pain. Uncomfortable to mobilise. Not using analgesia. Told [by Dr Capewell] not to use paracetamol so as not to mask fever. Back pain. Prolonged nose bleed on Sunday. Moving slowly and uncomfortably.

The registrar pulled his stethoscope from his coat pocket and listened to Sarah's chest. For a while, Sarah had a coughing spasm and he had to wait until she could breathe normally again. He wrote into the clinical notes that she had diminished air entry into the left lung base and abnormal wheezing sounds in both lung fields. When the doctor had finished, Di helped Sarah put on her fleecy top again.

Mark waited for the doctor to return to his desk before handing him the letter from the clinic.

After hastily reading it, the doctor cast the letter aside.

'Couldn't we put the next round off until she's a bit better?' asked Mark.

The doctor looked frustrated. 'Just because Sarah isn't well is no reason to stop it', he answered. [27]

Both parents looked bewildered. 'But Sarah has only been this sick since the treatment', said Mark. 'She had no real pain before that and ran around the paddocks at home. We're really worried about her chest. Is it possible to check that out?' Mark asked.

'Bring her back tomorrow for chemotherapy', persisted the registrar.

Mark realized, he was getting nowhere with the registrar, who was probably under instructions from the oncologist – who incidentally wasn't here to see how sick Sarah was. He had noticed that no one in the hierarchy of doctors had ever disputed the oncologist's views.

'We disagree, but because of the court orders, we will see you tomorrow', said Mark. 'But I insist on having the rest of Sarah's clinical records today'.

The doctor fished around his desk and produced a copy of Sarah's scan report, but refused to hand over any other material.

Mark felt stonewalled again. He told the doctor he would expect the rest of the documents and left him the contact number at Ryde, where they would be staying the night.

The family returned to their friends' home at Ryde, where they went out later that evening to do some Thursday night shopping at the local mall with their friends. They brought Sarah with them, and took it in turns to stay with her in the car while the other parent attended to the shopping.

---

[27] This doctor contradicted his medical notes when he swore in an affidavit submitted to the Supreme Court 21 days later that Sarah's chest was clear and she was in no respiratory distress. Moreover, it is considered best clinical practice to postpone risky treatments for a few days or even weeks to resolve significant complications. (Preventing Chemotherapy Toxicities And Other Issues On Drugs Used In Oncology, Dr. Robert Ignoffo, PharmD, Clinical Professor, UCSF, Zoe Ngo, PharmD &Julie Schwenka, PharmD, UCSF).

Soon after the family left the hospital, the oncology registrar reported to Dr Capewell and briefed him about his consultation with the family. The oncologist was unhappy and concerned the parents would not return the next day. He told the registrar to do whatever it would take to get them back to the hospital immediately.

For the next several hours, the registrar tried to contact Mark by phone. He tried the Ryde number, but there was only the answer machine. It was already past 9 pm when the doctor called Ruth at Gloucester. When she could not help him, he called the number at Ryde again and left a message on the machine. When Mark came home and got the message, he phoned the hospital. After several attempts, the switchboard finally put him through to the registrar after 11 pm. The doctor asked him to bring Sarah back to the hospital that night. By that time, Sarah was fast asleep and Mark told him he was scheduled to bring Sarah to the hospital in the morning in any case. The registrar told them to be at the hospital before 10 am.

The next day was 4 July. Mark battled the city traffic to the hospital and the family arrived at 9.30 am, in plenty of time for Sarah's admission to the ward. The nurse led them to a side room painted bright yellow. After the staff filled out the routine admission forms, Sarah sat on her bed wearing her favourite fleecy lilac jacket and waited for the chemotherapy. For the next two hours, a stream of doctors and nurses came in to examine Sarah, take observations and draw blood. Sarah's vital signs were normal and she sat up in bed looking alert, wondering when the chemotherapy would start.

Di leaned towards Mark. 'There wasn't this much fuss last time they did the chemo', she whispered.

When Mark's mobile phone rang, he moved into the corner to answer it. It was his Taree lawyer with the news that the department had contacted the judge for an urgent hearing that morning.

'What the blazes are they doing now?' asked Mark as he moved outside into the hallway.

'The department went to court early this morning claiming you didn't arrive at the hospital on time. They're asking for court orders to find you and take you in', said the lawyer.

'That's ridiculous', said Mark. 'We're at the hospital right now. We arrived at 9.30 this morning. They told us to be here by 10 am. We were early. Did they go to court just on that?'

The lawyer confirmed that someone in the hospital must have hit the panic button and, apart from that, there was no other issue raised. He said he would stay in touch.

Mark returned to Sarah's room to find a nurse posting a 'nil by mouth' sign above her bed.

'What's this all about?' asked Mark.

'Dr Capewell will see you later', she answered. 'Come with me, Sarah. I need to weigh you'.

Sarah went with her to the nurses' station. A minute later, a middle-aged doctor accompanied Sarah back to the room. Mark and Di had never seen this doctor before and wondered who he was.

'Guess what? I weigh 38 kg', said Sarah happily to her mother.

Di was relieved that all the home cooking had kept Sarah a healthy weight despite the ordeal of the past three weeks.

The doctor wrote Sarah's weight on to a graphed sheet of paper that contained a checklist. 'I'd like to have a look at Sarah', he said, as he removed his stethoscope from his briefcase.

Sarah unzipped her jacket and allowed the doctor to listen to her lung fields. He listened for a long time.

Di waited impatiently until he had removed the stethoscope from his ears. 'I'm worried about my daughter's chest. Could somebody please do an X-ray?' she asked the doctor anxiously.

'We will certainly do what's needed'. The doctor continued to fill out the checklist, but left unticked the box that indicated: *Anaesthetic (including risks) explained.*

With a weak smile, the doctor turned to leave the room.

Mark was bewildered. 'Which department are you from?' he asked.

'Anaesthetics. I might see you later', the doctor replied as he hurried from the room.

Di turned to Mark. 'What's going on?' she asked.

In his office, a few floors above the oncology ward where Sarah waited for chemotherapy, Dr Capewell was on the phone to the child protection department's manager at Taree. He told him he had postponed chemotherapy for a few days and instead planned an 'emergency splenectomy' on Sarah within a few hours. He now needed the department's consent. The oncologist further sought consent to administer a continuous morphine IV to Sarah, and sedation in case she did not co-operate with staff. He then asked the department's permission to give Sarah the next cycle of chemotherapy, starting only a week after her surgery. Then he planned to confine Sarah to the hospital for up to 10 weeks, away from her parents, until he'd finished the chemotherapy.

After the phone call, the manager at Taree contacted the Director General of DoCS. After being briefed, the Director General was of the view that the previous court orders were sufficient for him to consent to the emergency operation and other procedures without seeking prior consent from the court or anyone else. The matter was then passed onto a barrister at the Crown Solicitor's Office, who was serving as the department's legal representative. He was new on the case, replacing the female barrister who had previously represented DoCS in the matter. Around lunchtime, the barrister spoke with the judge informing him that an operation was planned, but providing scant details. Meanwhile, the decision to proceed with the surgery without patient or parental consent was made between Dr Capewell and the Director General. The Crown Solicitor's office did not schedule a court hearing to argue the merits of the operation, nor brief the judge, nor request the court's permission for the forced operation.

By early afternoon, the acting director of the Northern Region branch of the Department of Community Services faxed a formal letter of consent amounting to a carte blanche to Capewell's registrar.

While these major decisions were being made in the oncologist's office, Sarah sat in bed with a normal pulse and blood pressure, becoming impatient with waiting – blithely unaware she would be having 'emergency' surgery in just a short while.

Neither the parents nor their lawyers were aware of behind the scenes plans for an emergency splenectomy. Meanwhile, staff kept Sarah and her parents in the dark for the entire morning and early afternoon, even as the family sat and waited for someone to tell them what was going on.

The spleen issue confused almost everyone involved except the oncologist who wanted it out that day. The oncologist phoned a surgeon and gave him the perplexing history of Sarah's spleen, which he wanted the surgeon to come and urgently remove.

In children, the spleen is a bean shaped abdominal organ that sits in the upper left abdomen and is about the size and shape of a small kidney. It comprises a significant portion of the immune system, as well as producing red blood cells. Immunologically, it performs an essential role in infection surveillance and produces specialised anti-cancer scavenger cells capable of locating and killing active cancer cells in the body. The organ is sometimes surgically removed after traumatic rupture, an emergency condition not the case with Sarah. Splenectomy is also carried out on a non-urgent basis in individuals with certain blood disorders, which cause the spleen to significantly enlarge. Sarah did not have these conditions either.

In persons with a cancer like Sarah's, the spleen very rarely hosts a primary cancer, but may very occasionally become a site for a solid tumour metastasis (Carrington 90). When this occurs in conjunction with ovarian cancer, it is a confirmation that the disease is in stage IV. In such cases of advanced cancer with a poor prognosis, the spleen is often left alone to fulfill its remaining function (Yang 04).

Some cases of spleen enlargement are caused by a simple splenic cyst – a benign condition often simply monitored and managed non-surgically. Such a cyst can be present at the same time as an abdominal malignancy, and remain unrelated to the malignancy. One such case was reported by Yang et al., who describe a case involving a woman with ovarian cancer who also developed a splenic cyst unrelated to the malignancy. The splenic cyst had caused the patient no symptoms and had been managed non-surgically for a number of years (Yang 04).

In some cases, a surgeon will elect to remove only the cystic portion, leaving the rest of the spleen intact to perform its vital function as an organ of immune surveillance and blood cell production (Sink 82).

In a letter dated 12 June, Dr Capewell had reported to the court that Sarah's spleen had enlarged so rapidly, from either tumour or bleeding, that he had no doubt that she could suddenly die from this. Despite this, he did not operate on the enlarged spleen at that time. The following day, on 13 June, the oncologist had written another letter to the court alleging Sarah's spleen had further 'doubled in size overnight' and was now '14 cm below the rib margin'. He claimed the increase was due to 'bleeding' or some other 'tumour-associated phenomenon', which, if left untreated for longer than a day, 'may result in her death'. Yet despite his findings that the spleen was so enlarged as to be life-threatening, Capewell did not operate on it – even though Sarah had become a ward of court, and he had the power to request court orders to do so. For the next several weeks, Sarah had walked around in this purported condition without a word from the oncologist - and yet now, for reasons that remain unclear, he suddenly deemed it to be an emergency.

In medical practice, an emergency is a matter of life or death arising from an acute event, not typically a condition that has become chronic. Emergency surgery is usually performed after the patient has been resuscitated and had their vital signs stabilised. Sarah, on the other hand, was sitting up in bed with her street clothes on and showing normal vital signs – which, had the surgeon seen her, might have given him cause to wonder what the urgency is all about.

It was already afternoon by the time Dr Capewell had made all the arrangements, and only then did he venture downstairs to Sarah's room with the startling news. In front of Sarah, he told the parents that he had arranged for a surgeon to carry out an emergency operation on their daughter shortly.

'We're taking her spleen out', said Capewell. 'We have DoCS' permission and you have no rights in making these decisions'.

'What?' Mark was dumbfounded. 'Can you please tell us why you want to do this – and so suddenly?' he asked.

Di followed with several questions of her own.

The oncologist seemed irritated by the questions. 'I'm not obliged to discuss this with you. I've just told you what's going to be done and I already have the department's permission. If you persist, I'll see to it that you are escorted out of this hospital'.

The parents were shocked that someone could force an operation on their daughter without giving them a good reason or an explanation about it, and they took the doctor's warning seriously, about what would happen if they asked further questions. They knew that they had been effectively silenced.

The oncologist further informed them that he would give Sarah the first of many chemotherapy cycles a few days after surgery. This he would follow with a three-month stay in the hospital for a long course of chemotherapy. When the doctor was finished talking to the parents, he retreated to his office and stayed there while other staff handled the fallout.

After the doctor's visit, the parents retreated into the hallway outside Sarah's room to talk privately. They were stunned. Events were unfolding too quickly and they could not grasp the real reason for the sudden emergency spleen surgery. They worried about the anaesthetic when she already had a bad cough. However, the very real threat of being kicked out of the hospital left them with only one choice – even with their hands tied and silenced, they were more useful to Sarah inside the hospital than kicked out on the street or in jail for contempt.

In the hospital room, Sarah was in a blind panic after the oncologist's visit. The parents returned to comfort Sarah, but the events were geared to move even more quickly. It was 2.45 pm and the operating room was booked for emergency surgery at 3.00 pm. While the parents tried to calm Sarah down, a registrar came into the room.

'We're going to take you to the theatre', he told Sarah.

Sarah was now totally confused. She thought that meant she would be taken to a picture theatre to see a movie.

The registrar went on to explain that she would be opened up at the 'theatre' to have her spleen removed. With his finger, he traced on her tummy the long midline incision the surgeon would be cutting to access her abdominal organs in the 'theatre'. The doctor paused and looked around the room. Sarah looked as horrified as her parents. He stopped his medical lecture and beat a hasty retreat.

'What are they gonna do to me?' Sarah asked anxiously after the doctor had gone.

'They want you to have an operation', explained Mark. 'But we don't really know much about it'.

Sarah glanced from her father to her mother and then to the door. By then she knew that anyone could come through at any time and do to her what they wanted, and her parents could do nothing about it. She thought her only chance was to defend herself and she sat up in bed with her arms defiantly crossed.

The registrar returned a few minutes later with equipment to insert an intravenous cannula into Sarah's arm.

Sarah escaped to the far side of the bed. 'What are you doing?' she asked nervously.

Mark reflexively leapt from his chair to shield Sarah.

The doctor warned Mark off before turning back to Sarah. 'I have to insert this. You will need your spleen removed', he told her sternly.

'I don't want my spleen removed', she insisted.

Di turned helplessly to Mark. 'It's *her* spleen...' she pleaded.

Mark was incensed and paced the room silently.

The doctor was determined to stay in control. 'Sarah is having her spleen removed because we have permission from the Department of Community Services', he said firmly.

This did nothing to reassure Sarah or the parents; they'd been told no useful information and had no time to process the imminent surgery. By then the family took it as an additional insult to hear that a host of strangers had been informed and consulted while they were excluded from any decision-making.

Sarah, meanwhile, was incensed to hear that some strangers in an office had become her parent and now they wanted her spleen. She did not even know what a spleen was or why they wanted it, except that they would cut her open to get it. It was too much for her. She'd had no time to think about it, and she was desperate to stop them cutting her.

Without further explanations, the doctor attempted to insert an intravenous catheter, but Sarah still refused to lie down on the bed for the procedure. She put her arms up in a protective gesture. 'Get away from me', she warned the doctor. 'I don't want it and I don't want the surgery!' she shouted.

When Sarah made such an alarming fuss, the doctor beat another retreat to the safety of the nurse's desk. He phoned the anaesthetist to ask him how to subdue a kicking and screaming patient who refused surgery. The anaesthetist suggested they bring Sarah to the OR without her pre-op medication and he would use the induction mask to put her out.

Fifteen minutes later – just after 3 pm – several nursing staff arrived to change Sarah into an OR gown. She was terrified and resisted them, but they overpowered her and wrangled her into the cap and gown.

Mark found the scene unbearable and paced the floor with clenched fists.

When Sarah refused to be strapped into the wheelchair, Di lost control. 'Don't touch my daughter!' she cried out, but staff hardly heard her above the commotion and took no notice.

Shortly after the morning staff had manhandled Sarah into the wheelchair for the trip to the OR, the afternoon staff took over so the morning staff could go off duty. Among them was an experienced British nurse who had been allocated to Sarah that afternoon. She walked into the chaotic scene and expertly took control. She saw Sarah's terror and spoke to her in soothing tones, offering explanations about what was going on. Though her efforts came far too late, she was effective enough to calm Sarah down for the trip to OR.

The British nurse and the registrar wheeled Sarah down the corridor, and into the lift to the OR floor. The parents squeezed in next to their terrified daughter, who was restrained in the wheelchair. A few moments later, the elevator doors opened into a brightly lit OR corridor where swinging doors led into a row of pre-op cubicles.

Di was still dazed and stayed outside in the hallway while Mark followed into the anaesthetic bay. The nurse aligned the wheelchair with the anaesthetic bed but Sarah refused to get out of the wheelchair and onto the bed. She was unprepared for an operation she knew nothing about and had only known about for a short while, and she protested loudly. The anaesthetist heard the commotion and poked his head around the corner. He had never seen an 'emergency' patient turn up to OR kicking and protesting before. What kind of emergency was this when earlier he had taken Sarah's vital signs and they were normal? He suggested they bring Sarah into the OR, and with Mark in tow, the nurse wheeled her directly adjacent to the OR table. Sarah gazed at the overhead light, the coils of tubing and blinking machinery, and clung even tighter onto the wheelchair's armrests.

The British nurse urged Sarah to transfer onto the OR table. 'Come on Sarah, you have to do this', she said gently.

The anaesthetist in his scrubs clutched an anaesthetic mask and waited patiently.

Sarah looked to her father for help.

Mark mustered his most calming voice. 'You'll be all right. Your Mum and I will see you when you wake up'.

Sarah then allowed the anaesthetist and an OR nurse to guide her on to the table. Once there, she panicked again when she recognised a female resident doctor who was part of the group that had misdiagnosed her as being pregnant at the district hospital. The resident was rotating around the hospital system, and was presently completing her anaesthetic rotation in Sydney. She had then attempted to take Sarah's blood over four times unsuccessfully and when she came towards her again with a needle, Sarah refused to have the doctor near her. Mark apologised to the resident, reassuring her that it was 'nothing personal'. Finally, the anaesthetist intervened and waved the resident away. He had decided to dispense with the needles and intended to use the nitrous oxide induction by mask, allowing the resident to insert the IV cannula only after Sarah was under the anaesthetic.

Sarah looked vulnerable and scared lying on the hard and narrow OR table. Mark held his daughter's hand while she had a coughing spasm. The anaesthetist looked briefly concerned and waited until she had stopped. He had laid the mask near Sarah's face. She could hear it softly hissing, but was unable to see it. Now he showed the mask to Sarah and asked her to 'just breathe normally' as he slowly inched it towards her. At first, Sarah resisted the plastic mask near her face but gradually she allowed the anaesthetist to fit it around her nose and mouth in a tight seal. Her eyelids flickered slightly before she succumbed to the overpowering sleep of the anaesthetic gas.

Di paced the corridor outside the OR suites like someone caged.

The registrar, who had been in Sarah's room earlier, spotted her. 'I know you do not agree with this operation', he told her. 'But I think it is in Sarah's best interests and we are doing this with the consent of the Department of Community Services'.

Di searched the young doctor's face for any sign of compassion, but found only an intellectual frame of mind. It was not that she agreed or disagreed with the operation – the problem was that no one had told them about it, and her daughter was terrified out of her wits. In addition, she was worried that her daughter's chest infection would affect her ability to withstand the surgery, and no one had taken her concerns about it seriously. She also had a problem with the way her daughter had been manhandled into an OR kicking and screaming, to be opened up against her will and without a good reason or explanation. And finally, she had a serious problem with being prevented from asking questions on threat of being removed from the hospital. 'Where do you people learn your bedside manner?' asked Di.

The doctor walked away, not realising his comment had been far from helpful, and had in fact been taken as a further insult to the parents.

A few minutes later Mark returned from the OR looking ashen. 'They just ambushed Sarah', he said. 'What kind of medical treatment has to be done at gunpoint?'

Di agreed. 'Before her first operation, Dr Gilbert explained everything to us. He got our permission and even Sarah agreed to it'.

Mark shook his head. 'I don't know what this sudden surgery is all about. They've known about the spleen for over a month and they let her run around with it. Her real trouble started with those chemo side effects'. Mark rubbed his face in despair. 'In that American hospital she would have had the treatment without the side effects and I can't imagine any civilised place in the world where they'd drag a person into surgery against their will without telling them what was going on. If only they wouldn't have stopped us every time we tried to take her overseas'.

Moments later the British nurse emerged from the OR's swinging doors. She caught up with the parents and took them aside. 'What's going on?' she asked gently. 'Something here doesn't seem right'.

'That's what we'd like to know', answered Mark, before relaying a short version of their story, including the fact that someone in the child protection department had authorised the forced surgery without consulting them or Sarah.

She shook her head. 'Oh my God, that's terrible', she muttered. 'I am so sorry'.

Sarah went under gas anaesthesia at 3.30 pm, still terrified. It was her under-standing that some strangers at the Department of Community Services wanted her spleen and it disturbed her as nothing ever had before. In this, she was not alone. In time, the unusual situation came to disturb even some of the most emotionally detached professionals.

Before Sarah had arrived in the OR, the anaesthetist reviewed his notes. His job was to put patients to sleep during surgery, not to question why it was being done. Nevertheless, this seemed an unusual case of emergency surgery on a child with ovarian cancer with spleen involvement. That meant she had to be stage IV, but why the emergency? Metastases, if they are removed at all at that late stage, usually involve elective surgery, done at a convenient time.

The anaesthetist fished around the pre-operative paperwork. On the OR sheet was written a splenectomy code 30599 that applies only to patients who need surgery to remove a spleen that weighs over 1.5 kg. Since a normal child's spleen weighs only 50–80 g, roughly half the size of an adult kidney, the operation code 30599 indicated that whoever booked in the surgery was anticipating Sarah would have a massively enlarged spleen of up to 18 times its normal weight. Such chronically massive spleens sometimes occur in children with various types of leukaemia. They are surgically removed when they cause too many symptoms to be conservatively managed (Hickman 92). However, Sarah did not have the kind of condition that enlarged the spleen to that size.

On the other hand, a ruptured spleen after trauma is undoubtedly an emer-gency, but this girl had no history of trauma, and kids with a ruptured spleen are usually barely alive and not kicking like a mule.

This emergency operation also came with significant risk of post-op com-plications. On pre-anaesthetic examination, the girl had a moist cough and a partial collapse of her left lung base, and for the next several hours, those lungs would be exposed to a mixture of anaesthetic gasses and oxygen. The chemo she'd had previously prevented her from having therapeutic levels of oxygen, as this would place her lungs at risk of further damage or even lung fibrosis. This could become a problem during surgery if her blood oxygen levels dropped or if she needed resuscitation. In addition, she was already anaemic from the chemo and further blood loss would make it worse, especially during a blood-drenched operation like a splenectomy; and on top of this, her kidney function was impaired. Overall, the girl was not an ideal candidate for surgery at that particular time. He assumed that there were factors he was not aware of and that the oncologist had a good reason to want the operation. However, there was a chance things could get tricky and just in case, the anaesthetist called in another anaesthetic colleague to assist him. He also ordered several packs of cross-matched type O-positive blood from the blood bank and kept it close at hand.

Now that Sarah was lightly anaesthetized on the table, the anaesthetist waited for the female resident to finish inserting the IV catheter into Sarah's forearm, before he passed an endotracheal breathing tube through Sarah's trachea and connected her to a respirator. With the IV now running, he deepened the anaesthetic and injected a paralysing drug through the IV tubing. The drug did two things: it stopped the patient's breathing, allowing the ventilator to take over, and it relaxed the abdominal muscles to make it easier for the surgeon. Meanwhile, during surgery, both anaesthetists would monitor vital functions and blood loss carefully.

It was 3.41 pm. The patient was now deeply unconscious. The two anaesthetists sat at the head of the table while two gowned and gloved assistant surgeons spread sterile drapes over Sarah's abdomen. The remaining OR staff waited for the surgeon to arrive.

The paediatric surgeon, Dr Andrew Godfrey jogged to the scrub sink and adjusted the water temperature with his elbows. He was young and fit, but still out of breath from sprinting through the doctors' car park. The oncologist, Dr Capewell, had called him only a few hours ago and he rushed to finish surgery on another child in order to arrive on time to do the emergency splenectomy. The oncologist had given him a short briefing about the case: the patient was a ward of court and he was told to expect to remove a massive spleen from her. While he had the abdomen open, he was also to remove any obvious metastases from the ovarian cancer. The hospital's surgical registrar had taken care of the pre-operative details on Capewell's direct orders. There was no time to meet with the parents pre-operatively, and he was told everything had been taken care of.

A few minutes previously, Godfrey had heard the commotion in the anaesthetic bay and wondered what was going on. Emergency patients did not usually make noise in the OR; they were too acutely ill to raise even a mild objection. As he scrubbed, he wondered whether he should phone Capewell, but he dismissed the idea. The patient was already asleep on the table and he needed to focus on the operation now. He would find out shortly what the trouble was with the spleen.

Godfrey pushed the plastic swinging doors to the OR open with his shoulder while carefully keeping his hands upright to prevent water dripping back down his arms. With sterile tongs, the circulating nurse handed him a sterile towel to wipe his hands, before helping him on with his gown and gloves. Godfrey approached the table and greeted the anaesthetists and assistant surgeons.

Within seconds, the surgeon had made a clean midline incision down Sarah's abdomen from the tip of her sternum to the pubic bone. His assistants tied off the bleeders and retracted both wound edges for good visual access.

In a few minutes, Godfrey had exposed the spleen in the left upper quadrant of the abdomen, and was surprised to see a spleen much smaller than he had been led to expect. It was roughly only 9 cm in length, and was of a normal size and appearance on its anterior surface, with no sign of rupture or gross haemorrhage. However, on its back surface protruded what looked like a simple splenic cyst; the kind often best left alone instead of removed.

The surgeon paused for a moment. He now had to make a difficult call. He could leave the spleen alone and close her back up, or he could simply remove the cyst, or remove the spleen entirely. The last option was what the oncologist clearly expected.

Moments later, the surgeon told the anaesthetist that he might try a partial splenectomy, and if that wasn't possible, he would carry out a full removal.

The anaesthetist prepared for the considerable blood loss that always occurs during either of these procedures. He opened the IV full bore and asked the circulating nurse to bring him the first of several units of packed blood cells that he had ordered from the blood bank.

The IV packed cells (concentrated red blood cells) ran through at breakneck speed while Godfrey dissected the spleen carefully off the diaphragm and separated it from the surrounding ligaments and tissues. When the cyst came into view, he attempted to excise the bubble-like structure from the splenic tissue in order to spare the spleen and leave most of it intact. Unfortunately, he encountered sudden heavy bleeding from the incision into the blood rich organ. Unavoidably, this also ruptured the cyst, spilling its fluid contents into the abdominal cavity. In cancer patients, any spillage containing malignant cells is known to hasten the spread of cancer. For that reason surgeons are usually circumspect about operating on advanced cancer patients with metastases. The heavily bleeding splenic incision meant that the entire spleen would have to be removed to stem the blood-loss. This meant further bleeding from the splenic vessels when the organ was finally separated from its large vessels.

During the course of the operation, Sarah would lose a litre and a half of blood as a direct result of the procedure. This amounted to half her entire blood volume.

By 4.50 pm, Dr Godfrey was intensely focused on stemming the devastating blood-loss from the spleen.

At precisely the same time, the barrister representing DoCS was composing a letter to the judge of the Supreme Court. He was concerned about a number of issues surrounding the matter. In his letter, the barrister reiterated that the oncologist had earlier that day claimed that Sarah was in 'urgent need of an operation to remove her spleen', and that 'it was understood that Sarah's parents were at the hospital and were not objecting to the procedure (but that information was somewhat uncertain), that there was a possibility that Sarah might not survive the operation, and that the operation was expected to occur this afternoon'.

In fact, of course, the parents had not consented. The barrister was sufficiently concerned about the uncertainty surrounding the parents' purported consent that he attempted to establish the chain of consent and authority. He wrote: '...the Director General [of DoCS] took the view that the orders previously made by the Court were sufficient to allow the Director General to consent to the procedure...'

The barrister confirmed that the Director General himself had given sole permission for the potentially fatal procedure, without seeking permission from the judge, the parents, the child or, as far as anyone was aware, the child's legal representative.

Close to 5 pm, while dictating his letter, and while Sarah was on the OR table haemorrhaging, the Crown (DoCS) barrister hastily instructed Sarah's legal representative to re-contact Dr Capewell to establish whether or not the parents had in fact consented to the operation. When the legal representative contacted the oncologist, he apparently claimed, again, that the parents had consented to the operation. He did not mention that he had offered the parents no opportunity to give a written or a verbal informed consent to the surgery, and that he had warned them to refrain from any comments about the forced operation or he would have them removed from the hospital.

After speaking with the oncologist, the legal representative reported back the doctor's comments to the DoCS barrister, who included this information in his letter to the Judge:

> I advised that I would have an attempt made to confirm that the
> parents of Sarah had not raised an objection to the operation. I am
> now instructed (at approximately 4.50 pm) that [the child's] Legal

Representative, a solicitor employed by the Crown Solicitor, has spoken with Dr Capewell, who has advised her that he discussed the operation with the parents, that the parents had not objected, and that Sarah's father had expressed mild encouragement that the operation should proceed. I am further instructed that as at about 4.50 pm Sarah is in theatre and the operation is about to begin.

In fact, the operation had already begun an hour and 20 minutes earlier, and Sarah was now losing large amounts of blood. The judge was led to believe the parents had consented and that there was still time for him to intervene, had he wished to do so. He had no idea that the surgery had already progressed to a critical stage.

For the next hour, the surgeon focused intensely on tying off the splenic vessels and dissecting the spleen from its surrounding structures. This done, he lifted the spleen out of the abdomen along with the left adrenal gland, which had adhered to the cystic surface. Then he mopped up the abdominal cavity before he could closely inspect the remaining organs for the spread of cancer. He soon found several clumps of suspicious tissue around the intestinal vessels, which he carefully excised and sent to histopathology along with the spleen. Finally, he excised tissue from the liver and sent it to pathology. For reasons that are unclear, he left a large tumour metastasis in the groin intact and did not attempt to remove it.

After four hours, Dr Godfrey finished the surgery and left his assistants to close the wound. The surgeon disposed of his bloodied gloves and gown and retreated into a side room adjacent to the OR to fill out the routine post-operative paperwork. In it, he noted an average spleen with a simple splenic cyst attached to its rear surface. The rest would be revealed by pathology. It could hardly have been classed as an emergency. Even without the background story, he was beginning to wonder what was going on.

Just after 7 pm, OR staff lifted Sarah off the table and wheeled her to recovery. There, she required more blood and IV fluids to replace the blood loss from the splenectomy. She was cold to touch. With her abdomen open for hours, her core temperature had plummeted, sending her into hypothermia.

Sarah woke up moaning. Her first moment of consciousness was pierced by intense pain and shivering from shock and hypothermia. Recovery staff warmed her with heated blankets and gave her a substantial dose of morphine, which sent her to sleep. Sarah's long, vertical incision from her breastbone to her lower abdomen was held closed with subcuticular sutures – the sort that are not visible on the outside. The problems simmering in her chest would soon test those sutures, and Sarah's endurance, to the limit.

Several floors down from the OR, recovery and ICU suites, Mark and Di paced the floor, anxious to hear any news at all. Mark stared out of Sarah's hospital room window to the city traffic down below, while Di tried unsuccessfully to concentrate on needlework. The British nurse dropped in occasionally with reassurances and hot cups of tea.

Dr Godfrey came in to see the parents at 7.30 pm, still in his scrubs. He did not know what to expect of them, but was pleasantly surprised to find them obviously decent people who were very concerned about their daughter.

Likewise, the parents had not met the surgeon before and were immediately struck by his kind eyes and reasonable manner.

Godfrey shook Mark's hand warmly.

'How is Sarah?' asked both parents at once.

The surgeon seemed slightly bewildered. 'She came through the surgery and is stable in recovery at the moment. I'm not sure what you were told before the surgery – '

'Nothing' said Mark. 'We had no say in it'.

Di nodded. 'They just dragged her into the surgery. It was terrible'.

The surgeon looked down to the floor. 'I see', he said. He was starting to feel uncomfortable about this case.

'Was this surgery really an emergency?' asked Mark.

Godfrey looked uneasy and searched for the right words. 'Well, not your average one', he answered. 'The spleen had a cyst on it and I've removed the spleen and the cyst. Elsewhere around the intestines, I removed some tissue and sent it off to biopsy'.

'What happens now?' asked Mark.

'Do you mean after she recovers from the surgery?'

Mark nodded.

Godfrey looked at them both sympathetically. 'As far as I'm concerned, you can take your daughter home and give her a happy life'.

'Believe me', said Mark. 'That's exactly what we're desperate to do – along with finding another oncologist, a better treatment, and a different hospital. No offence to you or anything', he added.

The surgeon nodded as though he understood, before looking away awkwardly. 'Yes', he said, 'but I'm afraid you've got the oncologists to contend with'.

Mark gave the surgeon a knowing look before becoming thoughtful again.

'Doctor, you might think this is an unusual request', said Mark, 'but my wife and I have reason to be sceptical about this whole emergency spleen business. We were railroaded and told nothing this morning, but over the past weeks, we heard a lot of conflicting things about the spleen. We were wondering if we could possibly see the spleen for ourselves'.

The surgeon thought for a moment. 'I've never been asked that before', he said. 'The spleen is in pathology right now, but perhaps when it is finished there, you can have a look'.

Mark told the doctor he would ask again then.

Godfrey shook Mark's hand warmly and said goodbye to Di before leaving the room.

Three hours later, two recovery nurses wheeled Sarah back to her room. It was already late at night. The British nurse had gone off duty, replaced by the night staff.

Mark and Di were relieved to see Sarah again, even with tubes projecting from her. She had an intravenous drip flowing into one arm and a morphine infusion into the other. A gastric tube protruded from her nose, which drained blood-stained fluid into a plastic bag suspended from her bed. Di leant down to kiss Sarah's forehead and was shocked to find her cold to touch.

For a while, Sarah slept off the anaesthetic in relative comfort. Her temperature rose from the level of hypothermia and reached the normal range before continuing to climb into a raging fever. The nurses removed layers of blankets until Sarah had only a sheet left as cover.

In the rush before the emergency surgery, no one had thought to insert an indwelling catheter. Now staff woke Sarah frequently, urging her to use the bedpan and expecting to see a result from the several litres of IV fluids she had received. Each time they woke her, Sarah had a coughing fit and was in agonising pain from straining the sutures holding together a significantly large wound. The staff pushed Sarah's patient-controlled pain pump for her, but even then, Sarah needed more. This cycle was repeated into the early hours of the morning: being woken, the coughing fit, unsuccessful attempts on the bedpan, agony unrelieved by painkillers. It was torturous for Sarah to stretch, bend and sit after she had been run in half by a scalpel. For reasons unknown, staff did not insert an indwelling catheter after the surgery either, although it would have saved her from much of this pain.

Around 1 am, Mark decided to return to Ryde and try for some rest. After the truly horrendous day, Mark felt guilty for leaving Di alone, but he had a feeling the department would soon put on more court action and he had to call his lawyer in the morning before returning to the hospital.

Di was having the worst day of her life, but she urged Mark to go and assured him that she would sit up with Sarah all night.

Mark left the hospital and walked a few blocks to where he had parked his mother's car. Since the last episode with the over-interested car-park security guard, he had parked off the hospital grounds. The city was deserted apart from a few homeless people camped in the city park.

While walking in the dark, Mark had a bad feeling in his bones. Sarah looked deathly white. It was on the cards she could die. He wondered what was going on; that spleen business was not even an emergency. The surgeon had said it was a simple splenic cyst. It could have waited until she was in better shape, instead of risking her life with a tricky operation when she wasn't fit. Did somebody want her spleen? Would it end up in some tumour bank?

Events were converging from all directions and Mark wasn't sure if he could make a plan to cover all the bases. Right now, he had the feeling someone was playing with Sarah's life and that her future hung in the balance. These people had a lot of power and didn't mind using it. And what could he do about it? It was too late to avoid the trouble; they were too far into the system now. Although he wouldn't sweat the small stuff, Sarah's life was at stake and, despite the risk of being in contempt of court, he figured he had to stand up to the big issues.

Mark finally arrived at the deserted city parking station where Ruth's car stood alone. It was 1.30 am. He was dead tired and hoped to be in bed at Ryde in half an hour.

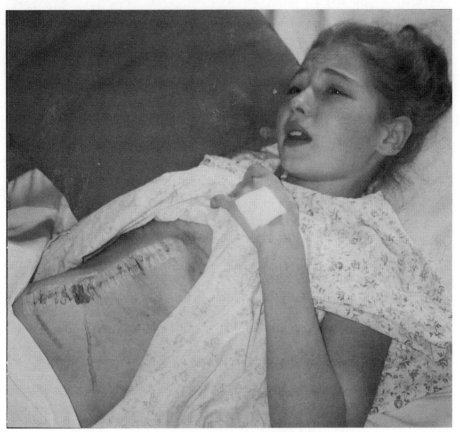

Sarah after forced surgery

BRUTE FORCE

Brute force – rough; uncivilized; unfeeling. The application of Predominantly physical effort to achieve a goal that Could be accomplished with less effort if more Carefully considered.

Webster's Dictionary, 1913

In Sarah's hospital room, Di kept a night vigil. It was just on 1.30 am, and Sarah was in a bad way. Di rigged pillows up to keep Sarah upright. Sitting up pulled on Sarah's sutures, but it was the only position that allowed her to breathe. She seemed air-hungry on room air, but was not allowed extra oxygen after the chemotherapy drugs she'd been given three weeks previously.

The nurses came in regularly to administer another bolus of morphine. When Sarah had reached her prescribed limit, she was still in agony. The coughing fits came regularly until Sarah was in a pain crisis. She begged her mother for help, but Di could only rearrange her pillows again and wipe her face with a moist washcloth. Soon Di noticed that Sarah had become a strange colour: pale and blue, like skim milk. Sarah was agitated and gasping for air. She reached out for her mother, wanting help to sit ever more upright. Di supported Sarah with her right arm while searching for the nurses' call button on the console behind the bed. Fortunately, she found the correct one and thumped it several times, before staring anxiously at the door. Di had raised the alarm just in time. Suddenly the pulse Oximeter alarm rang out from the machine sitting on Sarah's night table. The high-pitched sound unnerved Di, but she stayed with Sarah; by then she needed both arms to hold her upright to breathe. Di silently prayed for someone to come soon. If not, she planned to run from the room and shout down the hallway for help.

After an almost endless minute, the night nurse arrived and immediately noticed Sarah was in acute respiratory distress. She reached into the bin above the bed and uncoiled a set of oxygen nasal prongs. She attached one end to the wall outlet and lodged the prongs underneath Sarah's nose. The device was set to deliver only two litres of oxygen per minute, because of the oxygen restriction the chemotherapy drugs had imposed. After the nurse secured the nasal prongs, she reset the Oximeter to stop its alarm and sprinted from the room to call the night surgical registrar.

While the nurse was away getting help, Di felt alone and terrified again. She watched the red glowing numbers of the pulse Oximeter shoot up to 150 beats per minute as it registered Sarah's heartbeat. Meanwhile, the other numbers showed the oxygen saturation plummeting despite the nasal prongs. When the oxygen levels dropped to 75 per cent, from a normal range of 98–100 per cent, the monitor's alarm screamed again. Di looked from the machine to her daughter. Sarah was flaccid and slumped back on her pillow. Di raced out to the hallway and screamed for help.

Two nurses and the night registrar were already rounding the corner. The doctor listened to Sarah's chest and found no air entry on the left side. He immediately replaced the nasal prongs with an oxygen mask that delivered a higher percentage of oxygen. Normally people needing resuscitation receive 60–100 per cent oxygen, but 30 per cent was the maximum the doctor was prepared to give Sarah after the chemo she'd had, and then only for a few minutes. A quick check of Sarah's low blood pressure made him wonder whether she had burst an internal suture and started bleeding. It would be catastrophic if one of the ligatures the surgeon used to tie off the splenic vessels had blown off.

However, with the oxygen, Sarah came around and started a violent coughing fit. The doctor wondered briefly whether he should give her morphine to stop the coughing and pain or whether it would depress her breathing. Sarah made the decision herself, and between coughing fits, she begged for pain relief.

The doctor instructed the nurse to order an emergency X-ray. He then suggested they move Sarah closer to the nurses' station and monitor her carefully. If she deteriorated further, he would shift her up to ICU himself.

Just after 2 am, the X-ray technician wheeled in the cumbersome portable machine and X-rayed Sarah in bed; he had broken several speed limits getting to the hospital. A half hour later, he rushed the films up to the ward where the registrar waited. Sarah's left lung had been on the verge of collapse before the surgery, but now the left lung base was entirely collapsed and both lungs were compacted with full-blown pneumonia.

After speaking in whispers with the surgical registrar, the night nurse pulled Di aside into the hallway and advised her to summon Mark to the hospital immediately.

At 2.40 am, the phone rang at the house in Ryde. Mark had still been in the state halfway between sleeping and waking when the shrill sound jolted him fully awake again. He instinctively knew it was for him and hurried to answer the phone before it woke up the sleeping couple in the next room. He left Ryde at 3 am and sped through the deserted city, not knowing what he would find at the hospital.

At 3.30 am, Mark arrived to find Sarah struggling for each breath. She had a tag on her IV that indicated it contained antibiotics. He noticed something was different about Sarah. He had never seen such a look of resignation and despair in her eyes, as though she was ready to give up the struggle. Next to Sarah sat Di, looking sick herself but willing Sarah through each coughing spasm.

Sarah had been coughing non-stop since emerging from the anaesthetic and was too weak to shift the consolidated mass of infection sitting in her collapsed lungs. For the rest of the night both parents willed their daughter to live through each agonising spasm. It was a shocking experience for them; apart from childbirth, neither parent had ever seen anyone in so much pain before.

By sunrise the next morning, Sarah was able to cough up small amounts of sputum, which slightly improved her oxygen saturation. By then, the three were beyond exhaustion. Di collapsed into a chair. Her leg ached again and she was unable to stand on it. 'If only they'd X-rayed her before the op. Maybe they would have waited', she repeated like a mantra.

At 7 am, a team of physiotherapists arrived and inspected Sarah's chest X-rays before coming into the room. They were shocked at the sight of Sarah in agony and were afraid to impose more pain on her. Instead, they taught the parents how to carry out the physio on Sarah to unclog her lungs. Mark and Di took over the treatments for the rest of the day. They turned Sarah onto her right side, allowing her to cough up small mucous plugs from her left lung. The strain sapped everyone's strength, but in Sarah's case, her gastric tube still free-drained bloodstained fluid, making it impossible for her to eat.

When the chief pathologist came on duty that morning, he had a spleen and a large amount of tissue to examine from an 11-year-old girl with ovarian cancer. The pathologist weighed Sarah's spleen carefully before he sectioned it and checked it for cancer. A normal healthy adult spleen weighs 75–150 g, and a child's weighs slightly less. This spleen had a cyst attached, and the spleen with the cyst together weighed 81g – a normal average weight for a spleen. There appeared to be no significant spleen enlargement, and no evidence of gross haemorrhage that had occurred prior to the operation. The only evidence of bleeding that could be seen by the naked eye was on the spleen near the cyst, where a section was cut by the scalpel during the operation. Elsewhere, the spleen had a normal appearance. Predictably, however, the cyst was lined with malignant cells and tumour deposits of embryonal carcinoma. The liver biopsy also revealed malignant embryonal carcinoma cells.

Based on the pathology report it seemed reasonable to assume that the other abdominal organs could also be lined with malignant cells – even more likely after the cyst had unavoidably ruptured inside the abdomen while the surgeon prised it away from the surrounding structures.

After the pathologist had finished examining the spleen, he turned his attention to the several metastatic tissue specimens included in the tissue lot. Two were solid tumours consisting of high-grade yolk sac tumour and embryonal carcinoma. The cancer cells were still actively dividing despite the fact that Sarah had been recently treated with maximum-tolerated IV chemotherapy. It meant the response to the chemo was far from optimal.

With her normal-weight spleen now sitting in formalin, Sarah was missing a large part of her immune system and her main blood-making organ, while the cancer cells from the burst cyst were spread widely throughout her abdomen and seemingly not vulnerable to the chemotherapy she was prescribed.

By late afternoon, Di fell asleep in the armchair next to Sarah's bed and Mark went down the road to get her something to eat. On the way to the deli, his mobile phone rang. It was his lawyer phoning to let him know the department had scheduled a court hearing the following week. Mark was furious that the department was hounding them with endless litigation at a time like this, but realised he would have to prepare for it. The lawyer confirmed that the oncologist would start chemo on Sarah in a few days. Mark was horrified. He didn't want Sarah to have another round of the potentially lethal chemo just a few days after surgery when it wasn't certain if she would survive the complications – her collapsed lung and pneumonia.

When he returned, Mark saw how pale Di looked. Her leg was inflamed and swollen and she was running a fever. She desperately needed a break and some medical attention. He urged her to come with him to Ryde for the night, but Di refused to leave Sarah's side.

After reluctantly saying his goodbyes, Mark made a mental note to phone Ruth as soon as he arrived back in Ryde to ask her if she would travel down to

Sydney. He knew he was asking a lot. It meant she would have to farm out the rest of their children to other relatives, and leave his father alone to run the farm. But he saw no other choice. They were in a crisis. He would be back in court soon and Di's health wouldn't hold out much longer. And there was no telling what would happen to Sarah.

Like a one-woman army, Ruth alighted from the Country Link train that arrived at the Central railway station from Gloucester. After a cab ride to the hospital, she was a little afraid of what she would find there. She'd had to send some of Sarah's siblings to stay with Di's sister and the rest to stay with their other aunts and uncles. None of them knew what was going on with their sister; just that she was in a bad way. Before Ruth left Gloucester, the kids told her how sad they were, how they felt like their family was splitting up. They were confused and scared about it. No one could explain much to them, since things changed each day and the doctors kept the information to themselves. In the chaos, the children's school grades were suffering too. Laura had been doing her best to keep everyone together, but now the kids were scattered around the extended family. For all anyone knew the situation might be long term, and without information, the adults couldn't reassure the kids with any degree of confidence.

Ruth arrived at the hospital in Sydney to find Di slumped in a chair with her leg on a stool. Sarah, on the other hand, was in bed coughing and holding her stomach. Ruth kissed Sarah but she barely opened her eyes. She had never seen her granddaughter so lifeless or so thin – she hardly even raised a bump under the sheets.

Di anticipated what Ruth was thinking. 'I know. She's lost a lot of weight since the op', said Di.

'What does the oncologist say about it?' asked Ruth.

'He's gone on leave for a week. We haven't seen him since the surgery. And the doctors under him don't say much'.

'What about the doctor who did the op?'

Di smiled at the thought of Dr Godfrey. 'He's been very nice. He's the only one who seems to care'.

Ruth shook her head in dismay. 'And what does *he* say?'

'Every time he comes in here he looks sad and almost embarrassed. He's very kind to Sarah', answered Di.

Ruth shook her head and looked at Di's swollen leg. The nights sitting in chairs had finally taken their toll. 'I'm going to put you in a cab to Ryde. You need to see a doctor. Or maybe Mark can fetch you. Is he here?'

For once, Di put up no resistance. She was in obvious pain. 'Mark was in earlier today', she said. 'But he won't be back until tomorrow'.

After Di had said her goodbyes to Sarah, the two women stood in the hallway together.

'What was that emergency spleen business all about?' asked Ruth in a whisper.

Di steadied herself against the wall. 'We're very sceptical about it', she said. 'In the last month Dr Capewell told us a lot of different things. First he said Sarah's spleen was 10 times its normal size, and then he said it went down again to three times its normal size. Nobody could tell us how a spleen could go up and down like a yo-yo from one week to the next. Mark thinks he told the judge what was necessary to get the orders he wanted. Then, right out of the blue, the spleen had to come out straightaway. That's when they dragged her into surgery, against her will, screaming'. Di fought back tears before composing herself again. 'But Dr Godfrey told us her spleen only had a simple cyst on it and he didn't make a big deal about it at all'.

'Did Mark talk to anybody about it?' asked Ruth.

'He asked the surgeon if he could see the spleen for himself', replied Di.

Ruth nodded. 'Now, that sounds like Mark. When he doesn't believe something he's told, he wants to see it for himself. What did the surgeon say?'

'Dr Godfrey was good about it', answered Di. 'I think he could tell we weren't buying the oncologist's story. He told Mark, that as far as he was concerned, we could see the spleen when it came back from pathology. Mark asked his lawyer to request permission for us to have a look at the spleen for ourselves'.

Ruth reached out to comfort Di. The small, kind gesture broke Di's last reserve and she started weeping. 'Honestly, I know how desperate all this must sound', she sobbed.

Ruth found a tissue in her skirt pocket and handed it to Di. 'It's all right', she said softly. 'These are desperate times and you've been put into a desperate situation. Don't worry, now. I'll look after Sarah while you get that leg seen to'.

After Di left for Ryde, Ruth was determined to protect Sarah like a watchdog. Later that afternoon a nurse delivered a well-dressed visitor into Sarah's room, before quickly disappearing again. The woman introduced herself as Sarah's legal representative sent by the Crown Solicitor's office. She had come to speak with Mark and Di about the issue of consent. Clearly, that issue was still bothersome. Ruth introduced herself as Sarah's grandmother and told her that neither parent was at the hospital. On hearing this, the woman insisted on talking to Sarah alone; she said she had to find out Sarah's wishes before the next court hearing.

Ruth surveyed Sarah, who lay desperately ill in bed. 'I'm sorry', Ruth said, 'but Sarah is too sick for visitors right now and she is still on heavy painkillers'.

The woman inhaled deeply and stood more upright. 'I am the patient's legal representative. The Crown Solicitor's Office sent me and I am going to insist on seeing Sarah alone', she said firmly.

'She's still not well enough', insisted Ruth.

The woman faced Ruth off with a look that threatened unpleasant official consequences.

After an uncomfortable minute, Ruth looked at her watch. 'I'll give you five minutes', she said.

The woman waited until Ruth left the room and closed the door. From the hallway, Ruth peered through the window and saw her questioning Sarah and writing down notes.

Inside the room, the legal representative asked Sarah why she hadn't wanted the operation or the chemo.

'Because it makes me sick', answered Sarah before having another coughing fit. When it was over, she was in pain and clutched her stomach.

The solicitor reminded Sarah of her legal situation. 'It's been ordered by the court and that means you must have it', she warned.

'I have a right to say what I want', insisted Sarah in a weak voice.

'You're under age', replied the solicitor, 'and you don't get your say'.

Sarah turned away to look at the wall.

After exactly five minutes, the woman left the room. She gave Ruth a slight smile as she passed her in the hallway.

While Di was away, Dr Godfrey dropped in frequently to see Sarah and check on her condition. He always came alone and never with the other doctors on ward rounds. He had a way with children and Sarah trusted him. Of all the professional visitors, he was the one she occasionally smiled at. After his visit, Sarah often remarked to Ruth that he had 'kind eyes'. Godfrey, on the other hand, always looked concerned when he saw how sick Sarah was after the surgery and how slowly she was recovering. When the oncology team arrived, Godfrey usually left the room.

With Capewell on leave, the surgical and oncology registrars came in smaller groups, without the dozen or so others that usually accompanied the oncologist. Ruth told the doctors that Sarah was terribly weak and dizzy and suffered a bad case of diarrhoea from the strong antibiotics. She asked permission to give Sarah the pro-biotics prescribed by the clinic, but the doctors would not allow it without Dr Capewell's permission. Ruth wondered why such a simple remedy, available at supermarkets, would require a specialist's consultation.

Before Capewell left on his holiday, he had been concerned about Sarah and arranged for a paediatric psychiatrist to visit and discuss with her why she had been so 'uncooperative' just before the surgery. The psychiatrist visited Sarah twice and tried to engage her in a lengthy discussion while she was on a continuous morphine drip and too ill to respond. When Capewell returned, the psychiatrist reported that Sarah had been 'uncommunicative'.

During Sarah's post-operative week, Mark came to visit regularly. He assisted with Sarah's walks down the hallway and tempted her with special treats from the deli around the corner from the hospital. He told Sarah and Ruth that Di had been to the doctor, who had diagnosed cellulitis in her leg; she was prescribed antibiotics and bed rest. It had been coming on for months and since she'd had no time to have it treated for so long it had become severe, and would lay her up for a few days before she could return.

When Mark wasn't there, Ruth took Sarah for walks. The nurses were keen to get her out of bed and instructed Ruth to wheel the IV behind her. One afternoon, Sarah was inching down the hallway with Ruth when she had to stop to lean on the wall. Dr Godfrey had come to visit and watched from the nurses' station as Sarah struggled to stay on her feet. He noticed that during the post-operative week, Sarah had become visibly emaciated and had lost most of her hair.

He walked down the hall to greet her. 'Hi Sarah', he said crouching down on his haunches.

She looked at him listlessly.

'Are you alright?' he asked softly.

Sarah looked into his eyes and saw only kindness. It gave her the strength to shuffle back to bed.

Andrew Godfrey returned to the nurses' desk to review Sarah's charts. After that day, he seemed to be off the case and the family did not see him again.

When Di returned after a couple of days, she was shocked to see her daughter looking even frailer. Sarah had managed to hold on to her hair for weeks after the chemo, but now the surgery had caused it to fall out in clumps. Sarah was now almost bald with an unhealthy yellow complexion. Di had never seen her as sad as this. She kissed Sarah and got only a weak smile in return. Ruth had just fed Sarah some ice cream and jelly from the lunch tray and, despite having eaten; Sarah was stick thin under the sheets. Di pulled up Sarah's nightie and noticed her daughter's bones protruding sharply. Ruth and Di were both alarmed.

'Hasn't she been eating anything?' asked Di.

Ruth explained that Sarah had been eating a soft diet, but she was otherwise unwell with severe watery diarrhoea. She told Di she had raised her concerns with the doctors, but they were all waiting for the oncologist to return before making even the smallest decisions.

'What about the surgeon?' asked Di.

I haven't seen Dr Godfrey since the other day', Ruth explained. 'For all I know he's been pulled off the case. And by the way', she added, 'I overheard one of them saying that they were going to start another round of chemo on Monday when Dr Capewell gets back'.

Di was appalled. She went outside to summon a nurse. After hearing Di's concerns, the nurse weighed Sarah. Soon, everyone was shocked. At home, before the department's intervention, Sarah had weighed a healthy 43 kg. After the first chemo, she weighed still an average weight of 38 kg. The anaesthetist had recorded this weight on the anaesthetic sheet just seven days previously, after the nurse weighed her on admission. Now Sarah weighed 33 kg. During one week in the hospital, Sarah had lost around 15 per cent of her entire body weight.

On Friday, 11 July, staff at the Integrative Health Clinic took a phone call from Mark who relayed a message that he and Di were gravely concerned about Sarah since her forced surgery. He said he was afraid his daughter had lost the will to live and feared she would not survive the next planned course of chemo in a few days. He mentioned that she had lost a significant percentage of her body weight in the past week, and asked if we could do anything to help her.

On Sunday, 13 July, I travelled to Sydney to visit Sarah and her family. I arrived on the hospital ward in the early afternoon to find Sarah on her mother's lap with Mark and Ruth sitting nearby.

The double room was outfitted with biohazard disposal containers for che-mo. It contained two beds and a window that looked out over a main arterial city road. The second bed was empty. Along the shelves were numerous tasty treats the family had bought for Sarah: fruits, jellies, biscuits, nuts, rice crack-ers, and vegetable dips that Di and Ruth offered around regularly.

I greeted Sarah with a toy green frog, a box of chocolates, and some herbal skin lotion. She looked up only occasionally at the stuffed frog and folded her arms protectively around herself. Despite my attempts at conversation, Sarah seemed mainly mute. She wore a haunted expression that had set into her face since the last time I'd seen her. At the clinic two months previously, she had been chatty, friendly and lively, and it took only a mildly funny comment to start her giggling. Now, my attempts to make her smile were unsuccessful.

Sarah was nearly bald with just a few wisps of hair stubbornly clinging around the edges of her previous hairline. It gave her a wizened look. She had a pale yellow complexion and sunken eyes. Her face was particularly thin. When Sarah allowed me to see her tummy, I noticed it was concave with her hip and rib bones visible under her skin. Her long vertical abdominal incision was still livid red and reinforced with steri-strips. Over her torso were pigmented stripes in a random distribution that looked like a mass of lengthy, intersecting lacerations. I had seen Sarah several times before and yet I would not have recognised her. She looked like a child with severe malnutrition.

When hospital staff came through the door, Sarah became fearful and hy-per-vigilant, as if trying to read body language clues from them. Among them, she appeared to trust one nurse more than the others; the British nurse who had been on duty for several days postoperatively.

During the 10 years I had worked in paediatrics, I had seen thousands of children of all nationalities and backgrounds. Sarah's same demeanour was on traumatised refugee children just evacuated from war zones. Most notably, Sarah had lost her childish traits and was dealing with the world in a sombre, grave and flat manner. I had seen these same characteristics in people who had been subjected to severe physical and emotional trauma: war veterans, crime victims, torture victims. Sarah had been a ward of the State since early June. Prior to that, she had been an exceptionally happy child, despite her serious illness. It seemed that the five weeks Sarah had spent in the child 'protection' system had done her no good at all.

I soon realised that no words could pierce her protective wall, and I offered to massage her feet with the lotion. While staying on her mother's lap, she extended one foot and then the other for me to massage. While doing so, I felt the tension of her muscles. Even the tiny muscles in her feet and ankles were on red alert.

If anyone had asked my opinion at the time, I would have said that Sarah's most pressing problems at that moment were her shattered emotional state and her obvious malnutrition. I thought she could use some time at home with her family, followed by several weeks of three square meals a day – before any more 'treatment'.

Towards the end of my visit, I went downstairs to the hospital kiosk and bought a pretty diary with flowers on the cover. I returned to give this to Sarah, thinking she could find some solace in writing down her thoughts and feelings about what had happened to her. Unfortunately, I was wrong. In hospital, she could not let her guard down and reveal her innermost feelings. I hadn't realised then that staff rifled through her belongings routinely, and they would continue to so for a long time to come. In the end, I made like a ventriloquist, letting the stuffed frog say my goodbyes. Sarah gave me a reserved smile. It was one I would never forget.

The next day was Monday, 14 July. Ruth and Di were in Sarah's room when Dr Capewell came in with two oncology registrars.

Capewell looked fresh and well rested. 'The good news is that her tumour markers are down now and she is not anaemic', he announced in front of Sarah. He did not mention however, that Sarah had had half her blood volume replaced during the surgery, which had raised her haemoglobin. In addition, the donor's blood – clearly a person without a tumour – had made Sarah's tumour marker tests look as if they had suddenly improved.

The oncologist continued. 'The bad news is that we found cancer in the spleen and we're going to start chemo tomorrow'.

Sarah lay in bed looking nervously around.

Di shook her head and pointed to Sarah. 'She's in no condition to take that right now'.

Capewell glared at Di and turned to his registrars for support. He'd had about enough of this family.

The registrars looked embarrassed and searched for something helpful to say.

'I was in the hospital earlier this year', said Ruth, 'and they didn't start chemo before the wound had healed'.

One of the registrars came to the oncologist's defence. 'But we do that here with children'.

Ruth bolted upright. 'That may be so. But not with our child!' she insisted. 'Anyone can see she needs more time to recover. She's nothing but bones right now'.

Capewell refused to look at Sarah. 'I just told you her tests are fine', he maintained. 'And DoCS have told us to go ahead and do it'.

Di rose slowly to her feet. She took a deep breath and stood up straight to meet the doctor eye to eye. Her natural shyness vanished. She felt Sarah's life was at stake. 'If you do that, I'll sue you', said Di forcefully. 'What do you think another round will do when your last two treatments put her in this condition?'

Capewell was livid. 'That is not your decision. We will have to leave it up to the department to decide'.

Ruth glowered at the oncologist. She had no respect for a man who accepted no responsibility for his own decisions, and hid behind a government department. 'Coward', she muttered.

Capewell looked outraged at being confronted head on by these two women. He fidgeted and looked to his registrars uncomfortably. They remained silent.

'Anyway, I've got other things to do. You'll see the dietician tomorrow and we'll see what happens after that', said the oncologist, before beating a hasty retreat.

The registrars trailed behind him in embarrassed silence.

Moments later, back in his office, Dr Capewell phoned the Taree DoCS office.

Sarah woke the next day with a clearer head. She'd had the surgery 11 days ago. The first week was an agonising blur. The morphine had helped dull her pain but it made her feel dizzy, and itchy like the last time she'd had it. Without it, her eyesight was clear enough to count the rows of her mother's cross-stitch. At least she could now see the sky through the grimy window of her third floor room, but she still felt horrified that somebody could open her up and take a piece out of her body by force. A small relief had come the day the nurse had removed her gastric tube, and she'd been able to eat small amounts over the past several days since then.

The family hadn't seen Dr Capewell since they'd had a difference of opinion, but the hospital dietician had been around twice. On the first visit the dietician weighed Sarah and told Di her daughter was suffering of malnutrition and required a high caloric 'balanced' diet. Since then, sausages and chicken nuggets had come up from the kitchen.

At 8 am, the nurse brought Sarah's breakfast tray. Di sat Sarah up in bed and pulled the bed table close to her. Sarah lifted the aluminium cover. A pile of baked beans sat on the plate, edged by two slices of soggy white bread. On the side sat a cold sausage congealed in a puddle of white fat.

Di cut up the sausage and coaxed Sarah to eat, but she gagged after a few pieces. Since the staff had allowed her to eat again, it was an ordeal to get through a meal. She had asked the dietician for a bowl of porridge for breakfast, but it never came. The woman said that she needed a balanced diet specially created for her, to remedy her malnutrition.

After breakfast, the nurses routinely weighed Sarah, and the following afternoon the dietician paid another visit. She was shocked that Sarah was still losing more weight and took Di aside to ask her further questions about the diet Sarah was used to at home. Di told her about the anti-cancer regimen the doctors in Melbourne had recommended. This diet consisted of wholesome foods and included several servings of fruits and vegetables daily, along with beans, pulses, rice, chicken, fish and lamb. Di explained that it excluded artificial additives, junk food, processed foods and white sugar. The dietician asked Di which foods Sarah liked. Di told her that Sarah loved a wide variety of food that included rice, lamb, chicken, vegetables, stews, pasta, and wholegrain bread. She also enjoyed large helpings of her favourite soups like pea and ham, pumpkin and minestrone. Sarah ate veggies from the garden and she loved most fruits. Di explained that she baked homemade bread, cakes and biscuits, made with honey instead of sugar. 'We don't eat junk foods and takeaway', she added

The dietician took notes. About Sarah's diet at home, she wrote in the clinical records: *I know of no scientific basis for excluding these [processed] foods and see no need for these restrictions.* She then ordered a more 'liberal' diet for Sarah in the hospital than her diet at home, and noted: *Sarah is now Not following this diet since admission.*

It was clear from her notation that the dietician wrongly assumed Sarah had arrived in hospital malnourished. It is unclear why she came to this conclusion when a quick check of the anaesthetic record 11 days previously would have clearly shown that Sarah was a normal weight for her age when she arrived at the hospital for admission. From the composite notes, it was obvious that after her splenectomy, Sarah had been critically ill and unable to eat for much of the post-operative period.

To rectify Sarah's massive weight loss and malnutrition, the hospital dietician ordered processed meat, baked beans, chicken nuggets, sausages, ice cream and white bread – instead of the wholesome foods Sarah was used to.

Sarah found the fatty diet difficult to keep down and told her mother she craved vegetables and fruits. Di ventured out to the delicatessen near the hospital and came back with avocado and eggplant dips, rice crackers and an assortment of nuts, which Sarah hungrily ate.

It was just after 5 pm on 15 July when Mark came to visit. For a while, he and Ruth played a word game with Sarah to cheer her up.

After an hour, Mark looked at his watch. He had a feeling something was up and he didn't want to stay long. Mark leaned over to kiss Sarah goodbye and then asked Di to follow him outside. Ruth stayed with Sarah while the parents headed down the hall to the parents' room to talk in private. Both had been thinking that the past two days since Dr Capewell had returned had been far too quiet.

'Have you heard anything since you and Mum spoke with him?' asked Mark.

'Not a thing', she said. 'But the nurses seem a bit offhand since he's been back. Worse yet, the British nurse is due for some days off. I don't know what we'll do without her. On top of that', added Di, 'I think the dietician thinks my home cooking is responsible for Sarah's weight loss'.

'That's ridiculous', said Mark. 'She was a normal weight when we brought her in and she lost it all being put through the mill in here over the past two weeks'.

'I know that', said Di. 'But they still want to blame us'.

'They're just trying to cover their backs', said Mark. 'I don't know why these people can't be honest about things without making us into villains all the time'.

They sat with their own thoughts for a while, until the door opened and a young woman peered into the room. It was the oncology social worker. 'I've been looking for you', she said.

The parents froze like stunned rabbits.

'There's a DoCS conference scheduled for tomorrow at 1.30 and they want you to be there', said the social worker.

After both parents agreed to come, the young woman hurried away.

Di waited until the door had shut. 'Funny thing about that', she murmured.

'I might have guessed', answered Mark. 'I'll see you about lunchtime tomorrow then'.

The parents had correctly sensed a problem building behind the scenes. After Di and Ruth's encounter with Dr Capewell on Monday, he immediately phoned the child protection department complaining he'd been abused. He followed his call with a letter to the department stating:

> ...at the mention of further chemotherapy both mother and grand-mother rose and began abusing me and threatening me with legal and other retribution should we embark on chemotherapy. I reminded them I was acting in Sarah's interests ...nonetheless they pursued me with these threats.

He mentioned nothing in his letter about Sarah's forced operation, the terror it still held for her, the serious blood loss she had sustained, the post-operative crisis, the pneumonia and lung collapse or, finally, her startling weight loss and malnutrition – all in the space of two weeks. He told the department nothing about the parents being so alarmed by those developments that they didn't think their daughter was fit for chemotherapy. However, he did acknowledge Sarah's emotional distress since the operation, which he maintained was the parents' fault rather than the effects of a forced surgery and its serious complications. He wrote:

> I have a deep concern that the psychological ill-effects of their [the parents'] continued presence is having on Sarah [sic]...I believe it is extremely important that Sarah have a series of formal psychological assessments to ascertain her views of what has happened and what her views of death and dying are if she does not have any further therapy.

The oncologist then suggested moving Sarah back to the care of Dr Kotz, and then physically removing Sarah from her parents:

> I am unable and unwilling to continue her medical care...I believe that her care would best be carried out in the [regional hospital] and that it will not be possible for me or for that matter any medical person to deliver the chemotherapy that she still requires while she is in the care of her parents.

Finally, the oncologist was unhappy about the way in which Taree DoCS had handled the case. On this, he wrote:

I would also like to take this opportunity to remind you that your department has effectively been this child's parent for 1 month. I would also like to note that since Sarah has been seeing us here at this hospital, we have had no more than phone conversations with your office, mostly initiated by me. At no stage has an individual from your department come and assessed Sarah or her family, in particular Sarah's mental state, her wishes and how she is coping with treatment. These are simple measures which with the proper counselling and preventive maintenance may have altered the course of events and the parent's [sic] actions over the past month. I realise that funding for this sort of intervention may be difficult but note that her DOCS responsibility could have been transferred to a DOCS office in the East of Sydney.

This complaint came after Taree DoCS had granted all the oncologist's wishes; they had imposed at least six court cases on the parents to enforce the doctor's treatments, and had consented to the forced splenectomy and any other treatment he had deemed necessary.

Despite the complaints, the department was again at the doctor's service. The following day, Taree caseworkers planned a lengthy 300 km trip to Sydney to exert pressure on the family again.

Shortly before 1.30 pm the next day, the hospital social worker summoned the family to a conference room at the end of the ward. There they met the manager and caseworkers from Taree DoCS: Gary Boggs, Gillian and Judy. Gillian took notes that, the parents now suspected, would be rendered into affidavits for the next court hearing.

Di and Mark sat down on the brown vinyl hospital chairs that lined the parents' room, while Ruth sat further away. Sarah, now looking emaciated, sat on Di's lap. She had wanted to come with her parents rather than stay in the hospital room by herself. Gary and Judy sat opposite the parents while Gillian took notes from a vantage point from where she could see and hear everyone in the room.

Gary, looking slightly nervous, started the meeting by explaining its purpose: Dr Capewell wanted no more responsibility for Sarah and intended to hand her over to Dr Kotz at the regional hospital. The department now wanted the parents to agree to this arrangement in addition to giving a written consent to start immediate chemotherapy.

The parents thought the doctor was shifting the responsibility and they were still horrified by the brute force the department and various oncology staff had imposed on their daughter and the terrible toll it had taken on her over the past two weeks. They wanted the doctors and the department to include them in honest discussions, not the kind of talks that reappeared skewed and rendered into affidavits for the next court hearing as 'evidence' against them. The parents desperately wanted the doctors to hear their legitimate concerns about their daughter, to discuss the issues with them in a reasonable way, and to demonstrate a willingness to solve Sarah's present health crisis.

'Anybody can see that Sarah is too sick for chemo right now - it makes no difference which hospital', said Mark. 'Right now we want to be included in discussions and decision making instead of being ignored while doctors force treatments on our daughter'.

Gary Boggs asked Mark what he understood of Sarah's condition. Mark answered that they hadn't been told very much at all; instead, they were kept out of the information loop. Mark said it was obvious that his daughter was shattered physically and emotionally as a result of the forced treatment. The oncologist had been away during most of the harrowing post-operative period when Sarah had come close to death, and the remaining staff didn't discuss much with them.

Boggs waited for Mark to finish. Then he repeated that Sarah needed chemo; this time three months of it.

Mark was struggling to remain composed. 'This is exactly what I'm talking about', he said. 'You people aren't interested in having a proper discussion. You don't really care about our daughter. That's obvious by now. You just want your own way and you don't care how you get it'.

Boggs glanced over to the caseworker recording the session, before looking back to Mark. 'You realise by now, that we can go to court and get stronger orders', he goaded.

Mark had had enough of their repetitive legal action. He slammed his hand flat on the armrest and bolted from his seat. 'Frigging do it then! We are not going to be pushed around any longer. These meetings are nothing but a set-up. They've never resolved any issues. They only give you people more material for your affidavits'.

Boggs changed his tone and tried to keep Mark in the room by placating him. 'I understand your anger', he said with false sincerity.

'Oh no you don't', answered Mark bitterly.

'We're only trying to do what's best for Sarah', said Boggs.

The rest of the family stood ready to follow Mark through the door.

Di couldn't help herself. Now she had to speak her mind. 'This is her life we're talking about. I'm fed up with this too. We're not going to be bullied like this. You people don't care about her. Did you see what she looked like before?' she demanded.

'There are benefits to chemotherapy', insisted Boggs.

Di pointed to Sarah. 'Benefits? What benefits? The doctors can't even give us proof of that. Maybe you people have had benefits, but as you can see, there have been none for Sarah'.

Boggs reminded Di that there were still three months of chemo to go.

Di took Sarah's hand and prepared to leave with Mark. 'Another three months of this and she won't be here', she shot back to Boggs.

Mark had been standing at the doorway. 'Sarah had other cancer treatment options available to her, and you prevented her from having them', he added bitterly.

Di joined Mark with Sarah in tow.

Ruth followed Di. Near the door, she lingered and looked thoughtful. 'Just one last thing', said Ruth, who had been quiet up until then. 'The doctor at the regional hospital that you want to send Sarah back to has the same approach as this one here. We don't want Sarah there. Nothing would be different, would it?'

Mark left the room and the family followed suit.

The caseworkers left Sydney late in the afternoon and returned to Taree. Their office had the day before received a letter from Mark's lawyer. The parents did not want Sarah to return to the regional hospital but they consented to having Sarah admitted to a different hospital, based in Sydney.

Upstairs in his office, Dr Capewell was working late to prepare his report to the judge for the next day's court hearing. In his letter, he requested a psychologist's report on Sarah; for this, he had a particular psychologist in mind. He also stated his preference for having Sarah placed with a foster family.

By tomorrow afternoon, he wanted Sarah and her family out of his hospital ward and under the care of his colleague at the regional hospital, where he routinely visited.

The next day, on July 17, Mark was in the courthouse, briefing his barrister about the upheaval Sarah had suffered over the past fortnight.

In what was to be a lengthy hearing spanning most of the day, the judge heard the department's evidence. Dr Capewell had written a report claiming that Sarah's spleen had become larger and smaller over time, and that the spleen was found to have a 'large subcapsular haemorrhage'. His claim was not supported by the official pathologist's report, which made no mention of any such finding on close examination of the spleen. The oncologist's claim that Sarah's spleen was several times its normal size was also not supported by the weight listed in the pathology report, which was in the normal range. The oncologist did not release the pathologist's report, and in fact, it was not made available to the court at any time.

Further in his report, the oncologist alleged that Sarah's mother and grandmother had abused him, and claimed they continued making threats after he told them he 'was acting in the best interests of the child'. Mark was horrified to hear these allegations. He was equally disturbed by the doctor's failure to tell the court about the serious side effects Sarah had suffered from the forced surgery and her subsequent pneumonia and malnutrition. He turned to whisper to his barrister, and wondered when she would stand up and tell the judge about all the details that had been withheld, but she remained seated.

In his report, the oncologist went on to recommend that Sarah be placed in a foster home during the time she was not in the hospital being treated. He suggested she should be transferred to the regional hospital for immediate chemotherapy and then receive a full psychological assessment to explore her feelings about 'dying' in the event she did not have chemotherapy.

The next evidence came from Gillian, the caseworker who was present at the hospital meeting with the family the previous day. In her affidavit she stated that the family was 'strongly opposed' to the chemotherapy treatment, but did not mention that the parents felt this way because of Sarah's appalling condition since the forced surgery. Nor did she mention the parents' objections to and distress about being excluded from the information and decision-making process. Again, the judge had no information that shed light on the nature of the parents' objections and legitimate concerns. The family's barrister remained mute on the subject, with the exception of registering the family's objection to Sarah returning to the regional hospital.

During the court recess, a department caseworker attempted to locate a hospital bed for Sarah in another hospital located in Sydney. The head oncology professor in charge of the oncology unit asked for the background story. After the caseworker had briefed him, the professor asked how Dr Capewell had become involved in this type of controversy and then refused to take Sarah as a patient. Through the course of the day, the caseworker made similar enquiries to other hospitals, but was refused. It seemed the matter had taken on an unsavoury reputation and the only option appeared to be a return to the regional hospital. Dr Kotz had already discussed the matter with Dr Capewell, and had submitted his own letter to the court stating that he was only too happy to take Sarah back again for continued treatment, provided a number of restrictive rules governing the parents' access to their daughter were ordered.

By the end of the day, the judge ruled that Sarah be transferred to the regional hospital, where she would be subjected to psychological assessment prior to the next course of chemotherapy.

It was 4.30 pm when the hearing ended. Dr Capewell had written to the court stating: 'There simply will not be a bed available at the [Sydney based] hospital after this evening'.

When the judge adjourned the court, Mark rushed out into the hallway. He was devastated that the barrister had not told the court about Sarah's present situation. Since he had complained to her about this before, he had the urge to sack her there and then, but was stopped by his mobile phone ringing. It was Di. Back at the hospital, the nursing unit manager was about to unceremoniously discharge Sarah, but no ambulance was available to transport her to the regional hospital that night. In short, Sarah had to leave the hospital at once and they would be stuck without accommodation for the night. Di relayed that two caseworkers were there to take Sarah with them for the night and drive her to the regional hospital the following day.

Instead of talking with his barrister, Mark raced back to the hospital. In the middle of heavy traffic, his Taree lawyer called him on the mobile to tell him about the letter he had written to the hospital asking permission for Mark to see the spleen. The hospital had replied to his request; it seemed the spleen had been destroyed. Considering all the anomalies that had occurred lately, Mark didn't believe a word of it.

Mark was out of breath when he arrived at the hospital. Sarah had been put out of the room and sat in the lobby. Two caseworkers he had never seen before were about to leave with her when Mark stopped them. He reminded them that Sarah was still seriously ill and they had no medical training. He suggested instead that he and Di be allowed to stay overnight with friends who were medically trained. Mark was surprised when both women agreed that it was a sensible idea. In hindsight, Mark noted that it was the only occasion where he felt caseworkers acted out of genuine concern for Sarah's welfare.

The women phoned their office and returned to say they would allow them to stay with an 'approved' family for the night, before continuing the 300 km journey to the regional hospital – provided the parents agreed to have Sarah at the regional hospital before 10 am the next morning. The caseworkers had hastily prepared a document to that effect.

Mark and Di agreed and signed the undertaking. Silently they wondered why, again, the department had not allowed Sarah an ambulance with paramedics while she was still so ill – and when only the previous week, she had nearly lost her life.

PSYCHO·PROFILING

Psychologists avoid discriminating unfairly against people on the Basis of age, religion, sexuality, ethnicity, gender, disability, Alternatively, any other basis proscribed by law.

Australian Psychological Society Code of Ethics for Psychologists

Mark and Di arrived with Sarah at the regional hospital at around 11 am on July 18. They had stayed overnight with their friends and travelled the remaining long distance to the hospital that morning. It was two weeks since Sarah's major operation and pneumonia, and barely a week since she had been able to walk again unaided. At 33 kg, she was still malnourished, and hunched over from the still unhealed surgical incision spanning the length of her abdomen. The parents worried about Sarah on the trip, and were prepared to call the emergency number on Mark's mobile phone if necessary. They wondered why the department had airlifted Sarah while she was in vigorous health, but when she desperately needed medical transportation, it was denied her for a second time.

The regional hospital was as the family had remembered it from Sarah's first admission: a colourless, tiled building with a row of windows overlooking the car park and wooded area beyond. Sarah hadn't been outside for two weeks and paused to look at the gum trees. Di soon urged her on; they couldn't linger too long or DoCS would turn up if they were just a few minutes late. Both parents took Sarah's hand and led her through the yawning entrance. They didn't realise it would take months before Sarah was free to walk through that door again.

The receptionist at the admissions desk filled out the required forms and sent the family directly to the ward. A few nurses recognised Sarah from her first admission nine months previously. Some looked at her sympathetically, assuming her cancer had reduced her to skeletal proportions, not realising that the extreme weight loss had occurred in the previous hospital. At 11.15 am, a nurse admitted Sarah into a side room lined with hazardous-waste bins and biohazard protective equipment, reserved for children having chemotherapy. A few staff who recognised Sarah noticed a change since last they'd seen her. She was no longer happy and talkative.

All went routinely for the first hour. Nurses came in to take Sarah's vital signs and issue her with an ID bracelet. Mark and Di sat reassuringly nearby with their chairs out of the staff's way. The nurses were pleasant, and the parents responded politely.

During Sarah's admission, staff notified the oncology social worker, Caitlin Grimes, of her arrival. This was the same young woman who had a few months previously reported the parents to DoCS, wrongly alleging the parents were pursuing an alternative lifestyle and a religion that forbade medical treatment. The social worker came to the ward immediately, where she discussed Sarah and her parents with the admitting doctor and other staff. Next, she came in to interview the family. Sarah lay exhausted on her bed, while both parents were worn out from the drive, but still managed to answer the young woman's questions courteously. When Grimes had finished, she returned to the office to discuss Sarah's case with other staff again.

Subsequently, the admitting doctor noted the same incorrect information the social worker had repeated in many of her previous notations. He wrongly alleged in the medical records that Sarah's family belonged to a fundamentalist religious sect and that they insisted on 'alternative' treatments for cancer. This was a continuation of the prejudicial, stereotypical and incorrect information that had led to the family's present difficult circumstances.

Under the doctor's notation, the social worker made her own entry:

> *...family difficult to engage...had a conversation with [Gillian] of DoCS ...have asked for an informal meeting next week. If parents threatening to or actually remove Sarah from the hospital please contact me to access DoCS emergency pager. If parents' behaviour becomes unmanageable please attempt to diffuse situation with the assistance of social worker and security ...if unable to be diffused, the situation should be handled as per any aggressive clients in the hospital and the police may need to be involved. If Sarah's behaviour becomes unmanageable please contact social worker and a psych consult may be required. Then make a report to DoCS, if this could not be managed on the ward.*

Despite the family being polite and co-operative, and giving the staff no reason to suspect or anticipate violent behaviour requiring the involvement of the police, the social worker's notations set the tone for the rest of Sarah's stay. Professional staff became almost instantly offhand and unfriendly. The parents noticed the change in mood, but could not understand why until years later, when they saw the staff's notations in a batch of documents they had requested under the Freedom of Information Act. They were shocked to think this stereotyping went on inside hospitals and even more appalled to realise they were the victims of it.

To make matters worse, the admitting doctor wrongly noted in the medical records that Sarah was in stage III cancer when she was in the final stage IV. He wrote that her spleen had been removed due to rupture, which of course was also untrue. When Mark received these documents some years later, they were heavily edited and redacted. He felt this supported his earlier suspicions of a cover-up: it would have looked outrageous to impose three months of forced chemotherapy onto a stage IV cancer patient. He believed the court would never have approved it, had the judge known the truth. He thought that this explained why the doctors had consistently refused to release Sarah's clinical notes as well as her histology report, which would have confirmed that the cancer was widespread and included the spleen and liver.

To obscure matters more, a staff member made an error in the transfer sheet between hospitals, alleging Sarah had a 'teratoma', a usually benign tumour with a good prognosis.

The sum total of compounding errors, misrepresentations, stereotyping and profiling meant staff were misinformed from the beginning and unable to relate to Sarah as a terminal child with end-of-life needs that included kindness and compassion.

Later that afternoon, Mark decided to return home for the first time in two weeks. While Sarah was in hospital, the house had stood empty and they'd had to farm their other children out to various relatives. While Di roomed in the hospital accommodation to be with Sarah full-time, Mark looked forward to reuniting with the other children at home. The regional hospital was only an hour and a half from home, and now he could bring Sarah's siblings to see their sister regularly.

After Mark had gone, Di brought out her needlework. It was her way of re-laxing and it often unwound Sarah as well. After the long day, which had started before dawn followed by two hour drive to the hospital, Di thought

Sarah could use some peace and quiet. Sarah's bed was directly next to a large window and she was obviously enjoying looking at the gum trees outside while singing a few bars of her favourite song.

When a nurse walked past the room, she immediately veered inside and turned on the TV. Then she ordered Sarah out of bed, into a chair and gave her a book to read, before leaving again. The nurse returned to the office and wrote an entry into the records: *walked by Sarah's room, noted Sarah to be sitting on haunches at window rocking back and forth humming. Sarah's mum sitting on chair doing nothing. Encouraged Sarah to find a book to read – same done, now reading book in chair.*

Sarah had been at the regional hospital for three days when a clinical psychologist came to her room at 11 am on 22 July. Jean Sharpe was a middle-aged woman with a confident, blunt manner and an imposing physical presence. She had extensive experience in court procedures. Although touted as an independent psychologist, she had worked many cases for the department in the past.

Sharpe arrived with a bag of testing materials and told Sarah to come with her to an adjacent office for a psychological assessment. She instructed the parents to stay behind in the hospital room while she assessed Sarah. Later she would interview them, both separately and together.

In the side office, the psychologist briefly introduced herself before spreading her testing materials out on the table in front of Sarah. For the next two hours, Sharpe put Sarah through a battery of IQ tests. This included memorising long sequences of random numbers, which Sarah was asked to repeat in order. Then the psychologist told Sarah complex stories. She followed this by quizzing Sarah on the themes and hidden messages to see how well she was listening.

After that, Sarah was shown lengthy arrays of designs, pictures and puzzles and asked to analyse their meaning. She was required to perform the tests at top speed. Sarah was included in a group of normal healthy children without the burden of a terminal disease. It was predictable she would score lower than children in normal circumstances. At the time of the tests, Sarah had been off the continuous morphine IV for only 10 days, and still found it difficult to concentrate. Considering her uncharacteristically sombre mood since the forced surgery it was also possible Sarah was still suffering severe shock and emotional trauma. This could have diminished her capacity to concentrate and focus on intellectual tasks and mental problem solving.

Sarah was exhausted after the psychologist finished the extensive IQ testing, but the woman went on to conduct a prolonged interview. She asked Sarah questions about death and dying, what her religious beliefs were, what she thought about chemotherapy and how she felt about being taken from her home and placed into a foster home.

About chemotherapy, Sarah told the psychologist that she did not want any more of the kind of chemo the doctor wanted to give her because of the side effects, which she found difficult to endure. Like the last time she'd had it, she felt it would make her sicker than the cancer. Sarah also asked for her complementary treatments to be reinstated.

The psychologist then explored in depth how Sarah felt about going to a foster home, explaining that it meant she would be taken away from her family and placed with another family to live. Although the judge had refused this as an option at the previous hearing, Dr Capewell was apparently unwilling to let it go.

Sarah had never heard of such a thing as a foster home and she found that question unbearably painful. 'I just want to go home to live with my Mum and Dad', she replied sadly. 'I don't want to go anywhere else'.

Sarah was becoming increasingly upset, but the woman probed further, this time about death and dying. She asked Sarah whether she knew what death meant and whether she realised she would die without the chemotherapy the oncologist wanted her to have.

Discussing death and dying with children with cancer is usually a delicate issue, conducted with the utmost sensitivity and with only one goal in mind – to assist the child in coming to terms with the physical, emotional and spiritual aspects of their end of life journey. This involves lending emotional support to both child and family, whether they've chosen curative or palliative treatment options. Current best hospital practice requires staff to respect the cancer patient's and family's choices, values and wishes.[28]

In this case, both oncologists wanted the psychologist to ask Sarah whether she was prepared to die if she did not have their treatment. The question was posed as an ultimatum – either agree to chemo or die – and seems an insensitive question to ask any terminal patient, let alone a child. Moreover, Sarah had already been asked this question several times before; caseworkers had framed it the same way when they asked her what she thought about dying if she didn't have the doctor's preferred treatment. At no time were these questions posed in

---

[28] Behrman R. When Children Die: Improving Palliative and End-of-Life Care for Children.

context of Sarah's poor prognosis, her unlikely recovery from her particular type and stage of cancer, the existence of other legitimate cancer treatments, and the rights of persons with a terminal disease to accept or refuse any treatments.

To the psychologist's question about her death, Sarah answered quietly: 'When I die, I wouldn't be here anymore'.

Death was a subject Sarah knew a lot about. She had been close to death twice just over two weeks ago and was living under a death sentence from cancer. She'd heard the doctors say their treatment could kill her; then they said it would kill her not to have it – and then they said the cancer could kill her no matter what. On top of that, the staff around her insisted she would die if she didn't do what they told her, even though she would die of the cancer anyway.

Sarah told her parents later that she knew more about death than the staff at the hospital, but she didn't like having to talk about it all the time. Death wasn't what bothered her most; being put in a foster home disturbed her much more, and it also terrified her to have organs removed from her body by force. She just wanted to go home and be happy for the time she had left, and she wanted a treatment that would make her feel better and not worse than the disease she was suffering from.

When the psychologist had finished with her, Sarah returned to her hospital room, went to bed, and pulled up the covers.

Next, the psychologist called Di into her room while Mark tried to comfort Sarah after her two-hour ordeal. After seeing Sarah come out of the woman's office looking wrung out, Di was wary at first and kept quiet. She was asked about her religious beliefs and explained that she did not belong to a church or a particular religion. When the psychologist asked Di what she thought about placing Sarah in a foster home, Di was horrified. She shook her head forcefully. 'Why would you ask a mother that question?' she asked. 'I don't want Sarah or any of my children in a foster home. Not ever'.

Di had not been long in the office when the psychologist called a lunch break. It was already late afternoon when the parents took Sarah to the small cafeteria in the hallway outside the ward and ordered lunch for the three of them. Without being invited, the psychologist joined the family at the table and continued observing their interactions and making notes as they were eating. The family found this intrusive, but felt they could say nothing about it.

After the late afternoon meal-break, the psychologist called Mark into the interview room. When she asked Mark his views, he voiced his usual concerns, explaining when he'd asked the doctors to verify their claims of a cure with the treatment they were proposing, they couldn't or wouldn't answer. Instead, the doctors had involved DoCS and it made a total wreck of the situation. Without telling the psychologist what their plans had been, Mark attempted to explain that major cancer hospitals in the UK, Europe and the US offered newer cancer treatments without the side effects of chemotherapy. Unfortunately, the psychologist seemed sceptical. Mark sensed that she had never heard of any new mainstream treatments and thought he was talking about 'alternative' treatments.

Mark went on to explain that he and Di wanted the best cancer treatment available for their daughter including supportive and complementary treatments such as nutritional supplements and vitamin C. He said that he and Di resented the department's intervention, which prevented their daughter from receiving treatments elsewhere. He stressed his disappointment that the doctors had not engaged with them in reasonable and truthful discussions. As a result, the department had embroiled the family in stressful litigation and they hadn't been able to defend themselves because the doctors refused to release crucial medical documents, even when the court had ordered them to do so. He thought there were double standards; one for the doctors, who always got what they wanted, and the other for the parents, who never seemed to get a fair go.

The psychologist took copious notes before asking Mark about his beliefs about lifestyle. Mark told her of his interest in sustainable agriculture. His family's property had been handed down through generations and he felt a strong obligation to preserve the land in a sustainable condition for future generations. To that end, he applied the guidelines suggested by Allan Savory, a well-known wildlife biologist, author of textbooks on sustainable ecology and co-founder of the US-based Center for Holistic Management. Mark opened his briefcase and showed a laminated flowchart to the psychologist, but he immediately regretted it when she seized it and began to write prolific notes. By the woman's comments, Mark thought she had misinterpreted the sustainable agriculture chart and considered it some kind of alternative, hippy lifestyle rule-book.

The psychologist finished her notes about Mark's flowchart before going on to ask about the family's religion. By then, she had asked all three family members about their religious beliefs and each had told her that they did not belong to any organised religion. Mark explained this again, adding that any spiritual beliefs he might or might not have, posed no barrier to effective medical treatment. He had avidly researched mainstream medical options since Sarah was diagnosed with cancer, and was well acquainted with the current cancer treatments offered in major cancer centers around the world.

However, the psychologist persisted with her intrusive religious questions, even though psychologists are ethically required to observe either existing anti-discrimination laws and/or ethics governing such questioning and stereotyping.[29] The Code of Ethics as set down by the Australian Psychological Association requires psychologists to 'demonstrate an understanding of the consequences for people of unfair discrimination and stereotyping related to their age, religion, sexuality, ethnicity, gender, or disability'.

While being probed about his personal and religious beliefs, Mark wondered why health professionals couldn't simply discuss the facts of Sarah's treatment options with them, without psychoanalysing them, attributing a set of mistaken beliefs to them, accusing them of fictitious wrongdoing, and then stereotyping them in a way that demeaned them and destroyed their credibility. Finally, he had enough of the psychologist's questioning. He told her firmly that the only relevant issue was appropriate treatment options for Sarah and the scientific evidence to back them up.

After Mark's objection, the psychologist desisted, but remained frustrated at not being able to continue, while Mark was annoyed at having to constantly defend himself from staff's mistaken beliefs about their family.

The psychologist went on to ask Mark what he thought about Sarah staying in hospital for months until the chemotherapy was over.

'I don't think she'll come out of it very well', he answered. 'Sarah's not the kind of kid you could shut in for long in a place like a hospital'.

The psychologist chewed on her pen thoughtfully.

'What would you think of putting Sarah in foster care for a while?' she asked.

Mark did not like the way the interview was going. 'Why on earth would you ask such a question when we have done nothing wrong?' he asked tensely. 'It's not an option. Absolutely not'.

The woman asked how he thought Sarah was coping.

'Remarkably', said Mark, still shaken from the previous question. 'Considering what she's been through and the fact that the staff keep telling her she will die if she doesn't do what they say'.

---

[29] Under the *Anti-Discrimination Act 1991* (Qld) ss.124A, 131A; *Anti-Discrimination Act 1998* (Tas) s.19; *Racial and Religious Tolerance Act 2001* (Vic) ss.8, 25. Vilification based on 'religion' is against the law in Queensland, while vilification based on 'religious belief or activity' is against the law in Victoria and Tasmania (the Tasmanian provisions also cover vilification based on 'religious affiliation').

The psychologist noted Mark's answer and then asked him whether he had any requests. Mark told her that since DoCS had become involved his family had been suffering from various forms of harassment including phone tapping, and he wanted it to stop. He added that DoCS had also imposed heavy costs and hardships on them, expecting them to bear the travel costs over long distances to see doctors of the department's choice. The department was embroiling them in several court cases each month and now their entire family was suffering, including the other children, whom they hadn't seen on a full time basis for months. Mark requested some travelling reimbursements, a carer's allowance for Di, and a district nurse to assist them at home with Sarah's needs.

With that, the psychologist ended the interview. It was now dark outside.

Mark returned to Sarah's room. They all looked exhausted after spending the entire day with the psychologist, and Mark was beginning to get a bad feeling about where it was all headed.

Jean Sharpe had only three days to prepare the extensive psychological report for the court. To save time, she interviewed Dr Capewell by phone, and caught up with Dr Kotz in his office at the regional hospital.

During this interview Dr Kotz again claimed Sarah was in stage III cancer instead of the terminal stage IV she was actually in. None of this was accurate, but unfortunately no one other than Kotz and Capewell knew the truth at this point and the inaccuracy could continue in the system that had no checks and balances.

When the psychologist asked the oncologist what he would do in the event of another relapse, he maintained he would consider using an even higher dose of chemotherapy, but added that there wasn't 'a lot of data on this.'

Some years later, Mark read that comment in light of new information. He came to believe that the oncologist intended to give Sarah only chemotherapy in ever increasing amounts until the end of her life, because he had no other treatments to offer.

When asked about the chemotherapy's necessity, the oncologist added he was certain without chemotherapy 'she will have another recurrence of the tumour within 4 to 6 months'.

Later that day, the psychologist phoned Dr Capewell. He repeated his previous complaints, alleging the mother and grandmother had abused him when he wanted to start chemotherapy a few days after Sarah's surgery. He made no mention of the fact that the family had objected to the chemo because Sarah was still suffering severe post-operative complications and malnutrition. Instead, the doctor explained it was the grandmother's fault, alleging she was an 'influential force within the family'.

About Sarah's extreme weight loss, the oncologist alleged: 'it is because her spleen was ten times its normal size and was sitting on top of her stomach, which meant she did not want to eat for days on end'. This, of course, was inaccurate: the pathology report had noted Sarah's spleen to be in a normal weight range, and the weight loss had occurred entirely while Sarah was in his ward – after the spleen was removed. The doctor further claimed Sarah was bleeding internally from the spleen prior to surgery, (which was also contrary to the report), and maintained the parents had been reluctant to consent to the surgery, when in fact they were upset about not being consulted about it.

The oncologist then complained that DoCS had been 'un-supportive' and failed to organise a psychological assessment on Sarah to prevent his problems with the family. He said he'd had to organise his own consultation with the in-house psychiatrist, but twice the psychiatric professor had visited Sarah and she had been 'uncommunicative'. He made no mention that the psychiatrist had attempted to assess Sarah while she was in serious post-operative condition and required high doses of narcotics for pain.

The oncologist told the psychologist that he expected her to 'ascertain Sarah's views on what she wants and whether or not she understands and is prepared to die [without chemotherapy]'. To the court, the doctor advised: '...the Court needs to decide whether they are prepared to allow her to die, as that is the only alternative to treatment'. He then alleged any other treatment was 'complete quackery'.

Finally, he strongly recommended Sarah should be removed from home and placed in foster care over the months of future treatment.

After all interviews were completed, the psychologist had only three days to prepare the report for the next court hearing, listed for 25 July.

The day after the psychologist's marathon interviews, Mark brought Sarah's siblings in to visit. The other children inched into her room not knowing what to expect. They were glad to see their sister again, although they had never seen her so withered and shrunken. Laura had brought a dozen carnations and put them in a vase to cheer her sister up. Clara stayed behind Di until she was used to the medical setting. Both the little ones, Leah and Josh, took a while to get used to the strange sight of their sister.

Sarah ignored her siblings' shocked responses, and smiled for the first time in weeks. Before too long Hannah incited Sarah to mischief. Soon Sarah was showing off by blowing up rubber gloves from the dispenser above the sink and making balloons out of them. The other kids followed her lead and everyone laughed when Sarah made the inflated gloves look like cow's udders. The strenuous laughter caused Sarah coughing spasms, but it didn't stop her.

Laura took photographs of the family and tried to remain serious, but eventually warmed up to the fun. It was a welcome relief from the stress they'd all been through during the previous months.

Later that evening, Sarah's aunts, uncles and cousins visited, along with some friends from Gloucester. Finally, Sarah's spirits were lifted.

On the afternoon of July 24, I visited the hospital to cheer Sarah up. I paused for a moment outside her room. Through the open door, I saw Sarah in bed folding coloured paper. She was making cards for her sisters and brother. Occasionally she looked out the window. A woollen hat was perched high on her head. Di sat at the bedside quilting. She looked stressed, while Sarah seemed somewhat happier than the last time I'd seen her after the splenectomy.

Sarah smiled when she saw me juggling a huge fruit basket. Di invited me in. For a while, we sat together chatting, before Sarah knelt on the bed and started playing hairdresser with my hair. She fashioned it into a punk style and giggled at her creation. Occasionally she lent over, chose another piece of fruit and devoured it. When she offered me an apple, I declined, saying it was meant for her. Then she opened the top drawer of her bedside table; it was barely able to slide and filled to the brim with lollies and chocolate bars.

'The nurses give me these all the time', announced Sarah as she munched on the apple from the basket.

Di looked up from her quilting. 'They want to put weight on her quickly'.

'Yea', confirmed Sarah enthusiastically. 'They give me so many lollies and chocolates here that I've made up lolly names for all the nurses'.

'What about your main meals?' I asked.

Sarah made a face. 'Every morning they bring me bacon and cream. Eeeew!'

I watched as she polished off the apple before disposing the core in the plastic bag taped to her bedside table.

When a nurse came into the room to check Sarah's vital signs, she carefully eyed the fruit basket. On her way out, she turned on the TV. After she had gone, Sarah reached for the console and turned it off again. When I asked why the nurse inspected the basket, Di explained that staff looked in Sarah's belongings regularly, searching for contraband, such as vitamins.

Sarah returned to fixing my hair and soon I was set to walk out of the ward with an array of purple bows. I said my goodbyes and on my way out, I stopped at the nurses' station to ask if I could take Sarah and Di just outside the building for some fresh air. Sarah had been cooped up for weeks and I assured them as a fellow health professional that I would have them back in a few minutes.

The nurses refused my request without a moment's thought – perhaps because of the purple ribbons. When I left the ward that afternoon, I did not know that I would not be seeing Sarah again for a long time.

On the morning of 25 July, Mark paused in front of the imposing Supreme Court building. To steady his nerves, he took a deep breath and looked around. Behind the dour statue of Queen Victoria was the old colonial police station. Not far from there stood the barristers' chambers inside Victorian buildings with gargoyles adorning their upper storeys. The legal sector oozed old money and power. Mark could not imagine what it felt like to grow up with that kind of privilege: the best schools, the best of everything and doors opening automatically. He was just an ordinary bloke from an old Australian country family, and he had never thought he'd end up in court defending his family's rights.

Mark scanned the morning crowd for a glimpse of his barrister. He wanted to tell her about the psychologist's all-day grilling and ask her whether she had seen the report. He was feeling uneasy about it and to top it off, the psychologist had phoned him the previous day and wanted a copy of his affidavit. He didn't think psychologists normally tried to extract legal information from patients' families. He thought perhaps she was helping the department's case.

Mark wondered whom he could trust these days. He half expected to find his barrister arriving with the DoCS barristers from the Crown Solicitor's Office. Last time he'd spoken with her, he wondered which side she was on. When he reminded her that the hospital and doctors were in contempt of court for failing to produce the medical records, she told him that she would not pursue it against such respectable parties. When he complained about the department's bully tactics, she told him:

'You'd better do what the department wants or you'll lose all your kids'.

Mark wondered whether the department had read his barrister the riot act just as it had done with his lawyer in Taree; at least his lawyer didn't fold under their demands. Day after day, Mark did his own legal work. In court, the barrister scarcely put up a defence, while charging $5000 per day. At this rate, Mark would soon be out of money. To pay the legal fees, he'd sold all the cattle and had gone through their life savings.

By mid-morning, the hearing was underway. The barristers were at their respective tables before the judge. Mark sat behind his counsel and watched the DoCS barrister pass the psychologist's report over to Mark's barrister. She in turn passed a copy on to Mark. It was the first he had seen of it. For the next hour, the DoCS barrister made a speech while Mark scanned the report. Soon, he could not believe what he was reading.

Mark first scanned the psychologist's CV and noticed the department had employed her in the past for over five years. Didn't that disqualify her from preparing this report? He read on to find she had written a half page about Mark's goal of maintaining ecological sustainability on his property. She referred to his interest in Allan Savory's books on wildlife biology and sustainable ecology as: *He [Mark] did appear to have an extremely strong belief system that appeared to be derived from a number of sources that were not mainstream in origin.*

Mark thought this defied belief; if reading books on environmental sustainability made him alternative, then the whole world was alternative along with him these days.

The next page was devoted to the family's alleged religion. The psychologist seemed frustrated at not being able to religiously stereotype the family. She stated that if given more time, she would have explored the issue further. Of Sarah's illness, she incorrectly stated:

> *She has been diagnosed as suffering from Stage 3 germ cell cancer. Conventional medical opinion apparently gives the possible cure for the cancer as being in the realm of 80–85% with 4–6 cycles of chemotherapy being the standard form of treatment.*

Further in the report, the psychologist noted Sarah to be a stressed child, but attributed this to her parents' alleged belief systems, claiming that Sarah wanted only to please them when she said she didn't want the chemotherapy. She reported that Sarah 'believes that further chemotherapy will harm her' and that she 'cannot seem to make sense of why the doctors are trying to give her chemotherapy if it is going to hurt her, and she appears to be struggling to integrate this information'.

No wonder Sarah was confused when the oncologists made diametrically opposing claims. First, they told her she would be cured and live to be a ripe age, then the cancer would kill her without chemo, then the chemo could kill her too, and then that even with the chemo she could die. Mark thought this circular argument was enough to confuse anyone. That's why he had wanted hard scientific evidence the treatment would work in Sarah's case. However, Sarah wasn't confused about the chemo's side effects at all; she had already endured them and she knew she wanted no more.

About the parents, the report said: *Mark and Dianne do not appear to be suffering from a mental illness, however they appear to have an extreme belief system that is unable to be swayed by clinical evidence...*

Mark wondered what kind of extreme belief system could lead doctors to force a patient to have a treatment that was shown by their own studies to be unsuccessful on that type of advanced cancer.

He looked around the courtroom. The DoCS barrister in his wig and robe still talked about Mark's family as if they were some kind of way-out hippies, and waved the psychologist's report around to prove it! Mark forced himself to ignore the Orwellian courtroom scene and continued reading the report. Even more damaging was the psychologist's assessment of Sarah. She wrote:

> *Of particular note during the current assessment was Sarah's poor performance the subtest of the WISC-III that assesses her ability to integrate information and make sense of her environment. At a chronological age of 11¾ years, Sarah's abilities were commensurate with a 7½ year old. This obviously affects the degree to which her wishes should be taken into account versus decisions to be made in her best interests...*

Mark was no psychologist, but this test compared Sarah – who had gone through the worst things a kid could endure – to average kids who were under no significant stress. It hardly seemed a fair comparison. In addition, because Sarah did not score well on her IQ test – taken just after major surgery and seven days on a morphine drip – she could lose the right to decide what was done to her own body!

Mark continued reading. The psychologist made recommendations about Sarah's care. One option she listed was foster care: '...given the right foster parent (preferably a childless woman or a childless couple) foster care may be able to provide a more 'normal' environment for Sarah where she would be able to attend mainstream schooling between treatments'.

Mark wondered what this school issue was about when it had never arisen before. They had always sent Sarah and their other kids to the local public school for 'mainstream' schooling. The only time Sarah didn't attend was when she was too sick, and then her grandmother gave her the school lessons at home. After all, Sarah had a serious cancer, so why should she ride on a bus for two hours a day and undertake a full workload when she wasn't up to it? Mark felt insulted by this reference to mainstream schooling and the implication that their home was not a 'normal environment'. He knew his family had good standing in the community and were not a family of kooks as this report was portraying them.

Mark looked up again. The barristers were now discussing where Sarah would be staying during the chemotherapy. The judge listened intently to the DoCS barrister. He had the psychologist's report in front of him and referred to the sections the DoCS barrister wanted him to read. Mark's barrister rose occasionally to make a mild defence, instead of challenging the misinformation from the other side. The child's legal representative, who was supposed to represent Sarah's wishes and views in court, suggested that the parents and family should have restrictions imposed on their visiting rights. Where did she get that idea? It was no surprise DoCS wanted this, but Mark wondered why she supported it. Sarah would be horrified to find that her legal representative had suggested to the court that they should keep her own family away from her. The scene was surreal. He could hardly believe they were saying these preposterous things about his family while he had to sit there like a bump on a log. Where was justice? Had the world gone mad?

The judge ordered a short recess. Mark asked his barrister what was going on. She admitted things were going badly in court but thought Mark should be grateful the department had not taken the other children. He wondered whether she believed what was in that report.

After a five minute recess, the judge returned to issue his orders. He could only form an opinion based on what he had been told. First, he accepted the results of the psychological testing, meaning the court was not required to take Sarah's views into account. This denied Sarah her right to express her wishes, needs and preferences – a devastating position for a late stage cancer sufferer to be in, and one unlikely to have been imposed had the judge known that Sarah had little chance of surviving with or without the chemo.

The judge went on to grant most of the department's requests. Sarah was to be an inpatient at the hospital and have several rounds of chemotherapy, starting on Monday, 28 July. The oncology team had permission to administer any treatment they wished.

Next came the court order compelling Sarah to eat the hospital diet recommended by the hospital dietician. This diet consisted of bacon, ham and other processed meats, cream, ice cream, meat pies, soft drinks, lollies and chocolates. Not only did it seem inadequate in view of Sarah's existing nutritional deficiencies, but also, interestingly, it appears to have been the first time in Australian legal history that a Supreme Court had issued orders compelling someone to eat a junk food diet.

The next order prevented Sarah having complementary treatments. This meant she was allowed no nutritional supplements to correct her existing malnutrition.

Next came a court order preventing the parents asking any questions or disputing the necessity for the treatments the oncologist was giving.

In another devastating blow, the court ordered that Sarah's parents and all other family members were restricted to a cumulative period of two hours of visiting per day. Visits were at the staff's discretion, with the staff also empowered to impose all existing court orders with the force of the law. (The two hour restriction, in effect, meant that Sarah's time on the telephone was deducted from visiting time, and friends were not allowed to visit.)

Finally, the court ordered that failure to observe any of these orders meant the department and Sarah's legal representative would be empowered to act immediately to remove Sarah to a foster home.

Mark sat in the courtroom immobilised by disbelief as the judge adjourned the hearing and left. The DoCS barrister packed up his folders and headed home. Mark's barrister glanced over her shoulder at Mark before returning to her task of putting her papers into a briefcase. 'I'm sorry, but it's the best that could be done under the circumstances', she said.

'No. I'm sorry', replied Mark, 'you've said that before, and I disagree. More should have been done, and wasn't'.

Minutes later, Mark walked out of the Supreme Court building alone. For a while, he stood outside the main entrance gazing at the seal of Australia, cast in stainless steel, overhanging the entrance. It symbolised the country he loved, one his family had helped build from the time it first became a nation – a nation whose Constitution and rule of law guaranteed rights and freedoms to all Australians. How much more mainstream could his family be? And where was this nation headed?

Standing before the seat of justice, he wondered how his daughter could have 'lost' her human rights in that courtroom today. She no longer had the right to discuss, question or decide who should have access to her body. In the eyes of the law, her views didn't count because she didn't score high enough on a test! And now he and Di were deprived of their parental rights to voice an opinion. They couldn't even ask hospital staff a question about their daughter's treatment.

The only place Mark could speak up on Sarah's behalf was inside that courthouse – a task he had entrusted to his barrister. Now his money was spent, his family's rights had been disregarded, his back was against the wall, and he had nothing more to lose. However, he still held a deep conviction that human rights are inalienable and cannot be dispensed or withdrawn by any person. Now he had to find a way to reclaim his family's legal rights. Mark finally realised that his only hope was to represent himself. He knew nothing about being a lawyer, but he knew how to speak the plain truth.

Half an hour later, Mark sat in the rush-hour gridlock. He would be lucky to get out of the city in under an hour. Then it would take another three hours to get to the regional hospital. He reached for his mobile phone – then put it away again. He had to break this kind of news in person.

In the children's ward of the regional hospital, staff members were beginning to get edgy. They were in the office waiting for news from court.

At 4.30 pm, Di sat at Sarah's bedside wondering when she would hear from Mark. Sarah seemed content decorating cards for her friends and family. She occasionally looked out of the window to see if her father's car was in the hospital car park. Darkness fell by 5 pm and the car park disappeared into the shadows.

Earlier the dietician had been in, asking how Sarah liked the hospital diet. Sarah told her the bacon and cream every morning made her feel sick. When Di asked the dietician for more fruits and vegetables in Sarah's meals, the woman explained the diet was meant to be 'nutrient dense' to put weight on Sarah quickly. Di thought there were more nutrients in vegetables. Later, the dietician recorded Di's request for more fresh produce but noted she would leave Sarah's diet unchanged.

At 5 pm, Dr Kotz received a call from the department. Later, he came to the staff office and wrote in the notes: *Awaiting faxing of formal court orders – in essence; chemotherapy to start next week, limited access for parents, inform DoCS if any problems.*

The social worker, Caitlin Grimes had met with the staff most of the afternoon. In meetings, they had been discussing whose responsibility it was to explain the court orders to the family and how to eject the parents from the ward if necessary. Now these plans would go into effect. Staff members were made aware that the parents could question nothing about Sarah's treatment and that their directions to the family were legally enforceable. The nurse in charge alerted security staff and briefed them of the possibility that they might be called on to throw the parents out. Nurses could refuse anyone entry to

Sarah's room and have visitors ejected at their discretion with the full force of the law.

Grimes' main concern was about Sarah finding out who was behind the court orders. She thought a DoCS caseworker should tell her about her parents' restricted access. She noted that Sarah should not be told about the orders by health staff, in case she found out who was responsible for her family not being able to see her. 'If this occurs then the process for all parties will be transparent', Grimes recorded in the notes.

As it turned out, Sarah had no doubt about who was responsible.

By 8 pm, Mark arrived at the regional hospital. Staff saw him coming down the hall and reported his arrival to the others on duty. He sensed the staff watching him as he headed towards Sarah's room and it made him uncomfortable.

Once inside the room, Mark greeted Di and hugged Sarah. They were both relieved to see him, but soon saw Mark was white. He motioned for Di to come with him to the parents' room to talk privately. On the way, staff peered at them through the nurse's office window.

Is it that bad?' asked Di after Mark shut the door.

Mark nodded and told Di what had happened in court.

Soon Di was faint and asked Mark for water. He went to the water cooler and filled a paper cup for Di and one for himself.

Di took a long drink. 'Where did they get the idea that we don't feed Sarah properly, home school our kids, are part of a fundamental religion, don't go to doctors, and live like ferals?' she asked.

Mark put down the cup and scratched his head. 'I don't know where they got it from', he said. 'But it sure is working for them. Once they make us look like nutcases, they don't have to answer any more questions or produce any proof about what they're doing. They've even convinced the court to gag us'.

Di baulked. 'Couldn't we just tell –'

'They've shut us down. We're forbidden to speak about the treatment', said Mark. 'And after today, they effectively own Sarah. They can do whatever they want. She has no rights over her body'.

'But –'

Mark looked at his watch. 'We have to leave this place quickly. The two hours' visiting is up for today. Their word here is law and they can have it enforced by the police'.

Mark headed for the door, while Di stopped to look at a poster taped to the wall. Something had caught her eye. She called Mark back to look at it. It was the UN Convention on the Rights of the Child. Australia had become a signatory to the international Convention and it entered into force for Australia on 16 January 1991. The parents read the lengthy wall poster. Article 9 states:

> *3. ... Parties shall respect the right of the child who is separated from one or both parents to maintain personal relations and direct contact with both parents on a regular basis, except if it is contrary to the child's best interests.*

while article 12 states:

> *1. ...Parties shall assure to the child who is capable of forming his or her own views the right to express those views freely in all matters affecting the child, the views of the child being given due weight in accordance with the age and maturity of the child.*
> *2. ... For this purpose, the child shall in particular be provided the opportunity to be heard in any judicial and administrative proceedings affecting the child, either directly, or through a representative or an appropriate body, in a manner consistent with the procedural rules of national law.*

The parents were completely bemused. When this human rights document existed to protect children's rights, how could Sarah just have been stripped of hers? It obviously meant nothing and it evidently had no power.

At 9 pm, Mark and Di gave Sarah a brief goodbye and hurried from the ward. Their visiting time was up.

After her parents left, Sarah sat on her bed looking scared and confused. At 9.30, a nurse came in to explain the court restrictions. Sarah could not understand the meaning of it and asked whether this applied to her parents. When the nurse confirmed that it did, Sarah told her it was 'pointless'. She knew the doctors would give her chemotherapy, even without her consent, but keeping her family away was far worse. Sarah pressed her nose against the window and peered into the darkness.

'How do you feel?' asked the nurse.

Sarah blinked and wondered how the nurse would feel in her position. 'Sad', answered Sarah obligingly, but she was in complete turmoil and couldn't think straight. Over the past days, they had talked a lot about taking her away from her family. It scared her more that anything ever had.

The nurse turned the TV on and left Sarah alone. In the office, she wrote in the clinical notes: *Encouraged to talk to staff about feelings + emotions. When asked how she felt re Court's decision she shrugged shoulders + said "sad".*

That night Sarah was awake until midnight. Her mind was too noisy to sleep and without her mother beside her, the world was scary. When she finally fell into a restless sleep, she had a terrifying nightmare that was more real than her waking reality. They were coming for her. The ladies were taking her away from her family and into a dark and cold place where she would die alone. She screamed and struggled and tried to stop them, but they came anyway.

The night staff patrolled the side-rooms every hour after midnight. Sarah had the night terrors the entire night. The night nurse reported: *Quite a restless night. Lots of talking in her sleep. Becoming quite loud at times, quite verbal...*

Sarah woke up the next morning, still shaking. The fear clung to her and she desperately wanted to phone her mother. The nurse told her she could not until the oncologist gave his permission. Meanwhile Di arrived at 11 am and stayed for two hours before she had to leave again. Sarah spent the time on her mother's lap and cried when her mother left. She watched from the window as her mother waved from the car park.

From the road, Di saw Sarah sitting at the window looking lonely and distraught. Di could barely stop herself crying. She hurried into the family van and quickly drove off before she was tempted to return to the ward and give the staff a piece of her mind for subjecting her daughter to this kind of cruel and inhumane treatment.

Later that afternoon Sarah's grandparents and aunt arrived. Sarah's hopes were raised when she heard their familiar voices down the hall. Then she felt devastated again, when she heard the nurse turn them away. Sarah spent the afternoon looking out of the window to see if they were coming back, but no one came. She was inconsolable for the rest of the day.

At 6.30 pm, Harry Kotz arrived. He greeted Sarah happily and told her he would start chemotherapy in two days' time.

'Go away and leave me alone', she said.

He persisted in trying to explain to Sarah that he was doing all this in her 'best interests'. Sarah was unimpressed. She missed her family.

The nursing staff wrote of Sarah that day: *Quiet girl. Interacting with staff when engaged. However, making little effort to engage.*

That night Sarah was afraid of the terrible dream and it took her a long time to fall asleep. Only after midnight did she finally doze off.

The night nurse reported: *Observed to have nightmares overnight – calling out in sleep.*

The same nightmare had come again. It would torment her for a long time to come.

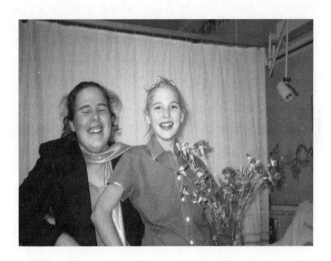

Sarah looking pale and thin - still suffering of post-operative malnutrition after transfer to regional hospital, but joyful to be reunited with her sister Laura and family again. That joy ended not long after the picture was taken when new court orders placed severe restrictions on family visits.

HOW COULD THEY DO THIS TO HER?

Regardless of society's attitudes, ensure that you do not counten-
ance, condone, or participate in the practice of torture or
Other forms of cruel, inhuman, or degrading procedures
Whatever the offence of which the Victim of such
Procedures is suspected, accused, or convicted.

Australian Medical Association Code of Ethics

July 27 was a cold winter's day, with a stiff southerly blowing up the east coast. I was just whipping up a Sunday morning pancake breakfast at home when the phone rang with a call diverted from the clinic. It was Mark. He said that since the restrictive court orders had come into effect two days ago Sarah was having constant nightmares, and he was afraid she was heading for a breakdown. She'd become more depressed each day since staff refused to allow her friends to visit and limited her immediate family to two hours. Mark said that on days when other relatives had already visited for the two-hour quota, staff had turned him and Di away. Moreover, the court orders prohibited them discussing Sarah's health or wellbeing with the doctors and staff, and they desperately needed outside help.

Mark said the family planned to visit Sarah at the hospital around 3 pm, and asked whether one of the clinic's practitioners could come along to assess the situation and perhaps play a role in helping Sarah. I told him I would discuss it with the others and it was likely someone from the clinic would be at the hospital that afternoon.

After breakfast, I had discussions with Dan Tyler, a practitioner at the clinic. As a medical doctor, Tyler was the best candidate for the job of liaising with the medical staff at the hospital. He was middle-aged and thinning on top, with an unassuming manner. Tyler had a good working knowledge of nutritional medicine, and while he was at the hospital, he planned to assess Sarah's current nutritional status, an issue the parents were concerned about.

For the clinic staff, visiting the hospital would not be without its perils. The clinic team wanted to check on Sarah without irritating the hospital's medical team. On one hand, we had a responsibility to Sarah, who was our patient, and on the other hand, we were obliged to maintain cordial relationships with fellow professionals. It would not be easy in this case where tensions already existed between the parents and hospital staff.

At around 4 pm that afternoon, Dan Tyler arrived at the regional hospital. He found Sarah in her room looking fearful and on the verge of tears. The nursing staff had just ordered the family to leave at the end of restricted visiting hours. When the grandparents left the room with Sarah's four sisters and brother, Sarah became anxious at the prospect of her parents leaving next. She burst into tears and hung onto her mother's skirt while the nurses continued to order the parents out of the ward, reminding them that staff orders were now legally enforceable. The parents were only too aware that the staff's word was law but they were unable to unlatch their daughter from themselves. She had fastened herself onto Di's clothing in a blind panic. When staff continued issuing orders, Sarah became more distressed and clung more tightly to her mother. Di asked for a few minutes with Sarah to calm her down but nurses refused this and prised Sarah off her mother instead. The nurses then told the parents to leave immediately. Mark and Di scuttled out of the room and joined the other family members in the cafeteria just outside the ward's entrance.

After Sarah's parents left, staff ordered Dr Tyler to leave. As Sarah's doctor, Tyler was somewhat offended by this and was also reluctant to leave out of concern for Sarah who was in an obviously distressed state. He lingered long enough to offer some reassurances but Sarah was too agitated to listen. She rushed to the window and frantically searched for signs of her family on the road outside. Tyler had never seen a child so frightened before and wanted to stay long enough to offer further words of comfort, but the staff was adamant he leave immediately.

In the hallway outside the ward, Sarah's siblings were crying and the entire family was upset by the experience. The group sat down at a table in the cafeteria where the parents planned to comfort their other children before setting out on the long trip home. The adults were so shaken by the ordeal that none were able to drive a vehicle until they had calmed down. Mark ordered cups of tea for the adults and juice for the children. A few minutes later, Dan Tyler joined them after emerging from the ward, looking somewhat ruffled himself.

While the group was in the cafeteria, the nurses tried unsuccessfully to interact with Sarah in her room but she would not leave the window, from which she frantically searched for her family outside. Staff turned on the TV as a distraction and left Sarah alone in her room, assuming she would forget all about her family and watch a show. As usual, TV did not work on Sarah. Instead, she became more agitated, feeling claustrophobically confined in her room. In no time, she had an uncontrollable urge to escape from the hospital. She wanted to catch up with her family and go home with them. Soon Sarah gave in to her impulse and burst full speed from her room. As she bolted down the corridor past the nurse's desk, the head nurse clutched her arm, but Sarah pulled away.

'Leave me alone. I want to go home', Sarah screamed as she sprinted toward the children's ward exit.

While two other nurses chased behind Sarah, the head nurse phoned hospital security and told them to come to the children's ward urgently. Then she called the social worker at home, who immediately phoned the after-hours DoCS caseworker. After placing the calls, the head nurse followed the other staff down the corridor.

Once through the ward doors, Sarah had turned left and headed down the corridor toward the hospital's main entrance, which led out into the car park. While darting past the cafeteria, Sarah was surprised and relieved to encounter her family there. She ran to them and buried herself in her mother's lap. 'Please don't leave me here', she cried. 'I don't want to go to a foster home. I don't want to be alone'.

Sarah huddled in Di's arms while Ruth and Jim protectively gathered up the two terrified youngest children, Leah and Joshua. The siblings were distressed to see their sister in such a state. They had seen what happened to their sister and they wondered if staff might lock them up in hospital too. Laura tried to comfort Hannah and Clara while Mark and Di worked to calm Sarah down.

Moments later, several nurses converged on the group. They demanded Sarah return to the ward immediately and repeated that their instructions were the law and must be obeyed. Mark wished they could be left alone for just a few moments to calm their daughter down. He was sure they could persuade Sarah to return to her room if only the staff would tread more softly. Instead, the nurses were behaving like a riot squad, with not one using any common sense.

Dan Tyler sat at the table watching Mark tensing up. He leaned towards Mark to suggest he should make himself scarce to avoid trouble with the staff, who clearly felt over-empowered. Tyler said he would try to calm the situation in his absence. Mark agreed, but it took him every ounce of willpower to leave the scene and make his way into a quiet alcove. From his vantage point, he watched staff surround Sarah while shouting their previous orders and threatening to have security remove the family from the hospital. Each loud threat worsened Sarah's terror. In despair, Mark looked away and glimpsed a painting on the wall. The large canvas, painted by an Iraqi artist, depicted images of emaciated and sad-looking children behind barbed wire. The scene was of a desert detention centre, typical of the ones that had sprung up around the Australian outback under the Howard administration, where illegal immigrant detainees were imprisoned for years while waiting for their visas, which in many cases were never granted. This haunting image, combined with his daughter's cries and his other children wailing, would be burnt into Mark's memory for life.

The tension escalated as more staff arrived and tried to prise Sarah away from her mother. Two burly security guards joined the group. Without introducing themselves, they started pulling on Sarah, but she clung even tighter and let out screams. The violence terrified other visitors to the cafeteria, who moved away from the scene.

Since Sarah did not know who these men were or what they intended to do to her, she tried to fight them off. 'Leave me alone or I'll kill myself', she cried while gripping more tightly onto her mother.

The guards grabbed Sarah's arms and dragged her from Di by force. The men then tried to manhandle Sarah back to the ward but she struggled loose and stood facing them off in the hallway. The nightmarish scene playing out in the hospital corridor for the public was of a tiny frightened girl being ripped from her mother by two guards, who then tried fending off the men herself.

Sarah's siblings were horrified and the littlest ones wailed and shouted to the men to leave their sister alone.

Dr Tyler watched the face-off between the two guards and Sarah and placed himself between them. Once there, he volunteered to take Sarah back to her room. The guards seemed aggressively opposed to his suggestion, but when Sarah was surprisingly willing to accompany him, they pulled back from further physical action. Sarah told the nurses she would return if they allowed her to say goodbye to her family. The nurses weren't happy about it, but reluctantly agreed. Moments later, Dr Tyler accompanied Sarah back to the ward – closely followed by the two unhappy security guards and a bevy of disgruntled nursing staff.

Once Sarah was back in her room, staff unceremoniously told Dr Tyler to leave. Despite receiving marching orders, he stayed long enough to watch the staff rifling through Sarah's belongings. They searched for any object she could have used to commit suicide. They found only children's books and stuffed toys, coloured paper and glue. They confiscated the handicraft materials Sarah had used to decorate the cards and letters she wrote to her family – her last source of comfort – and also the vitamins and minerals that had been prescribed by the clinic doctor as part of her nutritional support protocol when she had first arrived there as a patient. When they'd finished, the staff moved Sarah to a room next to the nurse's station where a 24-hour special nurse was assigned to watch her closely. The day after tomorrow she was scheduled to have chemotherapy, and the staff would allow nothing to interfere with that.

The family drove the long trip home in the mini-van, still reeling from shock. The grandparents sat next to the two youngest children, whose faces were tearstained. The older three girls were stunned and on the verge of tears themselves.

'That's the first time I've ever seen guards stand over a child in this country', said Ruth from the back seat. 'It's disgusting. She just wanted a minute to say goodbye to her parents'.

After arriving home that evening, the parents' first task was to comfort their other children.

'Is Sarah in jail?' asked Hannah.

No. She's in a hospital', replied Di as she prepared a light supper.

'How come they won't let her outside then?'

'Good question, Grub', replied Mark on Di's behalf. 'It's one we don't really know the answer to'.

Both Mark and Di struggled to explain why their daughter was a detainee in a hospital and treated like a prisoner – manhandled, deprived of her liberty, refused open access to air and exercise, prohibited her normal diet and denied the comfort of her family and friends.

The parents got little sleep that night.

'Do you know what Sarah asked me today during our visit?' asked Mark in the middle of the night.

Di was afraid to hear it. 'What?' she asked cautiously.

'She said she wasn't afraid of dying, only afraid of losing us. She only cared about being with us and nothing else mattered to her. She asked me what she had done so wrong that they would not let her see her family and friends'.

After talking until late Sunday night, Mark and Di resolved to phone the clinic the next day. They wanted staff to liaise with the oncologist and monitor Sarah's physical and emotional condition for the entire time she was involuntarily confined at the hospital.

The following day proved a busy one in the children's ward at the regional hospital. In her room, Sarah lay in bed feeling miserable, with a special nurse – allocated just to her – watching her every move. Staff had summoned the children's psychiatrist to assess her after her threat to commit suicide the previous day.

The next morning, the psychiatrist came to the ward and read Sarah's clinical notes. Since he was foremost a doctor who specialised in psychiatry, he would have gleaned from the medical information that Sarah had late stage metastatic cancer. This fact would have necessarily informed his approach to Sarah, since children with a condition expected to end their lives have special needs for compassion and understanding.

At mid morning, the psychiatrist conducted a lengthy interview with Sarah in her room. He started by asking her how she liked being in hospital. Sarah told him she missed her family, and that her friends were not allowed to visit at all. She felt cooped up in her hospital room. She was an 'outdoors' person who was used to being in a natural environment with fresh air, but the staff would not allow her outside, even for a minute. She also said she did not want the chemotherapy they were about to give her. The first three-day round of it had made her sicker than before and she was still sick from it. The doctor took copious notes and later wrote in the clinical records:

> *Believes that chemo makes her sick. Believes that she was given too much chemo in Sydney as she had been told that her nose bleeding for 3 days was an indication she had been given too much. Believes she nearly died during chemo with trouble breathing afterwards, weight loss, thought she would bleed to death or choke with her nosebleed. Worried about her skin markings. Had trouble with her back being bent forward and in pain with chemo, as well. Puzzled about the cancer in her spleen – how it could have grown so fast or was it seen earlier? Describes her family as a close family. She presents as a pleasant girl who is reluctant to have chemo because of its side effects and no guarantee of being cured.*

The doctor finished the interview, evidently without exploring Sarah's reasons for wanting to commit suicide the day before, when she had never before spoken of self-harm outside the hospital setting. Nor did he explore her feelings about having treatments physically forced on her.

To Sarah, it felt that all her wishes and views were invalidated – as indeed they had been, legally, by the Supreme Court – and that her basic needs and comforts were being denied. To Sarah the treatment felt like torture, and her family's comforting presence was something she could not imagine living without. Now that she was closer to home she had looked forward to seeing her friends again, but staff refused to allow them to visit. From her point of view, she was locked in a prison where those in power did whatever they pleased to her. Her sense of powerlessness and the fear of losing her family were utterly terrifying.

By the end of the session, the psychiatrist did not indicate that he had assessed Sarah for post-traumatic stress disorder (PTSD), a likely possibility in view of Sarah's extreme circumstances and her symptom of nightly terrors. Instead, the psychiatrist's visit seemed designed only to facilitate the planned chemotherapy the following day.

That morning Dan Tyler arrived at the clinic still upset by the previous day's visit to the hospital. He had been initially sceptical when Mark contacted us on the after-hours number claiming Sarah was not having her most basic needs met. He had intended only to briefly check on Sarah and expected to find everything in order. To his surprise, he walked in on the most disturbing scene he had ever witnessed in a general hospital. From what he saw, staff had treated Sarah in a degrading and threatening way when a kinder approach was warranted for a child in her condition. He saw that Sarah was deeply distressed. She looked unnaturally pale and emaciated, and clearly suffered from malnutrition. This meant some urgent action was needed, but it would have to be the appropriate action for all concerned.

Later that day, the team at the clinic called a meeting to discuss the complicated issues involved in Sarah's predicament and to decide what could reasonably be done. On one hand, Sarah was a patient of the clinic and we had a duty of care towards her. In accordance with the Australian Medical Association Code of Ethics, we were required to consider first her wellbeing and to treat her with respect and compassion at all times, as we had done when she presented to us as a patient. However, now Sarah was involuntarily consigned to a specialist's treatment in a hospital and bound by a raft of court orders, which the oncologist interpreted in a manner that clearly caused torment to the patient and her family. This meant that theoretically, if not practically, Sarah was being detained as involuntarily as any prisoner. In that case, what were her rights? The parents were legitimately concerned about the conditions and treatment imposed on Sarah, claiming it denied her the most basic human and civil rights. On this legal issue, we could not comment, but on the medical issues, the AMA

Code of Ethics states that the patient's right to complain must be upheld and efforts made to resolve the issue. This gave us some encouragement to continue monitoring Sarah's condition. On the other hand, the AMA Code of Ethics also obliged us to report any suspected unethical or unprofessional conduct by a colleague to the appropriate peer review body. This option put us into a delicate situation of inviting unwanted hostility from colleagues at such an early stage.

By the end of the meeting, we decided on a soft and diplomatic approach. Dan Tyler would request an appointment with the oncologist and discuss the issues with him as a fellow professional in a calm and rational way and in a peer setting. Tyler made the call to the oncologist that afternoon. Dr Kotz reluctantly gave him an appointment in two weeks' time. Meanwhile, Tyler asked Kotz to provide him with a study that supported the efficacy of the chemotherapy he was intending to continue using on Sarah. Kotz referred him to a UK study, which he said supported his treatment.

The next day was July 29. The children's ward at the regional hospital was crowded with department caseworkers from both regional DoCS offices at Taree and Cardiff. In the two months since the department had been involved with Sarah and her family, scores of personnel from several offices – both regional and head office in Sydney – had been actively on the case. This included top-ranking department bureaucrats and even the Director-General himself.

The NSW (DoCS) child protection department has frequently complained of a lack of funds and resources, and requested additional billion dollar funding packages from the NSW State Parliament over and above its annual budget (the annual budget for the fiscal year 2010, for example, has blown out to over 1.6 billion dollars).

In 2003, when Sarah's situation occurred, the total population of NSW was 6.6 million. Of that figure, the number of children in the state aged between 0 and 15 came to 1 320 000. That year, the NSW child protection department was allocated a budget of over $803 million, with an extra 1.2 billion dollar grant in the pipeline from the state Parliament. This represents one of the highest per capita child protection budgets in the Western world, and it has in turn funded the legalistic, statutory enforcement-based system of child protection currently in force in NSW. This police-and court-orientated system has resulted in the state having among the highest numbers of children removed from their families and placed into State care in the Western world.[30] It means that NSW families who do not abuse or neglect their children are at the greatest risk in the developed world of having their children taken away by the State. This is the case if they encounter any type of crisis or stress or if they are simply reported to the department. And yet, despite these unprecedented numbers, a child in NSW is twice as likely to die from abuse or neglect as a child in neighbouring Victoria, a state that removes relatively few children from their homes into State care. In other words, in NSW, the children removed from their families are not necessarily the ones at risk of harm.

In Victoria, the child protection budget is primarily spent on prevention and supportive services for children and families in need or under stress. By comparison, the statutory enforcement-based system of NSW appears driven by an excessively powerful bureaucracy, which despite many complaints about it to parliament, has steadfastly resisted any change. The NSW model of child protection has already resulted in human rights violations being reported to the United Nations, and it is threatening to bring Australia into international disrepute if it is not effectively addressed. The United Nations Committee on the Rights of the Child has already registered its concern in October 2005 about Australia's: 'considerable increase in the number of children in out-of-home care in recent years...'

For the state of New South Wales' three million or so taxpayers, the billions of dollars in revenue consumed by DoCS annually has represented a heavy burden while its social value has frequently been questioned by various NSW authorities, including the Liberal party and the Ombudsman. The scores of DoCS caseworkers involved with Sarah all earned base salaries of between $51 000 and $70 000. These high-salaried personnel were allocated to force a treatment on a single 11-year old girl with a terminal illness, while over the same period 76 children in New South Wales died of genuine abuse and neglect after concerned persons made reports to DoCS about the children and they were not acted on. [31] These ill-fated children could easily have been helped but had no funds or resources allocated to their needs.

---

[30] Submission into the Special Commission of Enquiry into Child Protection Services in NSW by the NSW Parliamentary Liberals/National Coalition.
[31] NSW Ombudsman 2003.

Meanwhile, the department's focus on Sarah showed no signs of abating. At the hospital, the department scheduled three meetings in one day. The first meeting included caseworkers, the hospital social worker and nursing staff. Caitlin Grimes recorded the outcome of that meeting in the records. Her entry repeated her earlier ones instructing staff to call security to have the family thrown out should they pose any 'difficulties'. In that event, another court hearing would be scheduled to assess 'whether the parents can continue to visit'.

After a tea break, a second meeting was convened between the hospital social worker, DoCS caseworkers, and Di, Ruth and Jim, who drove a lengthy distance to attend it.

The third meeting was held immediately after the second and included the oncologist, who had refused to speak to the parents or grandparents alone without department caseworkers being present. The doctor had evidently requested the department's protection from Di, a tiny woman, and the two elderly grandparents, with 70-year old Jim being somewhat frail. Mark did not attend the session for fear he would speak his mind and pay for it.

Di recalls that the meetings included no two-way discussions. The staff and the oncologist merely lectured to them and when she asked the doctor a question, the caseworkers reminded her gloatingly that the court order forbade her to question anything the staff did.

After enduring this lengthy session, Di, Jim and Ruth were allowed to visit with Sarah for a short while. But staff cut this visit short by the number of minutes that Sarah, who had a desperate need to connect with people who loved her, had used up talking on the phone that morning. To make matters worse, a caseworker had been installed in Sarah's room to record each word and facial expression the family produced during their visit. Sarah was irritated with the caseworker for intruding on her privacy and her time with her family. She began to feel anxious long before it was time for family to leave. With the prospect of chemotherapy later that day, Sarah had no way of knowing whether a member of her family would be allowed to comfort her while they again forced the drugs on her against her will.

After the DoCS meeting at the hospital, Caitlin Grimes wrote up the clinical notes:

Outcomes July 29, 2003:

DoCS to attend the hospital twice a week for updates on Sarah's medical condition with Dr Kotz. This will be shared by DoCS Taree and Cardiff. These meetings will be an opportunity for Dr Kotz to meet with Sarah's parents. And discuss her treatment. Dr Kotz not to talk with parents unless DoCS present, as requested by Dr Kotz.

It has been decided that all contact between Sarah and her parents is supervised...Nursing staff will supervise this initially during Sarah's chemo and then DoCS Cardiff will provide supervisors. Nursing staff are not required to intervene during supervision of parent's [sic] visits in the next couple of days but must document any inappropriate comments.

Parents to provide a list of visitors that can visit Sarah. No one outside the immediate family can visit.

The two hours contact that Sarah has with her family is inclusive of phone calls.

Sarah to be seen by the social worker, psychiatrist, play therapist and to attend the hospital school. We will look at having Sarah monitored with youth workers.

Mark stayed away from the hospital meeting. Instead, he tried to catch up on the work that had built up on the farm in the weeks they were in Sydney with Sarah. Slowly he and Di were making a home again for their other children, but everything seemed different now. The kids were sad since their family's disruption and they constantly worried about DoCS coming to take them away.

Outside in the paddocks were no more cattle, except for Brutus who also seemed sad and lonely since all the other cattle had gone and the kids weren't around to play with him. Mark had had to sell the entire herd to pay the $38 000 legal bills. On top of that, his dozer was gone. He'd used it to create swimming holes for the kids and dams for the wildlife. It hurt him as much to sell the dozer as it did to sell the cattle, but he had no choice.

Later that day, he planned a trip to Gloucester to see the bank manager. He needed to borrow money for the constant expenses imposed on the family by DoCS. They'd tied him up in court for months and he suspected they planned more of the same. Even though he could afford no more lawyers or barristers, he still had to take the time off work to prepare his affidavits – and the family had to eat. Mark suspected that the DoCS barrister knew by then that he was at the end of his financial tether, which made him suspect the department would put the screws on even tighter. He would need this borrowed money just to survive the next few months. The rest of their savings and their cattle herd had been wiped out and had long since disappeared down the deep hole of litigation.

Borrowing money was foreign to Mark's conservative nature, which compelled him to save up the money before he bought anything. He didn't even know how to ask a bank manager for money, but he thought he would just tell it like it is and hope for the best. On his way home, he planned to pick up some gyprock sheets to finish the internal wall in a guestroom he'd started building at the beginning of the year when there had still been a sense of hope in their lives.

With his morning chores out of the way, Mark chained up Muttley and Pooch and returned to lock the house doors before setting out in the utility.

Half an hour later, he sat in the bank manager's office telling the man his story. The manager looked at Mark sympathetically. He had known Mark's parents since he was a boy, and had heard on the grapevine that something was going on with Sarah.

'You've got a good job, which makes you a good risk', said the manager. 'I'll extend you a line of credit. But there's a limit to the number of times I can do this, so I hope you find a solution to your current troubles as soon as possible'.

Mark left the bank feeling a mixture of relief and humiliation, but he felt even worse when he stopped at the hardware store for the gyprock sheets. He had to rack them up on credit until the fresh loan money showed up in his bank account. Just thinking about getting into debt made Mark tense.

With a load of plasterboard strapped to the utility, Mark returned to the farm. As soon as he drove past the mailbox, he heard the dogs making a racket. As if something or someone had stirred them up, they barked wildly when he drove up to the house. Over the noise, Mark heard the phone ringing inside. He sprinted up the veranda steps with his keys ready to open the deadlock, but the door was already ajar. He couldn't possibly have left that unlocked, he thought. Mark dashed to the phone and answered it gruffly. The kitchen clock showed 4.15 pm. It was Di. The edgy sound of her voice alarmed him even more.

'They're starting chemo in a few minutes', she said.

'How's Sarah?'

'She told them she doesn't want it. They said they're doing it anyway. Thank goodness they're letting me be with her for a while, but probably not for long'.

Mark felt raw. 'Tell her to hang in there', he said. 'Tell her we love her'.

After Di hung up, Mark stared at the open doors. He was enraged at those faceless bureaucrats who had brought this nightmare on his family. Infuriated, he rushed outside and leapt up on the back of the utility. From there, he hurled the plasterboard on the ground. He didn't care when several sheets broke; he was just so angry. DoCS was playing a terrifying game of wits with him and the stakes were his family. He should have taken them all overseas when he'd had the chance, or even fled to another state where they didn't have this insane system. He'd never heard of a child protection department operating this way: harassing families, wearing them down in court, breaking them up, bankrupting families instead of helping them and interfering with people's medical choices. The 'best interests of the child' seemed nothing more than a front for tossing out children's rights, human rights and family rights while the State made orphans out of children with perfectly good homes. Well, he wasn't going to allow it anymore.

Mark leaped off the utility and strode to the shed to fetch his chainsaw. From there, he tossed it on the back of the utility and let the dogs off their chains. Whatever had set them off put Mark in the same foul mood.

'Those mongrels are not going to come on my property again', he growled as he slammed shut the utility door.

With the dogs on the back, Mark drove the ute down the thickly timbered bush track, headed for a dead ironbark tree he had marked out for firewood. The tree had been hit by lightening and was half split and hazardous. Moments later, he revved up the chainsaw and cut the hardwood tree into pieces, making tidy work of it in under an hour. After the last cut, Mark was covered in sweat and sat down to rest on the stump. There, he wept out the rest of his bitter frustration. The dogs seemed to understand and lay quietly down beside him. When he was finished, he looked out over his property. The hills and valleys were silent now, devoid of their lifeblood cattle. The threesome sat there for a while. Mark felt something inside him changing and hardening. This was a fight for his family's life, and DoCS was as serious a threat to their freedom and survival as anything that had ever happened to his forebears. He was going to put a stop to it and find a way to free Sarah from their control. He made this solemn promise to his family and to Sarah before driving away with the dogs, leaving the timber on the ground to cure.

When Mark returned to the house, the children were just coming off the school bus. In the kitchen, Mark put the kettle on while the kids raided the fridge for an after-school snack. Laura made sure they each had something to eat and waited until the little ones were out of earshot before talking to her father.

'How's Sarah today?' she asked.

'They're giving her chemo as we speak', answered Mark.

Laura looked discouraged. Only days ago she had witnessed her sister threaten suicide, and she still wasn't over the shock of it. 'That's not what Sarah wanted. She wanted the treatment without the side effects. And she wanted to be at home with us'. Laura shook her head. 'How could they do this to her?'

At 4.15 pm, the nurse in the children's ward hung the first bag of intravenous chemotherapy while Sarah sat on her mother's lap looking anxious. Sarah told the nurse for the umpteenth time that she did not want it, but the nurse told her she was going to inject it into her anyway through the cannula in her arm. She added for good measure that if Sarah didn't sit still for it, her mother would be asked to leave.

In the corner sat a caseworker whose job it was to watch Di. Sarah resented the woman's stares and did her best to ignore her. The nurse turned on the IV. After a minute, Sarah looked at the IV bag curiously. It was different from the previous ones she'd had. This had no colour and when it flowed into her vein, it had little or no effect compared to the previous ones.

'I think they gave me just saline this time', whispered Sarah to her mother.

The caseworker became alarmed and ordered Sarah to stop whispering. A short time later, Di was told to go home and Sarah was left alone.

To soothe herself while the IV was running, Sarah lay on her bed and fixed her gaze on the grove of gum trees outside her window. The new room she had been transferred to after her suicide threat had an observation window adjoining the nurse's station. From there the nurses, the social worker or visiting caseworkers watched her constantly – when they weren't in her room peering at her. On the ceiling was a strange looking bubble that looked like an eye, and on the wall were perforated panels that looked like speakers. This new room felt creepy and Sarah asked the caseworker to return her paper and coloured pencils to her – she wanted to make drawings to cover the observation windows. The woman turned on the TV instead and insisted Sarah watch a sitcom.

The next day, nurses brought in the next batch of IV bags with chemotherapy. This time, when the fluid reached Sarah's vein she was overcome with nausea and vomited over herself and the bed. She'd had a stomach full of chocolate bars the nurses had given her to help her 'accept' the chemotherapy and put on weight. The staff was so intent on putting weight on Sarah that they often refused to interact with her until she had eaten a chocolate bar or lolly. For the rest of the day Sarah lay sick in bed. In the late afternoon, the social worker came to visit. Sarah always knew when Caitlin Grimes was approaching her room – her high heels made a loud clicking noise on the vinyl corridor.

The social worker looked pleased when she saw Sarah. She said she wanted to 'explore' Sarah's 'feelings'. Unfortunately, Sarah had confided in Grimes before and had found that everything she had told the young social worker in strictest confidence had been passed on to the oncologist. When Sarah didn't answer the social worker's questions, Grimes gave her a small cosmetic case with half a dozen lip glosses in it to help her with her 'acceptance'. Over the next few weeks, Grimes brought in presents of beads, toys, a cosmetic case, a school bag, and even a promise to send her to Disneyland (which never eventuated) if Sarah would only voluntarily accept the chemotherapy. However, Sarah never agreed.

The nurses came around regularly for the rest of the day to record Sarah's vital signs. When the TV was off, the staff invariably turned it on before they left. Sarah spent the remainder of the evening feeling sick to the tune of noisy commercials for breakfast cereal, mobile phones and laxatives in the background.

The next day, the breakfast tray came up with the usual bacon and cream to fatten her up. She felt nauseated by its sight and smell and quickly replaced the metal cover. Not long after, nurses came with another two bags of IV chemotherapy. As usual, Sarah told the nurses she wanted no more, but they routinely told her she would have it anyway. By then, Sarah was unable to move without pain and fatigue and lay listlessly in bed on the drip with the caseworker looking on.

Later that day the social worker came again. She talked to Sarah in an artificially happy voice, telling her how much better she was. Sarah turned her head away. Grimes told her that she was expected to go to the hospital school, now that he was better. Sarah told her she felt too sick to go to school.

'It will be good for you', said Grimes. 'I'll make arrangements for you to go down tomorrow'.

The following day, the nurse took Sarah down to the schoolroom. She looked so ill that the hospital schoolteacher felt sorry for her and allowed her back to the ward. The teacher wondered what was going on and went upstairs to Sarah's room a few days later. There, she coincidentally encountered Di and Sarah's sisters, who were visiting. While out of the caseworker's earshot, the teacher asked Di what was going on with Sarah. She asked why – when she was so sick and miserable – Sarah had been sent down to school. Di could only explain a fraction of the story before the caseworker intervened. This ended the conversation, but left the teacher with an expression on her face of shocked compassion for Sarah. This made no difference, however; the staff insisted Sarah go to school anyway.

While waiting for the appointment to see Dr Kotz, Dan Tyler decided to pay a visit to the hospital to monitor Sarah's health. The clinic team scheduled a meeting to decide how best this could be done. We knew the caseworkers' monitoring of Sarah would be so stifling that it would restrict her freedom to express her thoughts and feelings during our visit. Since my background is in paediatrics, I suggested Dan take a can of play dough with him and simply spend some time with Sarah engaged in a neutral activity.

Later that afternoon, Dan set out on the lengthy trip to the regional hospital. When he arrived in Sarah's room, he was shocked to find her looking obviously unwell and lying listlessly in bed. In the chair beside her sat the DoCS caseworker, who recorded each word and facial expression coming from Dan, from the moment he entered the room. Dan found Sarah almost mute and reluctant to communicate; due to the almost hostile presence of the caseworker, he found the experience more than a little unnerving himself. Dan was unaware however, that the department was in the process of preparing another court hearing to have him eliminated from the scene entirely. This would prevent him independently monitoring Sarah in the future.

Between chemotherapy rounds, Di brought Sarah's sisters to visit. On one occasion, staff gave Sarah permission to go the cafeteria located in the hallway just outside the ward's entrance for a hot chocolate with her sisters. Sarah shuffled down the hall with Laura, Clara and Hannah, who were all delighted to spend some time with their sister. Behind them followed the caseworker with her writing pad. When the girls sat down at the cafeteria table, the caseworker muscled in between them. While the girls tried to chat, the caseworker wrote furiously in her notebook about their body language and what they'd said. In a few minutes the girls' chatter subsided, with none of them having the courage to say another word. They all sat in stunned silence and finished their drinks. The occasion was ruined and the girls returned to the ward feeling sad and disappointed. Back in her room, Sarah pulled the curtains around her bed to give her a private moment with her sisters. However, the caseworker immediately squeezed inside the curtain with them and sat in the confined space, continuing to take notes. Di took Sarah's siblings home soon after and they paused in the car park to wave at the lonely figure of Sarah sitting at the hospital window.

The next three days of chemotherapy came around all too soon. This time Sarah suffered more serious side effects. On the first day, she was so ill that she refused to go to school. By the second day of chemotherapy, she was far too ill to complete her homework, even from her bed, and on the third day, she lay in bed listlessly looking out of the window. The present round of treatments had triggered painful migraines so severe that Sarah banged her head against the bed-head in an attempt to stop them. The staff offered her a paracetamol tablet but it had no effect. She declined future offers of the tablet since it was useless against the severe pain. Staff offered her no stronger pain reliever or any other medications for these agonising episodes.

Despite her obvious serious illness, nurses came in regularly to convince Sarah to attend the hospital school, but Sarah still refused to go. This annoyed the staff, who thought she was being deliberately disobedient, and they responded by putting her under more pressure to attend. However, Sarah insisted she was too sick and told them she had trouble concentrating – a likely problem in a late stage cancer patient undergoing a gruelling treatment. Despite this, staff raised the issue in the twice-weekly meetings with the DoCS caseworkers. As a result, the hospital social worker was called in to convince Sarah. During her visit, she told Sarah it was 'good' for her to go to school and that the issue was non-negotiable in any event – Sarah was legally required to attend school. When Sarah still refused, the social worker called in the psychiatrist.

Later that day the children's psychiatrist turned up to conduct a psychoanalysis session. Sarah told him she was too ill to go to school – a fact already obvious to many, including her family, the school teacher, and Dr Tyler. After a lengthy session of psychoanalysis, the psychiatrist concluded Sarah should go to school regardless how she felt. If she did not comply, he intended to phone her mother about it. About Sarah's explanations and feelings, the psychiatrist was clearly unmoved. On returning to the office, he wrote: *Sarah has at times been quite oppositional about school and sometimes quite lazy. Our school staff will talk to her parents.*

It was Di who took the psychiatrist's phone call at home. She listened intently as he told her that Sarah had been unco-operative about attending school in the past few days. Di was shocked to hear that the hospital had pressured Sarah to go to school when she was so obviously seriously unwell.

'Will you convince Sarah to co-operate with us on this issue?' asked the psychiatrist.

Di paused for a lengthy time. 'Well, if you ask me, I believe Sarah is too sick to go to school right now'.

'I'm disappointed to hear that', said the psychiatrist. 'In that case, we will have our staff speak to her about it'.

Di hung up and sat down immediately.

Mark had just come inside from mending the fences. 'Who was that?' he asked.

'The hospital'.

'What did they want?'

Di's eyes watered up. 'Every time I visit Sarah these days she's sicker and weaker than before. That girl is dying right in front of our eyes. Now they're forcing her to go to school. How sick does a kid have to be to get a day off?'

Mark took off his gloves and placed them on the kitchen table. He rubbed his hands over the iron stove to warm them up. 'It's disgusting', he said. 'This torment is shortening what life she has left'.

Back at the hospital, Sarah was forced to attend the afternoon session of school.

The following day Di was visiting under the DoCS caseworker's supervision. Di and Sarah both heard Grimes' high heels on the lino, and braced themselves. The attractive young social worker appeared in the doorway demanding to know why Sarah had not attended school lately and why she hadn't been to school at the Sydney-based hospital. Di explained that Sarah had become critically ill just after her admission to the city hospital and had nearly died as a result of the operation and its serious complications. However, Di's explanations did nothing to move Grimes, who wrote in the notes later that day:

> *Sarah refusing to go to school yesterday morning, however I understand that she went in the afternoon. I discussed the issue of Sarah refusing to attend school with her mother. Sarah's mum said that she had not gone to school in Sydney as she was 'too sick'. I explained to her that it was important for Sarah to keep up with her school work and that this had particular benefits for Sarah's self esteem. Mum acknowledged this however she did not appear concerned at Sarah's refusal. I invited Mum to attend a meeting with Dr Kotz and DoCS on Thursday at 1 pm.*

How Could They Do This To Her?

The following Thursday, Di attended the weekly meeting with the case-workers and hospital staff. She regretted it as soon as she sat down. The staff took it as an opportunity to lecture her again about Sarah's reluctance to go to school. The social worker talked about Sarah's self-esteem and said it would be higher if she went to school. It wasn't Sarah's self-esteem Di was worried about, however – she was concerned for her daughter's survival if someone in that hospital didn't start treating her with some humanity. Unfortunately, because of the court order, Di was unable to voice her concerns. She sat through the lengthy session and left as soon as she could. Unfortunately, when she returned to the ward she found that her visiting hours had been shortened by the amount of time she had spent in the meeting. Di was turned away and could only wave from the car park to Sarah, who stood at the window looking gloomy.

Behind Sarah, the caseworker sat silently in her chair watching and making notes.

The nights tormented Sarah most during the next round of chemotherapy. She missed her family and lay awake in pain and whimpering, just like the children who had been her roommates at the other hospital. She wanted the pain to stop, but it got worse with each bag of chemotherapy. Now she couldn't sleep because her skin was red and burnt. When she did fall asleep, the terrifying dreams came back. Each time, it was the same nightmare: they came to steal her from her family. She kicked and screamed and tried to stop them but they took her anyway.

That night Sarah felt trapped between the pain in her body while awake and the fearful nightmare she knew would come if she slept. She could find no way out of her dilemma and began to cry with deep sobs. It was 10 pm when the night nurse came in and asked her what the matter was. Sarah hadn't seen this nurse before. Late at night, there were no caseworkers sitting in her room and Sarah desperately needed to talk to someone.

'You can tell me Sarah. It's alright. I won't tell anybody else', said the nurse.

Sarah's physical and emotional pain was so intense that she momentarily opened herself to trusting someone with her feelings. It had been months since she had seen her friends or been outside in the open air and sunshine. She missed her family and the terrifying physical effects of the chemotherapy made her feel she was dying from the chemical treatments.

'I just want to go home and if you don't let me go home I will die', confessed Sarah. 'Last time in hospital I got very sick and when I went home I got better.

And now I'm getting sick again and I know if I go home and play in the fresh air with my friends I will get better again'.

The nurse tried to talk Sarah out of her thoughts and feelings and told her she needed the chemotherapy.

Sarah pulled up her pyjama top and showed the nurse her torso, which was criss-crossed with welts. Between the welts, her skin was red like sunburn. 'I'm allergic to that stuff. Look what it's done to me', insisted Sarah 'It's a poison and that's why you nurses have to wear all that gear while I'm having it'.

The nurse tried to tell Sarah otherwise, but the welts were so prominent, she had trouble persuading Sarah.

Sarah then became upset, as she always did when someone tried to convince her or force something onto her. 'Everybody has lied to me around here to get me to do what they want', she said angrily. 'I don't believe anybody here. Why do they want me to die?'

'Nobody wants you to die', insisted the nurse.

'The doctor told me the chemo can kill me. And when I'm having it, I feel like I'm going to die. So why does he want me to die?'

When the nurse returned to the office, she reported what Sarah had said and wrote it up in the notes.

The following afternoon, Dr Kotz came to visit Sarah. He looked different since he had grown a beard and at first Sarah didn't recognise him. He spoke to her from a distance without making eye contact. He had found out what Sarah had said to the night nurse and he looked unhappy about it. He tried to convince her that he was just trying to help her, but added that he could give her no guarantees of her survival. He said he was just being honest with her.

Sarah remained unimpressed. She pulled up her pyjama top. 'How would you like it if I did this to you?' she asked the oncologist as she showed him the stripes and red blotches on her chest and tummy. 'And how would you like it if I didn't let you see your family?'

The oncologist hurried from Sarah's room and returned to the office to write in the notes:

> I have had a discussion with Sarah this pm. She is very upset today. Keeps saying that I want her to die and that chemotherapy will kill her. She also said that if chemotherapy didn't kill her, then the separation from her parents would, and this was all my fault.

At the end of his entry, the doctor noted his suggestion that Sarah's telephone calls should be stopped. This meant that he suspected the parents of influencing Sarah during the phone calls, when in fact DoCS and hospital personnel had closely monitored the calls from the outset.

The oncologist mentioned nothing in his notes about the allergic skin reaction Sarah was having to the chemotherapy.

Two days later, DoCS and the hospital staff called the next meeting to review Sarah's 'behaviour'. The oncologist wanted the parents to draw up a short visitors' list of immediate relatives only. Of those, he would personally decide who would be allowed in. Sarah's phone calls were to be further restricted to close family only. Staff were to carefully monitor the calls and strictly log their times. If Sarah spoke to other relatives on the phone for two hours that day, she would be allowed no more visitors. The caseworkers did not tolerate whispering or close contact between family members. Staff watched even more carefully each interaction between Sarah and her family and banned anyone who had any kind of 'effect' on Sarah.

At times Sarah heard her parents' voices down the hall and then listened as the nurses turned them away. Those were her worst days, when she could not see her parents, even for a minute. The nurses constantly peered through the window at her. At every opportunity, the staff continued to pressure her to eat chocolates, lollies, soft drinks and chips. The dietician came to weigh her often and seemed cross when she hadn't gained enough weight on the high sugar and fat diet. The social worker forced her to go to school when she felt sick. The caseworkers were ever present, watching her every move and writing down every detail. Sarah was beginning to feel intolerably stifled by the intrusive surveillance and the coercive atmosphere that amounted to medical martial law.

At night, Sarah turned away from the observation port to face the window. She liked to look at the stars. On a full moon, she found comfort in the thought that her family could see it too from home. Late at night when she thought no one was watching, she folded her hands under the covers and prayed to be released from this place and returned safely home to her family.

Back at the homestead, Mark stepped up the security around the house and property to protect his family. He had hardened his attitude towards trespassers and adopted a no-tolerance policy. His family had been abused enough without having to be fearful in their beds at night. None of the UN covenants, or the civil and human rights laws had done his family any good. Now he had to protect his family and property by himself. For weeks, he had left both dogs off their chains at night to guard the grounds. Muttley, in particular, would not hesitate to attack an intruder; Pooch was second in charge and usually followed Muttley's example. Since the dogs patrolled the grounds at night, the doors and windows had stayed shut.

After several unsuccessful attempts to see the oncologist, Dan Tyler was finally able to schedule another appointment with him. Before he left for the hospital, we had a planning meeting at the clinic to support Dan. Most of us had a thorough working knowledge of nutritional medicine. A lot was riding on this meeting and we knew this might be our last chance to help Sarah.

We decided the most pressing issue was to ask Dr Kotz on what evidence he had based his treatment. The oncologist had provided us with the name of the study that he and Dr Conway had relied upon: the Mann study from the UK. Late one night, I located the study on the internet and paid for it online before downloading it from a medical information provider. I printed it off, made several copies, and handed the study around to the clinic staff and several outside colleagues for their feedback. I supplied a copy to a relative, who was a postdoctoral medical science cancer researcher, and to other doctor relatives. Those who analysed the study found it interesting, but were disturbed about it being used to justify a forced medical treatment. The study included both boys and girls with germ cell cancers. This proved a confounding factor since the prognoses were significantly more optimistic for boys with testicular cancer than girls with ovarian cancer. Despite this, however, there appeared not a single case of a girl with the type of ovarian cancer that Sarah had. This meant that no conclusions could be drawn from this study specifically regarding Sarah, and certainly, no forced treatment could be based on it. Nothing in the study supported forcing a treatment onto a late stage cancer patient, especially when such force was out of line with normal clinical practice.

These findings were troubling enough, but we were not yet aware of the French (Culine 97) study, which Dr Conway had finally handed over to Mark after he had made several requests for clinical studies to support Sarah's treatment. This study showed that the only child with recurrent cancer similar to Sarah's had in fact died despite receiving the treatment currently forced on Sarah.

The second issue needing discussion was Sarah's current state of malnutrition. Her court-mandated hospital diet almost totally lacked fresh fruits and vegetables, a necessary source of micronutrients. At the same time, it was high in trans-fats, sugar and processed meats, which were associated with higher incidences of cancer (Sinha 04, Stattin 03). To make matters worse, staff were denying Sarah the nutritious diet she was accustomed to and preferred, while a court order forced her to eat the junk food the staff urged on her. Not only was this inadequate for her needs, but it also threatened to worsen the malnutrition she had been diagnosed as having after the surgery and severe post-op complications that had caused her extreme weight loss.

According to the World Health Organization, acute malnutrition is a medical emergency that must be addressed immediately with specific nutritional protocols. WHO Treatment protocols for malnutrition prescribe a diet of fresh foods, protein and carbohydrate as well as extra micronutrients such as vitamins, minerals and specific electrolytes.

Sarah also had additional nutritional needs specific to her advanced cancer. Her diet at home had maintained her at a normal weight for her age despite the first round of chemotherapy and advancing cancer. Her nutritional needs were higher while receiving chemotherapy. The longer her malnutrition continued without treatment the greater risk she had of developing chronic malnutrition. According to the National Cancer Institute, 20–40 per cent of cancer patients die from causes related to malnutrition, not from the cancer itself, while 80 per cent of cancer patients develop some form of clinical malnutrition. According to Dr Katz at Yale:

> *Cancer may kill, in part, by causing starvation and conventional therapies may actually exacerbate this aspect of the disease. While these treatments can effectively attack the cancer, they also take a toll on the patient. There is thus a need to combine effective assaults on cancer, with effective nurturing, and nourishing, of the body. Optimizing nutrition during and following cancer therapy is unquestionably a vital element in overcoming the disease, and reclaiming good health.*

The National Cancer Institute advises nutritional supplements for cancer patients having chemotherapy. According to best practice, this means that Sarah should have had nutritional supplementation before her chemotherapy and between chemo cycles, which is entirely compatible with chemotherapy. Unfortunately, the court order the department sought not only prevented Sarah having an optimum diet, but specifically forbade her the very nutritional supplements which were necessary to treat her severe malnutrition.

Sarah's splenectomy also meant she had extra nutritional requirements. During surgery, she had lost her main blood-making organ and also a large portion of her immune system that was capable of finding and destroying cancer cells (Herberman 81). To compensate for her missing spleen, Sarah required a diet rich in green leafy vegetables and fresh meats containing iron, B12 and other blood-making nutrients, to assist her bone marrow to replace red blood cells in the spleen's absence.

Finally, since Sarah had not been allowed outside for several months, she was at risk of developing vitamin D deficiency. This is an essential vitamin with anti-cancer properties, normally manufactured by the skin in the presence of sunlight (Deeb 07). Furthermore, while the staff did not allow Sarah outside for sunshine, they also refused her vitamin D supplements.

The next issue for discussion with the oncologist concerned Sarah's stress levels. Her incarceration and forced treatments had clearly had devastating effects on her emotional and physical health. Many studies have proven that stress accelerates the spread of cancer cells. Researchers at MD Anderson Cancer Center in Texas have clearly shown that chronic stress and low social support accelerate ovarian cancer, while reduction of stress reduces tumour growth (Sood 04). Studies also show that along with relief from stress, laughter and happiness has a direct effect on increasing the body's killer cells, which destroy cancer cells (Benett 07). Yet for Sarah there was no laughter and no outlet for her stress.

One way of lowering stress and its damaging effects on tissues is exercise. Canadian researcher Dr Sai Pan reports that moderate physical activity lowers the risk for ovarian cancer. However, during the several months of Sarah's incarceration, staff consistently refused Sarah any of the outdoor or indoor physical activity that usually gives cancer patients much comfort, a sense of wellbeing, and quality of life.

Finally, the chemotherapy drugs forced onto Sarah were in themselves carcinogenic and known to cause secondary cancer a few years later.

At the clinic, we were concerned Sarah may not have had enough resistance or nutritional capacity to fend off her disease. We feared that all these risk factors combined would set Sarah up for a major cancer relapse after the chemotherapy.

The following day Dan Tyler arrived at the regional hospital with a list of issues he wanted to discuss with Dr Kotz. The oncologist had called in the hospital paediatric department head for support and Dan found himself face to face with both of them. Once brief formalities were over, Tyler started with Sarah's diet and asked the oncologist to allow her to have nutritional supplements to address her serious malnutrition. He asked the oncologist to consider reinstating the nutritious diet Sarah was used to eating at home. The oncologist seemed dismissive and claimed the diet at the hospital was adequate for her needs.

Next, Tyler raised the disturbing issue about the UK study. He stressed that it could not possibly be used to support the treatment he was forcing on Sarah. The oncologist denied this and refused to discuss it further.

When Tyler tackled the issue of Sarah's human right to comfort from friends and family, outside air and sunshine and gentle exercise, the oncologist became irritated. He had stonewalled Tyler on each issue and refused to discuss it, claiming instead that everything was in accordance with the rules. He said there were court orders in place that legally sanctioned his treatment and management of Sarah, and that he was within his legal rights to carry on whatever he felt was appropriate.

Finally, Tyler raised the issue of the parents' concern about Sarah's emotional welfare since she had threatened suicide. They felt the psychologist's report reflected the interests of the doctors and the department and did not consider Sarah's needs. The parents wanted an independent psychologist to assess and support Sarah to ensure that, in her present intolerable circumstances, she would not carry out her suicide threat.

On hearing this, the oncologist became angry and made it clear that the meeting was over. After Tyler left, the oncologist wrote in the clinical notes:

> 1.   He [Dr Dan Tyler] does not believe the (Mann) article proves anything and does not indicate prognosis and cure.
> 2.   Psychologists report was: 'biased' and whether parents can request a psychological assessment. I suggested Sarah was having sessions with our child psychiatrist, and if they wish further input for the parents to discuss with him.
> 3.   My observation is that Sarah is having a reasonable paediatric diet.
> 4.   Explained that when she is discharged, if Sarah takes anything other than what I prescribe then it will be a Court order violation.

The following day, Tyler arrived at the clinic with the bad news. The oncologist had been unwilling to consider any differing point of view – even from a professional colleague. We had attempted to resolve Sarah's predicament in accordance with the AMA Medical Code of Ethics. Unfortunately, the oncologist was clearly resistant to discussions and entrenched in his position, despite being shown compelling evidence to the contrary. This should have been a time for all parties to review the validity of their treatments and make adjustments. Instead, the oncologist used the power of the State to entrench himself further into his position.

Later that day Mark phoned with the news that the department had commenced proceedings to prevent Dr Tyler (or any other practitioners from the clinic) from making any further visits to the hospital to monitor Sarah. The department's caseworkers had converted all their detailed notes, gathered during their close surveillance of Sarah, into affidavits. This included such material as what expressions or body language the caseworkers thought Sarah's visitors might be displaying. This would now be subject of the next court hearing.

So far, we had conducted ourselves entirely by the rules of medical ethics, with the welfare of our patient foremost in mind, and with polite consideration for our colleagues. However, a statutory bureaucracy was about to bludgeon us on behalf of a doctor who did not want to consider valid scientific evidence from a colleague. It was not long before we too received legal correspondence from the Crown Solicitor's Office, who represented DoCS. In addition, we began to receive correspondence from the department, from no lesser a person than the Director General himself, who signed the letter in his own hand. We were now up against the raw power of a department that wielded police powers.

For us, this development marked the first time the matter had left the medical framework and entered the legal and human rights arena. We subsequently wrote to the department stating that it was the clinic practitioners' belief that Sarah's human rights and dignity were being violated. We wanted it known that no one at the clinic endorsed the medical treatment she was currently receiving. We objected strongly to her current involuntary incarceration, which denied her the most basic human rights. We wanted these rights reinstated and advocated she receive the emotional comfort of her family and friends, an appropriate diet, exercise, outdoor air, compassion, and freedom of speech. Most of all we wanted appropriate, evidence-based treatment for Sarah's current health issues, which included treatment for her malnutrition.

Apart from complaining to the department, we wondered whom we could go to about these blatant violations of Sarah's human rights when Australia had no Constitutional Bill of Rights, as did the US, guaranteeing basic rights and freedoms. Our only option would have been to approach the Human Rights and Equal Opportunity Commission, but this would have taken far too long; Sarah urgently needed immediate relief from her current, intolerable situation, which we believed put her in DoCS' own words – 'at risk of harm'.

We had tried all known avenues by then. It would have done no good to report the doctors to the relevant professional boards, since court orders were on foot that endorsed what they were doing. (This indeed turned out to be the case when Mark lodged a complaint to the Medical Board and HCCC some time later. Both organisations informed him that the court orders made his complaint invalid.)

The parents had also exhausted all possibilities and were currently gagged by a court order. We also found ourselves scrutinised by a bureaucracy with police powers, which now had our clinic in its sights ever since we had tried to resolve a medical issue with the oncologist. With all the normal channels exhausted, the problem was spinning out of control.

It appeared the only way left to help Sarah now was to go public.

IN THE PUBLIC INTEREST

**If this [DoCS] Bill currently before NSW Parliament
Is passed, we will head in the direction of a
White Stolen Generation.**

**Former Shadow Attorney-General,
The Hon J Hannaford MLC
To NSW Parliament in 2000**

When Mark phoned the clinic to ask for an appointment with me, it was not had to guess what it was about. I invited him into a quiet room at the centre of the clinic to talk. We sat down in two comfortable chairs. He told me he did not know what motives the oncologists had for forcing their treatments on his daughter without evidence but he thought the court had been misled into authorising their activities. Worse yet, he believed the social workers and caseworkers, who were not medically trained, were now forcing Sarah to follow their own medical recommendations and orders in addition to the oncologist's orders. This, Mark thought, had led to his daughter living under a medical dictatorship instead of therapeutic environment, and he felt sure it was bound to end in tragedy for her.

Mark looked disillusioned when he reminded me that the usual channels had all failed him. He had exhausted every legal and bureaucratic avenue and still received no help. He knew that I wrote articles on health issues and asked me if I would write one about Sarah's desperate predicament in the hope it would bring an end to her plight, if made public.

To a freelance writer, this extraordinary situation was a hot potato. Since I was also involved with Sarah as a health care practitioner, I didn't think I should be the one to write her story. Worst of all, the department has a policy of veiling its deeds in secrecy. The whole of Sarah's matter had a court-issued gag order over it from the first hearing, preventing anyone from publicising it, particularly in a way that would reveal Sarah's identity. Anyone contravening this order would be in contempt of court and could receive a jail sentence.

On the other hand, I was absolutely convinced that Sarah's forced treatment and incarceration were far out of the ordinary professional practice standards and that they imposed such extreme hardship on her that something had to be done about it urgently. I was also sure the story fulfilled the gold standard journalistic criterion of being in the public interest, which is legally defined as: *whenever it is such as to affect people at large so that they may legitimately be interested in or concerned at what is going on or what may happen to them or others.* I believed that this standard applied in Sarah's case – that she and her family had been damaged by individuals, policies, and administrative decisions that were also a potential threat to others in the community.

I assured Mark I would think about it and make some enquiries. Later that afternoon, I phoned a few of my journalist contacts. They agreed the story had huge merit as news, but none would touch it for fear of the gag order. It seemed no one was willing to risk going to jail. By the end of the day I had run out of options; I didn't want to spend time behind bars either, and dreaded having to tell Mark that nobody would help him.

I went to bed that evening still feeling unsettled. Graphic nightmares disturbed my night, as shadowy people forced surgery on me and injected me with drugs. I woke up in a sweat the next morning, overwhelmed by the realisation of what Sarah must be going through. Still feeling rattled, I sat up in bed and decided then and there to write the story. I figured that even if the court locked me up for writing it, it would still be nothing compared to the torment Sarah was suffering each day. I had to be careful though, to write in such a way as not to identify Sarah.

When I phoned Mark later that morning, he seemed happy with my decision. It was his last hope to help his daughter. I asked him for consent to reveal various medical details and I wanted Sarah's blessing before I started. She'd already had too much done to her without her consent. This meant a family member had to get past the censors at the hospital, a problem needing some creativity to resolve.

Almost immediately, Di and Sarah's sisters sprang into action. During their next visit, they tried to get Sarah alone for just one minute but the caseworker prevented close contact. Sarah knew intuitively that her mother wanted to talk with her. She told the caseworker she was going to the toilet and wanted her mother with her.

In the narrow space between the flush bowl and the sink, Di asked Sarah her views on the idea and Sarah understood immediately that it could help her. Her only stipulation was that her own name be used in the article.

'My name is Sarah', she reminded her mother.

Unfortunately, it was one wish I could not grant her. But with her blessing, it now felt right to start writing.

Before beginning the article, I pored over the available documents, and noticed Sarah's was not merely a human interest story. It raised serious legal, medical and ethical issues, and I had to question what level of public interest this story might capture. Would it make the public worried about the standard of medical care in hospitals? If children have a right to participate in decisions about their medical treatment under the UN Convention, why is this ignored or ineffective? What are the ethics of forcing surgery on any patient – let alone a late-stage or terminal cancer patient – without their consent?

Then there were issues that arose from the effects of these medical and legal decisions on Sarah's life and health. Did the forced treatments help her or harm her? To what extent did the interventions abuse her human rights?

Treatment aside, I had no doubt Sarah regarded her present conditions as intolerable, possibly even cruel, inhuman or degrading. Some might define them as intimidation, or even torture. The Wiki dictionary definition of intimidation is:

> *The practice of compelling a person or manipulating them to behave in an involuntary way (whether through action or inaction) by use of threats, intimidation, trickery, or some other form of pressure or force. These are used as leverage, to force the victim to act in the desired way. Coercion may involve the actual infliction of physical pain/injury or psychological harm in order to enhance the threat. The threat of further harm may then lead to the cooperation or obedience of the person being coerced. Torture is one of the most extreme examples of coercion where severe pain and suffering is inflicted.*

I wondered what Australian laws guaranteed human rights. For over a hundred years, Australia has been the only common law country in the world without a Constitutional Bill of Rights. No amendments or special entitlements were added to the Australian Constitution because the founders believed the rule of law would guarantee all citizens their legal rights.

Recently, individual Australian states have taken steps to implement their own Bill of Rights (a charter) at the state level. However, this does not guarantee the comprehensive rights and protections contained in the American

Constitution and its ten amendments known as the Bill of Rights. Instead, the state's Bill of Rights originates from the United Nations in the form of international law. Victoria is to date the only Australian state to enact a charter of rights. It took effect on 1 January 2007, when the Victorian Parliament passed the Victorian Charter of Rights and Responsibilities. This requires state and local government and other public authorities to consider human rights when making laws, setting policies and providing services. Other states have also considered implementing their own charter – with the exception of NSW. The NSW Council for Civil Liberties has been lobbying for a state charter since the 1960s, but its efforts have so far been largely ignored by the NSW Parliament.

However, even if it had been in effect at the time of Sarah's illness, it is difficult to say whether such a charter would have offered the parents an additional legal avenue in any case. Mark believes in hindsight that it would have made no difference, since the United Nations Convention on the Rights of the Child had been of no help to Sarah either, even when he'd raised it in court. He remains certain that the only remedy left to him was to make Sarah's story public.

By late August, my feature article was ready for release. I had used pseudonyms for almost everyone and removed all the details that could potentially identify Sarah or her family. Sarah became 'Lisa' in the article. Out of courtesy, I also withheld the doctors' names. A Melbourne-based magazine acquired the article free of charge, which reserved my right to release it on the internet into the public domain. The editor told me she would publish it in two parts because of the feature's length.

Meanwhile at the regional hospital, staff continued to administer the chemotherapy to Sarah. For a few days, she also had a roommate, as another girl was admitted to Sarah's room for chemotherapy. Her retching and vomiting kept Sarah awake at night, and when Sarah fell into an exhausted sleep early each morning, her recurrent nightmares came again. Night staff recorded in the notes that Sarah had complained about being kept awake half the night, and when she finally fell asleep, she cried out in her sleep for her mother. Over the few days, Sarah had made friends with the girl just before the girl was allowed home – leaving Sarah alone in the room again with only the caseworkers watching her.

Even though Sarah was suffering severe side effects from the drugs, she became optimistic again, when she found out the article had been released. Like all detainees, she hoped others would soon know about her plight. She brightened up and visited other children in their rooms. When they were having chemo, she comforted them and gave them the gifts of beads, lip-gloss and other presents the social worker had given her. The staff noticed the change in Sarah and wrote glowing comments in the records, noting that she had finally 'accepted' her treatment. One notation read: 'Sarah bright and happy this afternoon. Playing with staff, and talking to other patients. Eating well – mostly junk food'.

The dietician also visited regularly to weigh Sarah. Despite the high fat and sugar hospital diet, Sarah did not fully regain the weight she had lost at the city hospital. She craved fresh fruits and vegetables and fresh (non-processed) meats, and she continued to ask the dietician for these foods. She told the woman that perhaps so many lollies and chocolates weren't too good for her, especially if she had cancer. However, the dietician explained that Sarah's diet had nothing to do with cancer and she could eat whatever she liked (evidently, that didn't include fresh food).

However, Sarah's blood tests showed severe abnormalities. She was still malnourished, and her body could not replace damaged tissues or process toxins without sufficient essential nutrients. Her liver function tests were grossly abnormal, indicating her liver was struggling under the load of chemicals. Her bone marrow function was depressed, and her haemoglobin had dropped to the point of anaemia. Sarah struggled for breath even after mild exertion because her lungs were hardening with scar tissue. This lung fibrosis is a common side effect from Bleomycin, one of the chemo drugs the oncologist was using to treat Sarah. Her kidneys also struggled with the chemicals, leaving waste matter in her blood.

Each time they visited, Mark and Di saw how much sicker Sarah was becoming, and they desperately hoped she would soon be set free.

Within days of its release, my article travelled around the globe on the internet and appeared on dozens of websites and in newsletters. Meanwhile, the Melbourne-based magazine featured the first part in its monthly edition. This brought an unprecedented response for the magazine, with readers contacting the editor with their emotional responses to the story.

Following the article's internet release, I was inundated with over 100 e-mails a day. They flooded in from Europe, the United States, Canada, New Zealand, South Africa, Asia, and South American countries. I rerouted many to Mark, who also received more correspondence than he could reply to.

Unlike most articles, which usually raise a mixed reader response reflecting differing points of view, incredibly, all who contacted me expressed overwhelming support for Lisa (Sarah) and her family, with not one negative response among them. I was completely unprepared for the emotional intensity of people's outrage at hearing the story. They came from many cultures and backgrounds, but all were united in their beliefs in family rights and freedom of choice. I was also surprised to hear from many professionals who had worked, or were still working, in the medical, police or child protection system. I admired their courage for lifting the lid on the system.

A senior police officer and father of three wrote that nothing surprised him after child-protection went 'out of control' in the late 1990s, which is when the mandatory reporting of child abuse came into legal effect in NSW. Since then, police have been required to notify DoCS when responding to each domestic incident. He agreed that there were many children who needed protection, but since mandatory reporting, he felt the department was removing too many children from their homes when the domestic problem was minor or had been resolved. After an initial domestic call, the department often called on him to return to the home with a DoCS worker to take the child from the parents, even though the parents seemed quite reasonable and obviously loved and cared for the child. The worst part of his job was seeing these parents and children crying and screaming when DoCS came to take the child. Increasingly, caseworkers were taking children from schools to avoid the emotional scenes.

Another police officer told me he had responded to many domestic violence calls to foster parents' homes. He knew of people fostering six or more kids and drawing thousands of dollars a week from the State. Many of these foster homes were in disarray and the subject of frequent complaints from the neighbours when the kids ran amok. Sometimes the foster children looked genuinely abused, neglected or out of control, but he said nothing is ever done about it since the children are already State wards. According to him, some of these kids are on so many behavioural medications they look and behave like zombies. They're classed as having 'special needs', for which the foster parent can receive up to $600 per week per child. Although he realised there are many terrific foster parents giving kids good homes when they really need one, in his opinion many foster children would be better off at home with their own parents. He felt that, with mandatory reporting, too many kids are routinely reported, and end up being taken from good homes while the ones at risk often are left in dangerous homes. Meanwhile, the department is lost in a sea of paperwork so deep they cannot even tell when a kid genuinely needs help anymore.

Several teachers also wrote to me about their experiences with the department. One middle-aged high-school teacher told me that before mandatory reporting she and other school staff treated students with simple kindness and understanding while they dealt with temporary problems at home such as their parents' divorce. Those who needed extra support were referred on to school counsellors. In those days teachers reported only what they believed were genuine cases of abuse or neglect, whereas now teachers are legally required to report so much as a bruise on a student. While she admitted that there has been an increase of drinking and other risky behaviour in kids in recent years, she argued that parents usually want to be informed and deal with it themselves. The teacher had been shaken to hear about Sarah, whose parents were trying to make responsible decisions, but then she read shocking reports about DoCS in the papers almost every day. Lately, she told me, she has become more reluctant to report children to DoCS: the department has lost its credibility with the public and she suspects its involvement with some children makes their lives worse instead of better. She has seen an upsurge of foster children and not all of them, she suspects, come from bad homes. She is concerned the system is creating a new generation of 'lost children' in New South Wales.

Nurses, too, wrote to me expressing their outrage at the family's experiences. One nurse who works in paediatric oncology at a Sydney hospital said, 'Lately, I'm seeing more kids having chemo forced on them'.

She added:

> *Personally, I wouldn't force any particular treatment on anybody with a chronic disease. In an emergency, you have to act fast sometimes, and the patient or parents cannot always give their consent. But recurrent cancer is a different story. I've seen kids with poor prognoses go through endless painful 'curative' treatments. To them it feels like torture and they just want to be left alone in the end. I've even had a child ask me to let him die. I don't know what stage Lisa was in but, in late stage or terminal cancer, I think the kids and the parents should get the final say whether they want any more chemo. The last time I had a kid with a court order on my ward [to force chemo], I didn't have the heart to do it. I asked to be reallocated to another patient. It's terrible what they did to Lisa [Sarah], and I can't understand why the nurses didn't take that kid outside for a play, or let her mum bring in some home cooked food. It doesn't take a genius to figure out how much comfort that would have given Lisa.*

Another nurse who worked in the emergency department (ED) of a large Sydney hospital told me she was not surprised the child protection system netted Sarah, especially after doctors had wrongly diagnosed her as being pregnant before they had done the necessary testing. In her area, mandatory reporting had turned the ED into virtual DoCS induction centres since every bruise, fracture, burn, graze, minor cut and sprain is technically 'risk of harm' under the legal mandatory reporting requirements. She said she is required to report even normal kids with great parents who just happen to have had an unavoidable accident. She recalls the time before mandatory reporting when staff used their professional discretion to report those children they genuinely suspected of being abused or neglected.

Of all those who contacted me, my greatest surprise was the number of ex-DoCS caseworkers among them. One caseworker told me that she had personally witnessed hundreds of children being taken from their parents. It was a simple matter of DoCS lodging a care application in the Children's Court with a supporting affidavit stating what the caseworker thought or even suspected was wrong with the parent. When I asked her whether caseworkers ever deliberately misrepresented the facts in their affidavits, she answered 'all the time'. The Children's Court judge usually grants the care application based on what the caseworker has written, without the parent being present in court. The caseworkers then return to the home and take the child from the parents immediately – often permanently. She said few things are as administratively easy as taking a child away from its family. The parents turn up in court a few days after losing their kids, usually too devastated to defend themselves. Meanwhile the overloaded Children's Courts work at a snail's pace, and it might be years before parents get a hearing. Worse yet, their lawyers often sell them down the river by not putting up a strong defence. She also felt that the system is definitely not set up to reunite families. Once the children are in the system, they have only a slim chance of being reunited with their parents until they are 18. By then they have grown up without their family and had have lost their sense of identity.

Another caseworker told me it is common practice for many caseworkers to pressure the natural parents into signing consent forms. The parents are unaware they are unwittingly consenting to their children being removed from them, often permanently. The parents' signature effectively terminates their parental rights and allows DoCS to place children in foster homes or even into permanent adoption, without need of a court order. The caseworker said she'd often heard her colleagues boasting about duping the parents and saving themselves a trip to court. She told me she'd quit her job because she couldn't bear to watch the system destroy good families while having little to offer families in trouble. She added that the department had a huge staff turnover and she suspected that most sensitive caseworkers quit their jobs within the first two years, leaving the harder boiled ones who stay, while many, she said, enjoyed the power trip.

Another caseworker told me of a worrying trend. The department increasingly adopts children out quickly once they are removed from their homes. Even parents who suffer temporary problems are at risk of having their kids removed and put up for adoption almost immediately. To make matters worse, DoCS receives a federal government-issued bonus for placing children into permanent adoptive homes. This terminates the parents' rights for life and often results in parents searching for their children for years, she said. 'There is huge potential for corruption', she added. 'Every case has a gag order over it'.

My own research confirmed this. The caseworker's threats to remove Sarah permanently from her home were no idle ones. The department had the power to adopt Sarah out to another family, because of the amendment to its Act[32] by the Permanency Planning Bill in 2001. The amendment allowed the department to take children from their homes and place them for immediate adoption. This included children who are in short-term placements of six months to give families respite during a temporary family crisis. It even gave the department the power to fine young people for telling their natural parents their whereabouts and revealing their foster or adoptive parents' address. The amendment also ensured that the courts were not required to consider any change in the natural parents' circumstances and their ability to care for their child before deciding permanent placement for adoption. Once adopted, children were to be deprived of contact with their natural family and their culture.[33]

While the Bill was wending its way through the NSW Parliament in 2001, it attracted some outspoken critics. Before his retirement from Parliament, the former Shadow Attorney-General, the Hon J Hannaford MLC, expressed his strong disapproval of the Bill by stating that the direction the legislation was taking would result in a 'white Stolen Generation'. Despite stiff opposition, the

---

[32] Children and Young Persons (Care and Protection) Act 1998.
[33] Community Services Commission, *Submission by the Community Services Commission to the Minister for Community Services in relation to the Children (Care and Protection) Amendment (Permanency Planning) Bill 2000*, September 2000.

Permanency Planning Bill was passed by NSW Parliament and came into effect in 2001.

While the article about Sarah (Lisa) was circling the globe on the internet and circulating in the print media, the oncologist scheduled another round of chemotherapy for Sarah. This time a routine blood sample revealed Sarah's bone marrow was too depressed and the doctor had to postpone it. Two days later the cell count rose high enough to give the chemicals and the usual routine was repeated. Sarah told the staff she didn't want the chemo but staff told her they would do it anyway. For a while, Di was allowed to stay and comfort Sarah. She dressed up in a biohazard plastic apron and rubber gloves to protect herself from her daughter's skin while she was having the chemo. Sarah sat on her mother's lap with the chemical infusion running through the cannula in her arm. After the nurse left the room, Sarah turned to her mother.

'I don't want that stuff in me. Can't I just undo it and let it go on the floor? When will I get out of here?'

Di saw that Sarah's skin was turning red again.

'Soon, I hope', said Di.

Most of the Gloucester community already knew of Sarah's plight, by word of mouth. However, 10 days after the article's release the Gloucester newspaper published a letter to the editor written by a local resident. This caused a wave of outraged readers' letters and inundated the community newspaper's office with an unprecedented flood of correspondence. The paper printed the entire letter:

Letters to the Editor: The brief article about Child Protection Week in last week's paper would certainly have raised the awareness of the need for constant vigilance by the community to ensure the welfare of our most vulnerable. Imagine my quandary, then, as a servant of these children required by law to report any apparent cases of child neglect or mistreatment, when I learn that the Government department charged with their protection has been the facilitator and driving force behind what I believe to be one of the most heinous and horrific maltreatments of a child and her family that I have ever in 37 years of teaching, parenting and grandfathering, had the misfortune to witness.

Lisa Eastley (that's not her real name but poor silly old blind justice in her wisdom determined she should not be known to the public) is a sweet, little 11 year old, one of a large and very respectable local family. In December 2001 Lisa's parents, worried about her lack of energy and general malaise, sought medical advice in Taree. The doctor's (and I use that term derisively) diagnosis was that; Lisa was 14 weeks pregnant.

DOCS was immediately advised and the child queried on intimate and personal details of her home life and activities. This trauma was soon swamped by the correct diagnosis that the child had a football sized tumour which required immediate removal. The distraught family, following a suggestion by a surgeon that chemotherapy would not be appropriate for Lisa, sought worldwide for another treatment and eventually found a reputable alternative in Melbourne. They advised the oncologist who had been put in charge of Lisa's case and began successful treatment in Melbourne. Imagine their shock when some months later the full onslaught of bureaucratic power play was inflicted on the family. Summonses in the dead of night, court case after court case, veiled and not so veiled threats of punitive action if the family attempted to fight the orders, and many other disturbing actions followed.

Little Lisa was made a ward of the State and eventually the gaggle of doctors and DOCS had their way, subjecting the child to the horror of chemo in a hostile environment from which her parents were legally excluded.

The horror continues to this day. Suffice to say I, and an increasing number of people made aware of the suffering this family has been subjected to, am disgusted and revolted by the treatment meted out by the bludgeoning hand of the authorities. I would ask you, as concerned citizens of our district, to read the full scope of this nightmare which you can find on the internet, and when you have finished weeping, rise up in wrath and begin writing ranting and raving to anyone you consider appropriate from DOCS to doctors MPs to radio commentators to help rescue this child and this family from the clutches of those who are inflicting such pain so needlessly.

'Log' Munro
   Gloucester. [34]

While Sarah stared mournfully from the hospital window, she had no way of knowing that thousands of people around the world were now doing whatever they could to help her. Some people overseas organised prayer groups. Doctors from foreign countries offered to help. One doctor from Kenya offered advice on vitamin remedies for children with malnutrition, while another from India also offered his assistance. A medical specialist from the United States wanted to liaise with Sarah's oncologists and offered to treat Sarah in Michigan. Several other overseas doctors also stood by, ready to help if Sarah could be brought to their medical facilities.

In the local community, people wanted urgent action from their Members of Parliament (MPs). They wrote dozens of letters, which their MPs in turn passed on to the MP responsible for DoCS. However, only generic replies came from the DoCS MP's office, cloaking the matter behind confidentiality. These non-replies only infuriated the public more.

Jim and Mark also contacted their local and federal MPs. While some were indifferent, others took a personal interest in the family's plight, among them Bob Baldwin, federal member for Paterson. The family also had a channel of communication to the prime minister's office. Through this, they had the article delivered to John Howard's office, along with a letter from the Westley family pleading for help. Unfortunately, however, someone else in the prime minister's office answered with a generic letter offering no assistance whatsoever.

Meanwhile, back in the ward, Sarah had begun some small acts of protest of her own. First, she persuaded the staff to return some of her handicraft materials. Immediately she started cutting out coloured paper for cards, which she decorated with drawings and sparkles. She pasted these onto the nurses' observation window, so preventing the staff from peering into her room. She then asked her mother to bring in her lilac bedspread from home. The colourful quilt transformed the stark hospital room into a pre-teen girl's bedroom.

Next, as a hint of her wish to leave the hospital, Sarah packed her bags and left them out for all to see. And finally, since the oncologist was forcing painful

---

[34] Reprinted with kind permission from Mr Munro, as well as permission from the Gloucester Advocate newspaper.

treatments onto her, she decided to refuse him the respect of calling him 'Doctor'. Instead, she started calling the oncologist 'Harry'.

'Where's Harry?' she asked the staff. 'I want him to let me out of here'.

While Sarah was still unaware that thousands of well-wishers all over the world were hoping for her release, she did notice some encouraging signs at the hospital. Four days after the article's release, the dietician recorded in the notes that Sarah was now 'allowed to have 1–2 pieces of fruit per day', and out of the vegetable group she was 'offered peas and potatoes'. The dietician noted that Sarah had been asking for salads and that she had 'arranged for Sarah to be offered some salads on her menu'.

Then, five days after the article's release, Dr Kotz noted in the records that soon he would allow the parents an 'unsupervised visit'. This foreshadowed a surprising turn of events.

When the article had been released, some of Kotz's professional colleagues had phoned him at home. After reading the article, they had wanted to make sure he wasn't the oncologist it referred to. When he admitted having Sarah as his patient, they had asked him what was going on. It was the final straw. The next day the oncologist came to visit Sarah. He seemed distracted and less confident than usual. For a while, he paced around the room, asking Sarah questions but not listening to her replies. He finally sat at Sarah's bedside and rubbed his face in exasperation before leaving again.

Not long after, an older doctor, aged in his sixties, came to see Sarah. He told her that he had 'heard about her', and asked to see her skin welts. On seeing them, he looked disturbed. Ruth was with Sarah at the time. She heard him whisper under his breath: 'what have they done to you?', before he left again, nearly in tears. She thought the man was the head of the department.

Later in the day, Dr Kotz called a staff meeting and made an unexpected decision. He would discharge Sarah immediately to a halfway house, located on the grounds of the hospital. There, she would be confined to a small apartment for another six and a half weeks. She was allowed one family member with her. Each day, she had to front up to the hospital for blood tests, school and chemotherapy. She had to obey strict rules or return to the hospital section. The social worker was given the task of breaking the news to Sarah.

A few minutes later, Sarah heard the sound of Grimes' high heels and braced herself. A minute later, she was ecstatic to hear the news, even though she remained under severe restrictions. As long as she could go outside, see her family and friends and never be confined to the hospital room again, she was happy.

When Di arrived for her two-hour visit later that day, the nurses told her to move Sarah into the apartment immediately. Di was unprepared for the move and felt slightly panicked. Sarah had spent most of the past few weeks in bed. She was now visibly ill from the chemicals and her leg and arm muscles had become wasted from malnutrition and lack of exercise. She'd become anaemic, partly deaf, and her lungs were damaged from the drugs, making her breathless after any small exertion. Di was frightened of caring for Sarah on her own at the halfway house and didn't think she was medically qualified to take care of her needs. She told the nurse she thought her daughter would require a level of medical assistance for a while. The nurse did not reassure Di – as might have been expected – that the hospital was just metres away and offer Di the staff's help whenever she needed it. Instead, she rang Caitlin Grimes, who came to the ward to deal with Di personally. The social worker told Di that if she did not take Sarah to the halfway house immediately, Sarah would be placed into foster care, as per the court orders. She added that Di and Mark were required to pay for Sarah's new accommodation.

After the social worker's talk, staff discharged Sarah from the ward and Di hurried to pack the rest of Sarah's belongings. Minutes later, without being offered a wheelchair, Sarah shuffled down the corridor behind her mother, who lugged her belongings.

Just outside the hospital entrance, Di and Sarah paused to catch their breath. Sarah squinted in the bright light as she slowly took her first breath of fresh air in many weeks. 'I'm glad they kicked us out', she said to her mother. 'I packed my bags a long time ago'.

They walked towards the halfway house on the hospital grounds. The trip took twice as long as usual, with frequent pauses for Sarah to catch her breath. When they arrived at the small apartment, Sarah explored the tiny kitchenette and two single beds. She beamed. This was her first step towards freedom and she already looked forward to the next step. It was three days before Sarah's birthday on 1 September, and she wanted to go home on that day.

As it happened, the next court hearing was scheduled for Sarah's birthday, and while Sarah was moving into the halfway house, Mark was at home preparing the necessary affidavits for it. He planned to ask the judge to remove all court orders so he could take his daughter home. This time Dan Tyler was also required in court, and we at the clinic were busy writing affidavits for him too.

In the meantime, even though Sarah's living conditions had almost miracu-lously improved, the department was spreading the battle into arenas it had never been before. After the Melbourne magazine had gone to press with part one, the article had created unprecedented nationwide interest, with readers contacting the editor wanting to know the story's outcome. The editor assured them the second part would appear in the next month's issue. However, a week later a lawyer from the NSW Crown Solicitor's office wrote the magazine a stiff legal letter. The Crown Solicitor acted as the department's legal representative and promised legal action against the magazine if it published the second part of the article. The letter also alleged I had made factual errors in the story.

The editor found the Crown's legal letter terrifying, but fortunately, she informed me of it immediately and faxed me a copy. After reassuring the editor that I had checked my facts, I immediately drafted a reply to the Crown Solicitor's Office, assuring the Crown that I had taken the utmost care complying with current court orders. This included giving pseudonyms to Sarah and most others in the story to protect their identity. I asked the Crown Solicitor to inform me within 14 days which of the facts were alleged to be incorrect. If I had received no reply by then, I added, I would assume that the matter was at an end and that the article's publication could be resumed without impediment. For the next few weeks, I waited for a reply from the Crown.

On the evening before Sarah's birthday, the family visited her at the halfway house. Ruth had volunteered to room in with Sarah, leaving Di to stay at home with the other children.

Some hospital staff had softened their attitude recently and organised party streamers to decorate the apartment. The family brought in home-cooked food and a birthday cake. Sarah revelled in the newfound comforts.

Mark told Sarah he was going to court the following day and asked her what she wanted for her birthday.

'I want them to stop tormenting us', Sarah replied.

The following morning Mark drove the 600 km round trip to the Supreme Court with Dan Tyler. When the court session began, it was noticeably different from the previous hearings. This time no barrister represented Mark and he was about to stand up for himself and defend his family for the first time. In his briefcase were bundles of documents of evidence the court had never seen before.

The DoCS barrister addressed the court first and presented a letter from Dr Kotz. The oncologist wrote to the court that he was very pleased with Sarah's progress. He claimed she had tolerated the chemotherapy well and that her hospital diet was entirely adequate. The only problem he mentioned was that one of the chemicals damaged Sarah's lungs sometime between the second and third cycles of chemotherapy. He stated he would omit the Bleomycin if her lung function continued to deteriorate. The oncologist claimed that Sarah had been so happy on the ward that she gave staff 'lolly names' and engaged with them in 'friendly happy banter'. He ended the letter by stating:

> *I am surprised to a degree and delighted that Sarah appears to have coped extremely well under the difficult circumstances. I hope this can continue in the environment of the [halfway house], however, if there appears to be a change in Sarah's psychological wellbeing or any increased side effects, then I would not hesitate to readmit Sarah for a further prolonged hospitalisation.*

When the DoCS barrister sat down after his submission, Mark began his own submission by listing for the judge a long inventory of Sarah's shocking hardships. Among them were the intolerable conditions of her incarceration at the hospital, her malnutrition, the severe side effects she had suffered from the chemicals, her isolation from friends and family and her threat to commit suicide.

Next Dan Tyler gave his testimony, explaining to the judge that the study the oncologist cited to support his treatments was not relevant in Sarah's case and could not be used to justify forcing a treatment. He then described the horrific scene he had witnessed in the hospital lobby when Sarah had tried to escape, first from the unbearable conditions at the hospital and then from the guards. He told the judge of Sarah's suicide threat when she had felt completely cornered and desperate. He said he could not imagine why Dr Kotz had omitted this fact from his letter to the court, since it would be a true indication of the stresses imposed on Sarah from the forced treatment and insufferable conditions. He told the court that he had visited Dr Kotz as a fellow colleague and virtually pleaded with him to allow Sarah access to her friends and family, outside air, sunlight, exercise, and appropriate food and nutritional supplements to treat her malnutrition. Despite all this, the oncologist continued to refuse her these basic needs and comforts. Moreover, Tyler told the court; subsequent to his meeting with the doctor, the department had banned him from monitoring Sarah's condition at the hospital.

In his letter to the court, Dr Tyler wrote:

Frankly, I have never been involved in a case where a patient has been deprived of their right to informed consent to treatment. As I understand it, informed consent is a legal requirement. I have never encountered in Australia a child held captive for weeks in a hospital without fresh air or sunlight, or friends and other familiarities. And I have never heard anyone apart from Dr Kotz describe the child's resulting suicidal behaviour as being 'normal' or 'happy' or 'well adjusted'. I cannot even hazard a guess as to the possible long term psychological damage this forced treatment and captivity might have visited on this child. I want to be on record that I do not approve or condone these methods and approaches as have been used in this particular case. It appears that this case deviates from the norm in a multitude of ways.

In conclusion, a number of colleagues have been consulted regarding this case and so far, all are in accord with the views I have expressed. With the greatest respect, your Honour, at the very least, I would strongly recommend that all chemotherapy be suspended and all planned treatment by Dr Kotz be ceased until such time as this matter can be closely reviewed by qualified medical specialists of the parents' choosing.

Tyler's testimony was the first time the judge had heard dissent among the doctors, and it weakened the oncologist's position.

Mark followed this by tendering another oncologist's letter to the court. The specialist was from another state and offered to take over Sarah's care and treatment, provided the court agreed to it. Furthermore, a Sydney doctor offered a report to the court in which he stated his opinion that the stresses and deprivations imposed on Sarah 'are likely to worsen her chances of survival'. He added that 'high quality nutrition and appropriate supplementation will increase her survival chances and minimise the risk of long term health problems arising from chemotherapy'.

The next report Mark submitted to the court came from an internationally known professor of medicine who had founded the first postgraduate medical course in nutrition in Australia. The professor wrote in his report:

...Dr Kotz has not made any entry into his medical records showing that he has fully informed the parents of the serious side effects of chemotherapy. The teaching of this College to its medical practi-

tioners is that the toxicity and side-effects of chemotherapy can be significantly reduced by attention to diet and the judicious use of appropriate nutritional supplements. There is of course scientific data available to support adjunctive nutritional support and Dr Kotz should inform himself of this information if he routinely uses chemotherapeutic agents. To my knowledge, Dr Kotz has no formal training or qualifications in Nutritional Medicine. He states in his notes that 'alternative therapies are not proven'. This assertion very strongly suggests that he is prejudiced against treatment, which may be helpful to a cancer patient but doesn't fit with standard textbook oncology. However, there is excellent peer-reviewed published literature to show that cancer patients benefit from 'other' therapies in many ways. For example, the concurrent use of antioxidant, vitamins, trace elements and fatty acids can reduce the toxicity of chemotherapy, and improve the prognosis and quality of life. Exercise, given during chemotherapy in patients with solid tumours or leukaemias, results in more energy less pain and fatigue, fewer blood transfusions and a shorter stay in hospital. Meditation is not uncommon practice in cancer patients and it reduces the need for analgesics, antidepressants and many other symptom relieving drugs. In fact, numerous teaching hospitals in the United States support the use of these complementary therapies as an integral part of cancer patient care.

I understand that Dr Tyler has been unable to successfully address concerns with Dr Kotz that Sarah is, in his opinion, suffering from nutritional deficiencies due to her cancer, the chemotherapy treatments, her significant weight loss and her loss of appetite due to the stresses imposed on her at this time. This is not a matter of applying 'alternative therapy', but rather it is best practice in medicine to address nutritional deficiencies. According to the National Cancer Institute about one third of all cancer deaths are related to malnutrition. It is extremely important that this child's nutritional deficiencies be allowed to be corrected by a wholesome diet and the appropriate use of supplementation. Failure to respect the reasonable requests of the parents is ethically unacceptable. Furthermore to ignore or refuse complementary therapies which are safe and potentially beneficial, especially in life threatening situations, constitutes negligence.

In conclusion, I would recommend a full assessment of Sarah's management including the suitability of the treating oncologist.

The DoCS barrister did not seem happy about the new developments. He was even less pleased when Mark next presented the article I had written and told the judge it had already been published and widely distributed. Mark also attached a number of photographs of Sarah taken at the hospital, depicting her serious post-operative condition and malnutrition. On seeing the photographs, the judge learnt for the first time in graphic detail the effects the forced medical treatment had had on Sarah. Mark's impression was that the judge looked increasingly concerned on learning of this and hearing the other doctors' testimony.

After Mark finished, the DoCS barrister gave a long submission disputing each point of Mark's argument, based on Dr Kotz's letter. He ended by arguing that the chemotherapy should be completed.

Following that, Mark asked the judge to revoke the previous court orders, and allow Sarah to go home without further treatment.

At the end of both submissions, the judge looked uneasy. He called for a recess and gathered up the large bundle of evidence Mark had just presented to the court, which he intended to read in his chambers. With the judge out of the courtroom, Mark paced the hallway for the next half hour with Dan Tyler. When the court session resumed, the judge sat down at his bench and briefly reviewed his notes from before the recess. He looked noticeably uneasy as he prepared to hand down his orders. Mark tensed in anticipation of the verdict. He had a feeling the judge was not gone long enough to review Mark's entire bundle of documents.

Finally, the judge prepared to address the court. He looked openly uncom-fortable when he ordered the chemo to continue until it was finished. This was based on the oncologists' claims that Sarah had a high chance of being cured with the chemo – an assertion that was, of course, entirely incorrect.

The DoCS barrister gave a brief but satisfied smile. The judge noticed this and gave the barrister a stern glance. 'I will not hear this case again', said the judge emphatically.

Mark sat at his defendant's table devastated by the verdict but curious about the judge's unusual statement.

The barrister rose and addressed the judge. 'Your Honour, this case is not finished', he said self-confidently. 'You will be hearing more of it as it becomes necessary'.

For a brief moment, it seemed to Mark that the DoCS barrister was in control of the entire case and not the judge.

The judge adjourned the session and hastily left the courtroom.

Mark walked from the courtroom with Dan. Neither of them could understand why the judge had ruled in the department's favour.

The following day Mark drove another 300 km roundtrip to break the news to Sarah at the halfway house. He dreaded telling her she had to endure the next six weeks of chemo until the treatment was over.

'Dad', she said, looking disappointed, 'then promise me: when I get home, I will never have to see them again'.

Over the next six weeks, Ruth stayed with Sarah at the halfway house. Each morning Sarah fronted up to the ward at 8 am for her medications. After that, she was required to attend school and eat the hospital lunch. On chemotherapy days, she stayed in the ward until the intravenous drip finished, and returned again the next two days until the three-day cycle was completed. After a short break, the chemo cycle would then start all over again. On weekends, her family visited and brought a load of Di's home-cooked food. Sarah ravenously ate it while playing games with her sisters. When nurses next weighed her, she had gained a kilo.

Just when Sarah was beginning to enjoy her privacy again, she had another reminder that she was still under scrutiny. One afternoon, Ruth took Sarah for a short walk on the hospital grounds. The season was changing to spring. The wattles were in bloom and Sarah liked to visit the trees she had looked at for so long through her hospital window. When they returned to the apartment, Ruth noticed a tiny black device had been stuck to the wall while they were away. Sarah looked at it curiously for a minute before climbing up on a chair, removing it, and taking it into the bathroom with her. It reminded her of the gadgets in the hospital room and she flushed it down the toilet. Ruth was ready to scold Sarah, but on reflection, she had to admit it was a bit strange for the thing to suddenly appear while they were out. In any case, whatever it was – it was history now. Ruth and Sarah were in fits of laughter over it for days.

By October, Sarah had spent four months in hospital, including three solid months of chemotherapy. The caseworkers and the regional hospital staff still conducted twice-weekly meetings, which none of the family wished to attend. As Sarah's release date neared, the department desperately wanted Mark to turn up to one of their meetings. They phoned him at home to pressure him into attending the next scheduled meeting at the regional hospital. Mark finally relented, and agreed.

On arriving at the ward, Mark saw a battalion of caseworkers and social workers with the oncologist and immediately regretted his decision. Before they started, DoCS workers cited their usual preamble – 'We're just here to help you' – but as usual, this statement only led into caseworkers reading him the riot act once more. Gary Boggs was there with Gillian and Judy. Mark counted several others he hadn't seen before, and of course, the hospital social worker was present. The group took turns repeating their previous warning that Sarah was not to have any vitamins, even after she went home. The caseworkers even extended this stipulation to the rest of their children, saying they too would be taken away and placed with another family if the parents gave them vitamins. Mark asked why they were imposing rules on their other children when they weren't the subject of any court orders, but Gary Boggs said the department was entitled to do this.

Mark turned to the oncologist. 'Do you have that ridiculous order forbidding Sarah proper nutrition still on foot?'

The oncologist answered defensively, claiming that it was not his idea but DoCS'. Mark was disgusted that Sarah was still refused vitamins when the top medical specialist in nutritional medicine in the country had reported to the court that Sarah needed her nutritional deficiencies treated. He waited for the oncologist's answer before realising the doctor would say nothing more.

'If that order still stands, then I have nothing more to discuss here', said Mark as he stood up from his chair.

Boggs raised his hand to stop Mark, reminding him that Sarah was also required to go to school on a regular basis. He added that DoCS caseworkers would visit their home to check on Sarah whenever they wished to make sure those orders were carried out.

Mark levelled his eyes at Boggs and gave him a warning look. 'I wouldn't be so sure about coming to our place', he said, before heading towards the door. Mark was about to walk out on the lot of them when he turned to deliver an after-thought. 'If you do come, you'll be as welcome as a family of vipers', he added before closing the door.

A SNAKE AT THE DOOR

Most families now would know that it is not sensible to contact DoCS Seeking help. To go to the department for help invites the Potential for removal of children and a life living with DoCS supervising every aspect of how you live.

FAMILY INCLUSION NETWORK NSW
Submission to the SPECIAL INQUIRY INTO CHILD PROTECTION SERVICES IN NSW 2008

In mid October, Sarah was sick when she fronted up to the hospital ward for her last round of chemotherapy. The chemicals had dropped her haemoglobin to a low of 8, whereas it should normally have been in a range of 12 to 15. This meant she was severely anaemic; a haemoglobin of 7, is the level at which doctors normally give blood transfusions to patients.[35] After the chemo, Sarah dragged herself to the hospital school. By the time Sarah returned to the apartment she looked so white that Ruth, rushed out to buy fresh fruit and vegetables from the local markets. She hoped the fresh food would boost Sarah's iron levels, since the court order was still in place that prevented her having vitamins and iron supplements to help raise her blood cell count. Most of all, Ruth hoped Sarah would be released home soon, as she feared her granddaughter might not survive much longer otherwise.

Meanwhile, the caseworkers were not happy with Mark. His early departure from the hospital meeting the week before had left them with a sense of unfinished business. Before Sarah's discharge from the hospital, the department wanted to impose a complicated care plan on the family in addition to the existing court orders.

---

[35] Torpy et al. *Blood transfusion* , JAMA 2004 292(14).

On an unusually hot October's day around lunchtime, Mark was just returning to the homestead, sweaty from repairing fences. The first of the searing weather for the season had brought every kind of animal out from its winter hibernation, looking for a feed. This time of year, kangaroos damaged fences while running for cover and rabbits burrowed under the mesh. When Mark arrived at the house, he noticed the mini-van was gone: Di was already on her way to visit Sarah at the hospital. He tied up both dogs and went inside to fix himself a sandwich. Just as he was about to sit down to lunch at the dining room table, the dogs started barking. He peered through the kitchen window and saw a white, compact government car parked in his driveway. Another quick glance towards the yard gate revealed two DoCS caseworkers heading toward the veranda steps. Mark did not intend to let the women in, since he had lost all trust in the department by then. From experience, he knew they would gather evidence at every turn. If he let them into his house, they would try to find any fault they could, then twist it around and use it against them in court. Since the department had become a risk to his family, his new policy was never to open the door to them. To ensure that the caseworkers never needed to come to his house again, Mark had asked Gary Boggs to put everything in writing in future, and he wondered why they had ignored this and what they were doing here now. As far as Mark was concerned, he would obey the standing court orders but this did not include allowing the caseworkers inside his home.

Mark barely had enough time to disappear behind a dividing wall when the two women knocked on the door. He looked through a narrow fissure to see the caseworkers peering through his windows into the living and dining rooms. From their vantage point, they could easily see his lunch on the table, untouched. They returned to the French doors and knocked for the second time. When they grasped the door handle, Mark tensed. For a moment, he thought they would come into his house. The women had a discussion on the veranda while Mark waited patiently. To his relief, they left after a few more minutes. When he saw their car heading down the driveway and turning onto the main road, he returned to his lunch.

Half an hour later, Mark was just enjoying a cup of tea when his father phoned. Evidently, the caseworkers had gone up to Jim and Ruth's house next. Ruth was in town that morning and Jim, too, was just sitting down alone for lunch when the two women arrived at his door. Jim peered through the dining room window where he discovered the department's white car parked in his drive. Like Mark, Jim had lost trust in the department and felt in no way obliged to open the door to these people after the trouble they'd caused his family, and he could think of no legal obligation requiring him to do so. Jim returned to the table to continue his lunch. From there he could see the women's silhouettes through the milky glass front door. He continued eating his tomato sandwich, and when next he looked up, he saw that the women were no longer there. He got up to clear the table and while taking his plate back to the kitchen, he heard another series of knocks on the door. He peered out of the dining room window to see the car had gone from the driveway. In that case, who was knocking at the door, he wondered. With his curiosity aroused, Jim headed towards the front door and saw no tall shadows behind the frosted glass. On the bottom pane was a section of clear glass Jim had replaced years ago when the frosted pane had broken. He crouched down to look through the glass and immediately saw the culprit. On the other side of the window pane was a six-foot black snake, writhing around the spot where the two caseworkers had stood only moments before. The metaphor was not lost on Jim. Immediately, he phoned Mark.

'I've just had a fiendish visitor', he chuckled.

'You too?' asked Mark.

A few days later, a caseworker phoned Mark again wanting to arrange a meeting.

'You're not coming on my property again', he told them sternly.

'Then where can we meet with you?' asked the caseworker, nonplussed.

Mark thought quickly. 'I'll see you at my solicitor's office'. He didn't think the Taree lawyer would mind hosting the meeting, even though Mark had been representing himself in court lately.

The following week, the meeting was convened at the Taree law office with Mark's lawyer present. This time Mark brought Di, while Boggs brought Judy and Gillian.

Inside the lawyer's office, Gary Boggs repeated all he'd said at the previous hospital meeting in the same official monotone.

'I've heard all this before', said Mark. 'I've already given you an undertaking that after Sarah comes home, we have every intention of taking her to scheduled hospital appointments for scans and blood tests to monitor her condition. We have always done this anyway'.

Boggs then fossicked around in his briefcase and brought out a document he had prepared. It was an undertaking he wanted the parents to sign, agreeing not to give vitamins to their other children or Sarah would be removed from the home.

Mark and the lawyer looked at each other. They both knew no court orders existed over the other children but it looked like the department wanted to extend its power over the family by agreement.

'Even if we gave our other children vitamins', said Mark, 'which we don't, because they don't need them, it would be between us and the health professionals who prescribed them, and nothing to do with you'.

Boggs was briefly taken aback but continued on another tack. 'And she will need to go to school', he added. 'We will monitor that by making regular visits to your home'.

The two caseworkers nodded in support of Boggs.

Mark stood up to his full height and glared at Boggs. 'In future, no one from the department is welcome on our property', he said.

Boggs looked livid. 'But we have a legal right to visit whenever we want'.

Mark stayed firm. 'You may think you have rights on my property, but let me spell it out for you. I've already told you that you people are not welcome and if you ever set foot on my property again you will be dealt with as trespassers'. Mark glowered at Boggs to ensure his message was understood.

The lawyer called a brief interval and asked the caseworkers to wait in the foyer while he discussed the issues with the parents in private. His secretary was out to lunch and he personally showed the three DoCS workers through the concertina door separating his office and the hallway, before leading them down the corridor to the outer waiting room. He returned to talk with Mark and Di in his office and pulled the folding door across. They had scarcely started when they heard scuffling noises. The lawyer put his index finger to his lips and got up from his desk. He flung open the concertina door and caught the caseworkers red-handed. They'd had their ears pressed to the door.

Mark stood up in disgust. He thanked the lawyer for his help before he left the legal office with Di. Outside in the car park, Di didn't know whether to laugh or cry.

'That's the mentality we're dealing with', said Mark as he unlocked the door to the mini-van. 'They're like a bunch of kids; except they've got police powers and they have our daughter's life in their hands'.

'What are you going to tell them?' asked Di.

Mark started the car and put it in gear so fast he left a coating of rubber in the car park. 'I've got nothing more to say to that mob', he replied.

A few days after the meeting, while Mark was at work and Sarah's siblings were still at school, Di and Ruth drove Sarah home from the hospital. Sarah's body functions had changed after the chemicals, and on the way home, she was carsick. When they turned into the drive, Sarah burst into tears. This is what she had been wanting for months, and yet the world looked very different now. Did she dare to be happy or would they come and take her away again? She used to feel completely safe at home, but now she didn't feel safe anywhere. This was why she had begged her father just a few weeks ago, to never let those people near her again.

Pooch and Muttley excitedly jumped on Sarah while she struggled up the few steps to the veranda. She paused to catch her breath and played with the dogs briefly while Di and Ruth brought in the luggage from the car. Sarah headed inside, while her mother sorted out her washing and her grandmother prepared her bed. Sarah stood in the kitchen and looked out the window towards Sarah's Hill. Although her home was happily familiar, she herself seemed so different. She knew she was too weak to run around the paddocks, and that a big part of her life now had ended.

Sarah opened the fridge. It was full of last night's baked potato and pumpkin. A small dish of roast chicken legs sat temptingly at the front. Sarah picked up a drumstick and sniffed it before taking a bite. She had almost forgotten what it was like to eat all the home cooking she wanted. When Sarah had finished, she felt suddenly tired. Fatigue replaced all the strain and vigilance of the past winter. For once, she could relax and stop worrying about what people might do to her or what they write into their notebooks about her. Sarah now craved only one thing: to go upstairs and get into the bed her grandmother had just made up for her. Under her lilac quilt, she wanted to sleep for a whole year.

Sarah was fast asleep when her siblings came home from school. They woke her up for a noisy reunion. Laura was doubly relieved her sister was home. She'd had the heavy responsibility of keeping the other kids safe at school, making sure they were all on the bus each afternoon and that none went missing. The other children had also been deeply affected by Sarah's absence. Clara, who needed a calm routine, had suffered terribly from the constant disruptions. In addition, Hannah and the two youngest, Leah and Joshua, who had idolised Sarah and thought she was invincible, now feared that whatever happened to Sarah could also happen to them.

The children knew little about Sarah's condition, since the doctors still hadn't given their parents much clear information. The kids thought that although their sister had a serious illness, she would pull through just as she had so many times before. In fact, no one in the family was told the full situation until some years later, when Mark issued Freedom of Information requests to DoCS and the hospitals. Even then, he received only a small fraction of the documents, many had been heavily edited or redacted, and it took the family and this author several years to piece together a clearer picture of what had happened to them.

Meanwhile, the children all remained traumatised and confused at the time. They had felt desperately alone while their parents had no choice but to devote most of their time and resources to fighting DoCS and caring for Sarah. Laura kept a diary and has written of that time:

We children had always striven to do the right thing towards those we didn't particularly like and we'd never [before] had a reason to hate anyone. But hatred was the only word that could be used to describe the feelings we had developing for the people who were ruining our family. It was beyond our young minds to imagine that there could be people in the world without thought or compassion for other human beings.

We could not comprehend why our family was being bullied and forced into things we didn't want to do. As children, we'd always been allowed to make our own decisions, with a positive influence from our parents, who always had our best interests at heart. Now even our parents were being manipulated into situations they didn't wish to be in. We didn't understand why Sarah was being forced to stay in the halfway house when she was perfectly well enough to come home. Why she was made to stay in the hospital, and have chemotherapy when she didn't want it, and it only made her sick. Why she wasn't even allowed to go outside for a walk around the hospital grounds. No amount of explaining could satisfy our minds, because none of it made any sense, even though the older children were teenagers. Not even our parents could answer all our questions.

We kids were beginning to become resentful of Sarah too. We were sick of our mum and dad having to spend all the available time and finances on Sarah. We knew that a lot of people were giving Sarah gifts, and we couldn't help but wonder why no one seemed to pay any attention to us. Our marks at school were gradually declining, because of the distractions we had at home, and we were all losing our normal enthusiasm for life. As children do, we felt unfairly treated, and were craving some attention from our parents. This of-

*ten resulted in the kids being moody and they would fight. It only
put more strain on the situation. Often we children would cry ourselves to sleep, because we were caught in a web of confusion and
frustration at not being able to understand what was happening to
us. We were constantly terrified and at times had nightmares of being torn away from our parents and all that we held dear. We loved
each other, our parents and all our other family members. We lived
under constant threat of losing all we knew.*

Now that Sarah had returned home worse for wear, each family member realised afresh the importance of being together. If anything, their terrifying experiences had strengthened their bond.

That night at dinner, Di and the children were reunited for the first time in months while Mark worked long overtime hours at the mine to catch up with the bills. Sarah's siblings could not stop staring at her. There was something very different about their sister. Sarah had always been tall for her age with a head of thick shiny hair. Now she seemed oddly stunted, with a stubbly regrowth on her head that made her look like an urchin. While incarcerated, she had not fully regained the weight she had lost in the city hospital – and she had not grown a single millimetre either. During her winter-long stint in hospital she had become so hunched over and puny that Hannah, who was two years her junior, was now taller and heavier than Sarah.

Their sister behaved differently too. She had picked up colourful language from the hospital and acquired glib street smarts. Laura, Clara and tiny Leah rolled their eyes each time Sarah dropped a clanger.

That evening, Di served up Sarah's favourites: a delicious roast, mashed potatoes and vegetables. The kids displayed their usual eating quirks. Hannah loved potatoes and created an igloo of mash with the roast hidden inside, before tackling her dinner. As usual, Joshua made himself a mashed potato sandwich as an appetiser before he finished the meat and veg on his plate. Sarah tore off hunks of freshly baked bread and used them to soak up everyone's spare gravy. In these familiar rituals, at least, Sarah found comfort that some things had stayed the same.

Attracted to the commotion was Brutus the calf. While the family ate dinner, he had ambled across the house paddock, peered over the yard fence, and begun to bellow. All winter he'd roamed sadly around the outer paddocks, missing the kids' company. The children ran from the table and greeted him at the gate. Like a frail old woman, Sarah followed them outside. The calf had grown into a bullock over the year but lapped up the children's attention, just like old times. He licked Sarah with his sandpapery tongue. While Sarah patted Brutus, the tough expression on her face softened. Her sisters were relieved that Sarah was starting to look like their sister again.

When night fell, each had their own fears. With Mark working long hours they felt vulnerable in their own home and wondered who might be outside looking through the windows. Since the department had intruded into their lives, strange things had happened around the house. While Mark and Di were in Sydney with Sarah, her siblings were farmed out to other family members, spending just a few hours at home after school each day before the relatives collected them. During this time, their belongings had been disturbed so often that Laura and Joshua had thought up their own security device. Before leaving the house, they sprinkled white flour on the floor near the entrance and in the study to check if someone had entered the house while no one was home. Hannah had even had the idea of spanning a thread across the outside of the door. When the children returned to the house two days later, the thread had been broken and there were adult-sized footprints in the flour.

In the same space of time, Laura had written letters to a friend describing the family's ordeal. She had hidden the letters her friend wrote in reply in her room. She was spooked when those letters went missing, but terrified when they turned up a week later in her mailbox after someone had reposted them. Together with the break-in at Ruth and Jim's, where documents had disappeared, and the car break-ins Mark had experienced, the odd happenings seemed more than just co-incidence.

For the first time in the children's lives, being taken from their home was a very real possibility, since the department constantly used this threat as leverage against the parents. They were somewhat relieved when their father told them that nothing had happened since the dogs had begun to patrol the grounds at night and that they were perfectly safe. That night, however, Sarah refused to sleep in her upstairs bedroom despite Mark's reassurances, and Di had to make a bed up for her downstairs. Only when the others were asleep did Sarah climb into it and settle for the night, on the proviso her mother slept with her. That night, and for months after, Mark came home in the early hours of the morning to find Di with Sarah. Most nights Sarah shouted and talked in her sleep. She still had the same recurring nightmare that had started in the hospital: they were coming to take her away to a dark place where she would die. For months, Sarah would not sleep until she was sure all the doors were locked and windows closed. Even on hot summer nights, she would not let Mark keep a window open.

The parents realised their daughter had been as severely traumatised by incarceration and forced treatment at the hospital as victims of war were by the extreme conditions imposed on them. They desperately wanted to take Sarah to a counsellor for help, but because of the mandatory reporting law in NSW, they knew the counsellor would be required to make a report to DoCS. They feared they would be blamed for the devastating effects the department's actions had had on Sarah and thought it would only worsen their current plight. [36] Sarah, on the other hand, was distrustful of counsellors since she had been emotionally probed so often by the social worker and caseworkers. The parents were therefore entirely on their own in dealing with Sarah's unusually severe emotional trauma, not to mention their five other traumatised children, who also needed comforting and support.

For the first week at home, Sarah was bone tired and did little more than sleep. She was pale as chalk with persisting anaemia, for which she was still not allowed treatment. Despite this, she was forced to attend school until the end of the school year in mid December.

Each morning Di was required to put Sarah on the bus for the jarring 45-minute ride to school. Then Sarah had to complete an entire school day before the long bus ride home over unsealed roads. Her day began at 7.00 am and ended at 5.00 pm. Once home, she headed straight up to bed and could not keep up with her homework. The next morning Sarah was so exhausted her mother could hardly wake her. Since the bus driver was at the mailbox at 8 am sharp and would not wait a minute longer, Sarah was often late for the bus and Di had to drive her to school. Once there, it was sheer torture for Sarah to sit in class and pay attention. She found it difficult to concentrate and often dozed off. She was embarrassed by her pallor and the stubble on her head. The hats she wore became intolerably hot in summer. At times, she wore a wig, but was embarrassed by its artificial look and the fact that it sometimes fell off.

In physical education, Sarah could not manage the exercises because of her damaged lungs. On one occasion, the teacher said to her: 'Come on Sarah, a little exercise isn't going to kill you'. Sarah was so upset she told her sisters on the bus that afternoon. On arriving home, she went straight to her room and shut the door. Sarah had never baulked at physical activity – once she could run

---

[36] A 1999 University of California study published in the American Journal of Public Health on mandatory reporting highlights the damage this policy has caused to therapeutic relationships.

for miles – but now she found even walking a strain. She had soft flesh where her muscles once were, her lungs had hardened and she could hardly breathe. The teacher's remark reminded her of the quality of life she had lost and how drastically her life had changed.

In the weeks leading up to Christmas 2003, Mark and Di were concerned about Sarah not coping with school. Day after the day the routine was the same: Sarah came home sick and went straight to bed. Di had to bring up a tray and wake her for dinner. Then at night, the recurrent nightmare would come again and she would wake up screaming. Di had to sleep in bed with her until she settled again. Di then usually woke up when Mark arrived home from his night shift, at which point she returned to her own bed. There the parents sometimes talked until dawn. No one got much rest.

'She can't keep going to school when she's this sick', said Di.

Mark was furious each time he heard about the continued hardships the department was imposing on Sarah. 'You wouldn't put a horse through this', he said. 'She can't take this anymore and neither can we'.

'What can we do about it? asked Di.

'Maybe we can still get her overseas for treatment'.

'How?'

Mark thought for a moment. 'I'm going to ask for a court hearing. We have to get her out of here', he said, 'before they kill her'.

On Mark's next day off, he and Di took Sarah to the family GP in Gloucester for a tumour marker blood test. The doctor drew the sample and sent it to the lab. In the hospital during the months of chemotherapy the tumour markers had decreased, but were never entirely absent from the blood despite the constant flow of chemicals.

Two days later, the results came in. Sarah's tumour markers were rising again. It meant the months of forced chemotherapy had been a complete failure: Sarah had relapsed for the second time. Her chances of survival were now almost non-existent. She was in the terminal stage of cancer.

Inexplicably, Mark and Di were not told of the lab results at the time or the implications of the rising tumour markers. Sarah was still required to go to school, even though she was terminally ill. The social worker had told them that 'school will raise her self-esteem', and the child protection department agreed. The oncologist Dr Kotz, who knew what the rise in markers meant, raised no objections to DoCS' strictly regimented plan for Sarah.

Three weeks before Christmas Mark phoned the clinic to ask whether we could help Sarah in any way. Since there was still a standing court order preventing Sarah having nutritional and supportive treatments, we could not do much at the time.

Mark asked me how we were going at the clinic. I told him I had finally heard from the Crown Solicitor's Office. After they had gagged the magazine and alleged I'd made factual errors in the article, I'd written the Crown Solicitor's Office a letter asking for a list of the alleged errors.

'What did they say?' asked Mark.

'They sent me an invitation', I replied.

'Where to?'

'A summons to the Supreme Court... the day after tomorrow'.

'I'm coming to that hearing to give you support', promised Mark. 'And I want to raise some of my own issues there as well', he added.

A CRY FOR JUSTICE

To be left alone is the first step towards freedom.
Anon

On a hot day in December, when Sydney teemed with Christmas shoppers, I was called to the Supreme Court to defend the article I had written in August. I stood waiting for Mark by the statue of Queen Victoria in front of the NSW Supreme Court building in the legal district of Sydney. The old queen had reigned during the Federation period, the time when Australia was released from its colonial shackles and emerged as a constitutional monarchy. The young country was bequeathed the British legal system and its guiding principle: the rule of law. This meant that all citizens, organisations and government departments were subject to the same laws of the land. I hoped that rule would apply today, since I had come to represent myself without a barrister and was up against a powerful government department. I had a bad case of nerves, which I treated with a dose of altruism. I felt I was defending both myself and also every writer and journalist who takes personal and professional risks to reveal important issues to the community. I'd had some self-litigation experience involving a number of social justice issues, but never in the Supreme Court.

I looked up to see Mark rounding the corner towards the court. He wore a grim, determined look. If he felt nervous, he didn't show it. He looked more like a man who'd planned decisive action towards a definite goal.

In fact, Mark was intent that day to secure Sarah's release from DoCS' control. The department had imposed its own strict rules on his daughter, and he believed they were damaging her health. At the very least, Mark wanted Sarah's malnutrition treated, or else he feared it would shorten her life even more. Furthermore, he now considered this to be his last chance to take Sarah overseas for a cancer treatment that would buy her time and quality of life.

We entered the imposing glass building together and checked the hearing list in the lobby before taking the elevator up to the equity division. The court session was held under the original suppression order and remained closed to the public. Apart from the legal staff, no one but Mark and I were allowed in.

We entered the courtroom and sat down at the defendants' table on the right side before the judge's bench. At the other table sat DoCS' legal representative. He was a youngish, enthusiastic barrister from the Crown Solicitor's Office, dressed in his black robe and horsehair wig.

The court officer announced the court was in session and we all rose. The judge was a bewigged, older gentleman bearing a dignified expression that gave away no trace of emotion. Once seated, His Honour wanted to deal with my matter first. He asked to hear from the DoCS barrister and then he would hear my submission.

The barrister began a long discourse alleging I had breached the suppression orders. He particularly objected to my mentioning Mark's occupation and the general region where the family lived, claiming this could identify Sarah. He asked the court to impose a series of harsh gag orders and punishments on me for having written and published the article.

The judge had been dealing with Sarah's matter over the previous seven months. He had already read my article when Mark had presented it to the court at the previous hearing. He now leaned forward to hear my response.

I stood to reiterate the points I'd made in my affidavit. I had taken particular care to de-identify the information used in the article in accordance with professional standards. I had given both oncologists the courtesy of withholding their names, even though they were used in the Supreme Court's own case-law website. When the judge seemed surprised to hear this, I showed him the proof I'd printed off from the court's website. The barrister was unhappy about this since it didn't help his argument.

Next, I argued that the article raised issues critical to the public interest. As a writer, I had found it particularly newsworthy that several of the oncologist's own professional peers found no scientific basis for his claims of a cure. The article's newsworthiness had only increased after a number of medical colleagues had opposed the oncologist's forced treatment and objected to his refusal to treat Sarah's malnutrition. Yet, despite his professional colleagues' serious concerns, the oncologist still continued his forced treatment and refused to address Sarah's nutritional deficiencies. I submitted that the article represented a family's cry for justice and raised professional ethics issues and human rights concerns to the community.

His Honour listened courteously to my submission. The DoCS barrister had earlier objected to my mentioning Mark's occupation and the general region where the family lived. The judge asked what I thought about removing these details and I readily agreed, since it made no change to the article's context.

On this issue, Mark stood up and volunteered that his entire family, including Sarah, had been consulted about the article before its publication and that no one had any objections to it. Furthermore, no family member minded if it identified them, since their plight had been broadly known in the community even before the article appeared. Mark added that as far as he was aware, the community widely disapproved of the doctor's actions and the authorities' handling of the matter.

I waited for Mark to finish before going on to discuss my correspondence with the Crown Solicitor's Office. I told the judge I had asked for a list of the factual errors the Crown alleged I had made in the article. I'd never received a reply and was still interested in finding out what the errors were. The DoCS barrister jumped from his seat to argue that errors were not the problem, quite the opposite – the article was too factually accurate for the department's liking.

After some deliberation, the judge made an order requiring me to change the details concerning Mark's occupation and delete a reference to the region in which the family lived. I told him I would happily change the hard copy but was not certain if I could do the same with the electronic copies that were floating around the World Wide Web. I explained that the article had already travelled around the globe to several other countries and was impossible to retrieve from cyberspace, which was not an actual place at all. The judge seemed perplexed by the concept until the DoCS barrister offered him a tutorial about the internet and reluctantly confirmed what I had said. For a while longer, the judge tried to integrate the wild frontier of the internet with the current laws governing publication. Finally, he accepted that once electronically released into the public domain, I had no more control of the article. He allowed me to continue to publish the article provided I made the changes to the hard copy. Just for good measure, I volunteered to contact those individuals who I knew had an electronic copy and offer them an amended copy. The judge seemed satisfied with this, while I was delighted with the judge's decision. It was a triumph for me and for the family, not to mention for other journalists and writers who tackled difficult issues.

With my hearing out of the way, the judge turned his attention to Mark. Since July, Mark had been battling the unusually restrictive orders the department had managed to obtain from the court. Since then DoCS had imposed a raft of additional demands; caseworkers had threatened to remove Sarah and her siblings, if they gave any of their children nutritional supplements. Since these supplements, such as fish oil, were in every supermarket and everyone else was free to include them in their shopping basket, Mark asked why the department was trying to interfere so irrationally in their lives. The caseworkers were not trained in health care, nutritional medicine or cancer treatments, yet they still insisted on practicing their own version of medicine on his family. Mark was concerned that these caseworkers would continue to prevent Sarah from pursuing genuine medical options and that she would die as a result of DoCS' misguided and uninformed views on what constituted appropriate health care and medical treatment. He believed only tragic consequences could come from non-medically trained staff in government departments playing doctor, especially when they made life and death decisions and misused their statutory power to force their uninformed opinions on people. He felt this had already visited endless hardship and misery on his family. In his submission to the judge, Mark told of the bribery and manipulation imposed on Sarah at the hospital. He detailed her terrible state of health since the forced treatment and her inability to sleep at night for fear of DoCS. Mark reminded the court of Sarah's desperate need to have her malnutrition treated with supplements. Even though several doctors, including a professor of medicine, had recommended this, for some reason, DoCS was still forbidding it.

Mark maintained that Sarah and the entire family needed to be left alone to find closure after a shockingly traumatic year. He wanted their rights reinstated to select their own doctors and oncologists. He asked for all previous orders to be revoked and for DoCS to have no more involvement in their lives. He wanted Sarah released from the State's wardship and legally restored to her family.

That day Mark believed that surely the judge must have by now read all the evidence Mark had put to the court in the previous hearing, and have enough material to reverse the restrictive orders. There were now four doctors on the court record who had expressed serious concerns about Sarah's welfare and had disapproved of the oncologist's treatment. Even more doctors had contacted Mark off the record and expressed the same views. He thought he had amply demonstrated to the court that a number of highly qualified clinicians were available to take over Sarah's care, if released, (including those in the world-class facilities of internationally known cancer hospitals).

After Mark finished his motions to the court, the barrister delivered his own lengthy arguments against Mark's requests. He reminded the court that both oncologists, Drs Kotz and Capewell, had repeatedly reported that Sarah would probably be cured with their continued treatment. Unfortunately, the court remained in the dark about Sarah's poor prognosis and the judge therefore still assumed Sarah could be cured. Though he appeared genuinely troubled once again by Mark's testimony outlining Sarah's hardships, the judge ruled to continue whatever treatments the oncologist wanted to administer. This meant DoCS would remain in the family's lives.

However, as a concession to Mark, the judge revoked the previous order banning Dr Tyler from Sarah's care. Lifting this order, meant Sarah was allowed to come to our clinic again as a patient. It was the only morsel of hope Mark took away from the proceedings and it rounded off 2003 as the worst year of their lives so far.

After the court hearing, Mark and I were both relieved to return to our respective homes, thankful that no litigation was scheduled for the remaining two weeks of the year.

I drove home pondering the stressful year and hoped 2004 would be quieter. We intended closing the clinic over the Christmas and New Year period and reopening in mid January. I looked forward to the rest. If we did see Sarah at the clinic in the New Year, it would pose a challenge, however. On one hand, we could not administer metronomic chemotherapy, since Australian oncologists had not yet adopted it. On the other hand, there still existed a court order prohibiting Sarah from having appropriate treatment to correct her nutritional deficiencies.

For Mark, the three-hour drive home was agonising. He had to break the bad news yet again that DoCS would remain in their lives. Worse still, they were still not free to take Sarah overseas for a cancer treatment that could extend her life. Their only allowed option was to attend the clinic for supportive treatments, but even that was impossible while DoCS insisted she go to school.

A few days before Christmas, the community of Gloucester pulled together and donated presents and financial help to the Westley family. For the second year running, various community organisations, a few private individuals, and even Mark's union passed the hat around for the family. Di recalls that without help, they would have been in for a lean Christmas. Although caseworkers had promised them financial help and practical assistance, it had never materialized.

Instead, DoCS' continued legal assaults that year had cost the parents over $48 000 to defend themselves. This was money that had been earmarked for Sarah's medical treatment, now wasted on litigation.

Mark and Di insist they will never forget the community's generosity. Help came when they needed it most. Not only did presents appear under the tree for the children, but the community support restored the parents' faith in humanity. Even with community help, however, the holiday season of 2003 was unsettled. Family members remained shell-shocked from the horrific year and the household was tense, bracing for the next onslaught.

New Years' Eve was hot and humid. At dusk, Mark opened the windows hoping for a cool breeze. After the kids were in bed, he poured a couple of ginger beers and sat up talking with Di. They discussed the previous New Year's Eve when they'd been so hopeful of finding Sarah the best medical care available. Now, instead of the life-extending treatment Sarah urgently needed, all the caseworkers were focused on was sending her to school. The parents sat on the couch forlorn. It was all so depressing. At 12 o'clock, the hallway clock struck in 2004. That year, even the chimes sounded like a bad omen.

In mid-January, we reopened the clinic. Soon after, Sarah's parents brought her in for a check-up. She had already been underweight, fatigued, and anaemic on her discharge from the regional hospital in October; then, after spending four months seriously ill in hospital, the department had forced her to attend school. This extra stress had made it impossible for Sarah to recover from her ordeal. Moreover, without being allowed nutritional supplements, she still suffered from untreated malnutrition. By January, she had gained weight on Di's home cooking. Sarah's face rounded out, but she still looked anxious, pale and obviously ill. She still suffered constant fatigue; her muscles still wasted from the devastating weight loss in the hospital.

By contrast, Sarah had been strong and well muscled when we first saw her at the clinic in May 2003, before the forced treatments. She had been in above average percentiles for both height and weight. Despite having cancer, her nutritional status had been excellent, with no trace of nutritional deficiencies, as she had been taking regular, prescribed nutritional supplements at the time. During Sarah's bout of malnutrition at the hospital, however, she had dropped to well below the average height and weight for her age. At the city hospital, her weight plummeted down into the tenth percentile. This meant that during the hospital admission, 90 out of every 100 children weighed more than Sarah. Mark and Di were concerned that Sarah's untreated malnutrition could shorten her life. These concerns were not unfounded.

There are two types of malnutrition. A chronic form occurs over months or years of under-nutrition while the acute variety – known as marasmus – is sudden and life threatening. It results when insufficient nutrition is coupled with a sudden and substantial increase of energy expenditure and essential nutrient depletion. This occurs in children suffering sudden trauma, major surgery, burns, major infections, severe diarrhea, and extreme stress. [37] Sarah had been subjected to five of these six intense stressors over a two-week period in hospital. At the same time, she had been too ill post-operatively to eat and replenish her calories and nutritional requirements. Under these extreme conditions, acute malnutrition can develop in a previously well-nourished child. Marasmus is accompanied by extreme and rapid weight loss and muscle wasting. It is a serious metabolic crisis causing the rapid breakdown of fat, muscles and body organs. In a virtual meltdown, the body consumes itself in order to survive. This cascade can reach a critical point that results in sudden death. Marasmus is known to occur in Western hospital settings and requires urgent treatment with hydration, nutritious foods, protein or amino acids, and a large variety of vitamins and minerals including iron and folate (Joosten 08, Pawellek 08, Rabinowitz 07). Yet Sarah was not treated for malnutrition; she was given chemotherapy instead. This posed an additional stressor and further depleted nutritional stores. Worse still, severely malnourished patients do not respond well to chemotherapy: their tumour growth is not diminished by the treatment. This was the case with Sarah, who had no apparent beneficial response to the chemo that was forced on her.

Moreover, those who survive marasmus are prone to long-term metabolic problems and damage to the digestive system and organs. Untreated acute malnutrition leads to chronic malnutrition. In cancer patients, this means a shortened lifespan.

If any child ever needed nutritional supplements, it was Sarah. Several medical colleagues agreed. It was clear she had no chance of battling her cancer while nutritionally deficient. However, her symptoms indicated that she was not absorbing food adequately and the nutrients would need to be administered through intravenous drips over a three-hour period. This would require two trips a week to the clinic over several months. We were aware DoCS forbade Sarah nutritional supplements, but we knew this was precisely the medical treatment she needed and felt it was unethical to withhold an appropriate treatment. For Sarah this meant a full nutritional loading protocol – 12 vitamins, dozens of minerals and trace minerals, amino acids and potent broad spectrum antioxidants to process the toxic residue left from the chemotherapy

---

[37] Simon S Rabinowitz, MD, PhD, Professor of Clinical Pediatrics, New York Medical College; Chairman, Chief and Medical Administrator, Department of Pediatrics, Chief, Pediatric Gastroenterology and Nutrition, Richmond University Medical Center.

and assist in detoxification. Some of these nutrients would be in an oral form while others were intravenous. In addition, Sarah required protein and nutrition-dense calories in high-quality foods, which she was already getting at home.

At the clinic, we could offer only supportive treatment to Sarah rather than treat her cancer directly. Metronomic chemotherapy is designed to treat the cancer itself and could have offered Sarah extra months of life. In the past 20 years, cancer treatments have changed to include regimens with fewer side effects. In his study of Gina, the young woman with ovarian cancer whom he treated with metronomic chemotherapy, Dr Riccardo Samaritani states:

> Not surprisingly patient attitudes to toxic chemotherapy regimens for advanced, platinum [chemotherapy] resistant, ovarian cancer are often negative, as the adverse effects of treatment often seem to outweigh any potential benefits. Thus, the introduction of newer approaches, having improved or at least equivalent efficacy but reduced toxicity, are highly desirable. Therapy must be individualized according to previous response, toxicities, and patient wishes.

Dr Samaritani had previously given Gina conventional chemotherapy, to which she had not responded. As a last resort, he prescribed metronomic chemotherapy (as a salvage treatment) in small daily doses, along with nutritional supplements. These were to address Gina's nutritional deficiencies and anaemia – side effects of both her cancer and the conventional chemotherapy she'd previously been given. Immediately Gina gained weight and her anaemia resolved. Three months later a scan showed that her cancer had not progressed further and her general condition had improved. Gina was feeling well and resuming an active life at the very time Sarah had her second relapse and was in desperate need of a salvage treatment to extend her life. We were disappointed we could not offer Sarah this treatment, as it was not available for use in Australia. We could only offer nutritional and supportive treatment in the hope it would improve Sarah's quality of life.

By the end of the visit the parents wanted to schedule a series of appointments for Sarah's intravenous treatments, but the new school year was due to start the next day and DoCS was still watching their every move. They would have to explain Sarah's frequent school absences, since the drive to the clinic and back, plus the treatment time, would take up an entire day. Mark was upset that DoCS was preventing his daughter from having proper treatment yet again, and promised to bring Sarah back for the appointments as soon as he could find a way around the restrictions.

The next day the new school year started. Sarah was in Year 7, her first year of high school. These milestones are stressful for any young girl but for Sarah, with terminal cancer, being forced to go to school was emotionally overwhelming and physically devastating.

At the end of February, Mark and Di took Sarah back to the hospital for further scans and tests. Her tumour markers were still continuing to rise at an alarming rate. It was the first the parents had heard of this discouraging news. However, Dr Kotz still did not advise them that Sarah was in a terminal phase of the cancer, nor did he correct his earlier claim of having an 80 per cent chance of curing Sarah. Instead, he offered more of the same chemotherapy he had already forced her to have. The parents asked him why he was offering the identical treatment when Sarah had had such devastating side effects to it and it had not worked in the first place. The oncologist said he could offer no more. The parents had on several occasions asked him about the smaller dose chemotherapy treatments, but he mentioned nothing of the metronomic chemotherapy as salvage therapy for terminal patients. Nor did he mention palliative care to the parents, nor the likely downhill course Sarah's disease would take in the next months. Indeed the parents left the consultation somewhat confused about the course of Sarah's illness.

With DoCS insisting Sarah attend school despite her terminal condition, she struggled on until March, at which point she became physically unable to continue. Mark and Di then decided to begin her intravenous therapy urgently at the clinic. When they told the deputy principal that Sarah would not be attending school again on a regular basis, he was sympathetic. He had seen Sarah struggling and felt sorry for her. He had offered Sarah help whenever she needed it – and as it turned out, she would soon require his assistance. After a few days' absence from school, Sarah's legal representative contacted the family. She told Mark to bring Sarah to an unfamiliar address in Newcastle early the next morning around 8 am. Mark thought the time seemed too early for office hours and became suspicious. He negotiated the time for later and reluctantly agreed to come.

The next morning Mark, Di and Sarah set out on the long trip to Newcastle. Mark's mobile was out of range until they drove through the small village of Stroud, when it beeped with a message. The legal representative left word that she was unwell, and instead of seeing her that morning, they were scheduled to see another person at the same address. On hearing the message, Mark did a U-turn and headed straight back to Gloucester.

'What are you doing?' asked Di.

'There's something fishy going on. We're going back home'.

Half an hour later they arrived home and Mark phoned the legal representative to ask what was going on. She picked up her office phone sounding far from ill. She explained that she had felt ill, but was alright now. Somebody else wanted to talk to Sarah in a teleconference. Could they bring Sarah to the high school, where the principal would preside over the conference?

Mark agreed to take Sarah to the principal's office later that day, but couldn't guarantee that Sarah would want to speak to them.

That afternoon in the high school office, Sarah explained to the deputy principal that she did not want to talk to her legal representative on the phone. The woman had come to see her in the hospital several times and had asked her what her wishes were. Each time Sarah told her what she wanted her to say in court, but the woman said she would say the opposite. Sarah believed her legal representative was partly responsible for the restrictive court orders imposed on her. Now Sarah did not want to talk with her again, and didn't want her representing her in future either.

When the deputy principal suggested she tell the woman on the phone what she had just told him, Sarah answered, 'They already know. Dad told them too, but they don't listen. I don't want to see them ever again'.

The deputy principal went into his office to relay the message. He told the legal representative that Sarah did not wish to speak with her and he didn't intend to force her. There was nothing more he could do about it.

After Sarah returned to the waiting room, Mark gladly took her home. He had only agreed to bring Sarah to the school because he trusted the school principal. Now, hopefully, the legal rep and DoCS would get the message that their services were not wanted or appreciated.

Meanwhile the article about Sarah had continued to circulate – this time with the required changes – and more and more people began to learn of Sarah's plight. Now, with the court's blessing, the editor of the Melbourne-based magazine put up the second half of Sarah's story on the magazine's website. By then, some readers were aware that Sarah had been released from captivity, but few knew that she was about to enter the final battle for her life.

THE CLINIC

We can no longer pretend that the patient's perceptions don't matter.
And we can't pretend that healing is something doctors do to a
Patient. Your mind is in every cell of your body. And
Your emotions are the bridge between the
Mental and the physical.

David Felten, PhD, University of Rochester School of Medicine.

On a Friday afternoon in late March, Mark and Di arrived at the clinic with Sarah for her first intravenous (IV) treatment. Sarah stuck to her parents like mud while they filled out the necessary consents and paperwork. Once we had briefed the parents about each aspect of the procedure, I showed the family to the spacious IV room and planned to introduce them to the other dozen patients who sat comfortably in recliners receiving various types of intravenous drips. At first, Sarah was too anxious to enter the room and I stood aside while her parents reassured her that this treatment was different to chemo. Even though the room was comfortably furnished, with soft Monet prints on the walls and medical equipment kept to a minimum, I was certain the scene reminded Sarah of the hospital chemotherapy rooms that she'd come to associate with feeling sick and vomiting. I wanted to let Sarah warm up gradually without pressure. Finally, she pushed the swing door open a fraction and peered inside. The other patients were chatting happily without a vomit bowl in sight. I explained that all those people were here because the treatment made them feel better and it might help her too. I'm not sure she believed me at first. She continued to watch from the doorway until she figured out the people were there voluntarily and none were being forced into anything. Only then, did Sarah enter the room and sit down in an empty recliner, insisting her parents sit on either side. She looked vulnerable and self-conscious with her stubbly re-growth of short, wiry hair.

Apart from being the clinic's co-founder, I had my own busy nutritional and complementary medicine practice based there, and in addition to that, my job included running the IV program and supervising several other professional staff in the IV room.[38] Occasionally Dan Tyler dropped in between patient consultations in his office. This time, he stayed out of sight until we had Sarah settled in. For a while Sarah sat in her chair, her arms defiantly folded, daring anyone to threaten, bribe or trick her into something she didn't want. She was wary of the staff and kept a safe distance from anyone with a needle, an intravenous cannula, or a pair of gloves. I explained that she could just sit a while, but if she decided to have the treatments, she might feel well enough to run around the paddocks again. She thought about it and looked around the room. The other patients smiled at her encouragingly. A nurse summoned Dan from his consulting room to lend support. Finally, Sarah presented her arm to let me apply the local anaesthetic before Dan inserted the cannula into her vein. After I started the IV, Sarah spent another few tense minutes until she realised the drip didn't make her sick. She finally folded back the recliner, put her feet up, and stared nervously at the door. Part of her wanted to relax but she was still afraid that a caseworker would arrive at any minute.

Our patients came to the clinic wanting IV treatments for various conditions. Many cancer patients wanted IV vitamin C, a powerful antioxidant, and immune booster. This does not interfere with chemotherapy when given between and after cycles, but it significantly diminishes chemo side effects, allowing many patients to subsequently breeze comfortably through the treatments (Smyth 97). Even though we did not use vitamin C as an anti-cancer treatment, some studies do suggest that high tissue levels of intravenous vitamin C can kill cancer cells and prolong survival times for terminal cancer patients (Jackson 05, Padayatti 06, Padayatti 00, Cameron 78, Murata 82).

We also administered intravenous glutathione, which is the most potent antioxidant known. It is an amino acid based protein naturally produced by cells, but is often lacking in people experiencing illness, malnutrition or an overload of chemicals, when the body's ability to naturally produce glutathione is impaired and it is necessary to replace it. When given as an oral supplement, the glutathione molecule is not well absorbed from the digestive tract. Until recently, when an effective oral glutathione accelerator has been formulated,[39] it needed to be administered intravenously.

---

[38] Since I had worked most of my professional life in intensive care units, I put hospital IV protocols in place in the clinic. This resulted in a 100 per cent patient safety record during the time the clinic was in operation.

[39] Max GXL.

Glutathione is used as an integrative treatment for people with Parkinson's disease, whose brain cells are found to be depleted of glutathione and damaged by free-radical oxidation (Johannsen 91, Sechi 96, Kidd 00, Merad-Boudia 98). [40] Other oxidation-damage neurological diseases benefiting from glutathione include autism, multiple sclerosis and Alzheimer's disease (Liu 04, James 08, Mann CLA 2000).

Glutathione is also used as an adjunct to treatment for many other conditions including chronic fatigue syndrome, liver disease, diabetes, and various forms of toxicity induced illness. Healthy people use it as an anti-aging treatment and athletes often take it to boost energy and endurance.

For Sarah, we prescribed glutathione for several reasons. Firstly, children suffering malnutrition are found to have lowered glutathione levels and it was essential to add glutathione to her vitamins and mineral protocol for her nutritional recovery (Ramdath 86).

Secondly, the four-month chemotherapy put Sarah's system under severe oxidative stress and, according to medical studies, glutathione reduces the toxicity of, and cellular damage by, the specific chemicals she received. This treatment has been shown to improve the quality of life of patients treated for ovarian cancer (Smyth 97).

It was obvious from the rise in Sarah's tumour markers almost immediately after the chemotherapy that her body was depleted and not capable of resisting the cancer. With supportive nutritional therapy that included vitamins, minerals, essential fatty acids, glutathione and vitamin C, we aimed to correct Sarah's malnutrition. We also hoped the supportive treatment would neutralise the chemically caused free-radicals, strengthen Sarah's immune system and coax it into fighting the cancer (Anderson 81).

Finally, we wanted to avoid the growth stunting that so often occurs in children receiving prolonged or high dose chemotherapy (Siebler 02). Although oncologists rarely give patients nutritional supplements to replenish the nutrients depleted by the chemotherapy, integrative medicine practitioners tend to do so as a matter of normal clinical practice. This makes the integrative approach beneficial to cancer patients – a practice now widely adopted in

---

[40] A free-radical is any atom or molecule containing a single unpaired electron in an outer shell, causing it to be highly chemically reactive. Free-radicals are caused by radiation, stress and chemical pollutants. They cause cellular damage and DNA damage that can lead to cancer and many other diseases. An antioxidant is a substance that neutralises free-radicals, thus preventing cellular damage.

cancer centres of excellence overseas (Senturker 97, Malvy 97, Thun-Hohenstein 92, Pietsch 00).

During her first session, Sarah sat in her chair shyly peeping over the top of an enormous picture book while the other patients smiled at her. Her IV was less in volume, but it took longer because of her smaller size. The adult patients finished their drips and left the clinic long before Sarah. But even on her first visit, we noticed that something about Sarah had softened the atmosphere. A cranky elderly gentleman, who usually complained in loud and spicy language about his aches and pains, had turned almost saintly with Sarah in the room. The man's wife collected him from the clinic and asked me what we were doing with him, since he had not been so nice to her in years.

At the end of the day, Mark and Di were relieved that Sarah had tolerated the vitamin IV well, and the three of them left for the two-hour trip home feeling hopeful.

Mark was scheduled to work the following Tuesday, and so Sarah arrived at the clinic for her next visit with her mother and oldest sister Laura. Laura was four years older than Sarah, sturdily built and openly nurturing towards her sister. Unlike Sarah, Laura had a mass of chestnut curls framing her face and she glowed with health.

To our delight, Sarah's skin colour had also improved since we had seen her the previous Friday. Di told us Sarah had been eating like a horse since the last drip. She had more energy and played outside with Brutus and the dogs over the weekend. This time, Sarah bounced into the recliner and presented her arm to us. She was keen to have the treatment again. After we started the drip, Sarah made Easter cards for her friends and family while listening to the other patients chatting amongst themselves. Her eyes widened when she heard two women with breast cancer discussing their baldness and flat chests. Just as the talk threatened to become graphic, one of the women lifted her wig and pulled a face until everyone in the room had hysterics. Sarah was determined not to smile at first but burst out laughing in the end. Laura blushed and covered her face with a magazine while giggling behind it. Even Di was beginning to relax and enjoy the three-hour sessions. She had brought her cross-stitch and started smocking cherry print fabric for the matching outfits she planned to make for the girls.

Half through her treatment, Sarah presented me with an Easter card which she'd decorated with a drawing of an Easter chick hatching from an egg. I thanked her and taped it onto the IV room window for everyone to enjoy. When the other patients praised her artwork, she let rip a series of giggles that became her trademark.

On their way home, Di allowed Laura to drive on her learner's plates. With the extra driving practice on the lengthy trips, Laura got her driver's licence in record time.

During the Easter school holidays, Di brought Sarah to the clinic with her sisters Clara and Hannah. They'd been curious about what went on there and wondered why Sarah liked it so much. Clara was two years' Sarah's senior and quietly sat down without a word. By comparison Hannah, two years younger than Sarah, wanted to know everything about the clinic and plied staff with endless questions. She let rip giggles identical to Sarah's.

This time, Sarah swung like a monkey from the clinic railing before wrapping the cubicle curtain around herself and letting out muffled giggles from inside the cocoon. It was a relief to see the real Sarah re-emerging. Her body and metabolic functions were also recovering. When I weighed Sarah that day she had gained another 2 kg and was fast approaching an average weight for her age. Her limbs were no longer stick thin. She had packed on some of the muscle mass she had lost at the hospital during her bout of severe malnutrition.

After we started Sarah's drip, our last afternoon patient arrived. Sarah and her two sisters watched the man limping in on a cane before plopping into the recliner reserved for him. The man rolled his trouser leg to the knee, snapped off a couple of bindings, and twisted his leg slightly until it came off. The girls watched fascinated as he propped the leg upright next to his chair, complete with a sock and a shoe attached.

'That is so cool!' squealed Sarah and Hannah in unison.

After I'd routinely recorded the man's blood pressure and vital signs before his treatment, he offered to tell the others in the room the story of his leg. Sarah and her sisters listened eagerly. It turned out to be a cautionary tale about smoking and ended in a redeeming message about taking good care of one's body – or, as in the man's case, what's left of it. Sarah's missing parts were internal, but she still related to the story. His honesty so inspired the other patients that they shared their own stories for the rest of the afternoon session.

The highlight of the IV sessions always came when Ann Smith arrived with Tupperware containers filled with home-baked gluten free pastries. Ann was a patient of the clinic who had became a volunteer. Instantly likeable, Ann is a grandmotherly woman who had endured 25 years of chronic illness. We had given Ann and others, who couldn't afford it, free treatment at the clinic. In time, Ann improved enough to resume her passion for natural horsemanship. She was a horse whisperer who had rescued and adopted several horses over the years. In return, the animals became her loyal friends. Ann gave riding lessons to the local kids, some of whom went on to become champion riders. Ann had donated her time to community service work despite her illness, but was so grateful for the improvement to her health that she volunteered at the clinic two days a week. She kept the patients' water jugs filled and entertained them with her occasionally off-colour humour, which she cleaned up in Sarah's presence. Between Ann's jokes and Sarah's antics, there came such loud laughter from the IV room that patients in the lobby waiting to see other practitioners at the clinic wondered what was so funny about the treatments we offered in there. Even our secretarial staff and the clinic accountant dropped in for morning tea and mixed happily with the patients.

The clinic staff and patients genuinely cared about Sarah and her family. It was the first time since Sarah's cancer diagnosis that she had encountered an unconditionally accepting healing environment. By then, the family desperately needed a positive medical experience.

After Easter, Sarah loved it when the cooler weather ripened the Shiraz grapes under the veranda of the family homestead. Without the burden of school, Sarah could now pursue some quality of life. She enjoyed sitting in the sun and going for slow walks again with the dogs up to Sarah's Hill. Di brought Sarah to the clinic twice a week, either alone or with Ruth, while the other kids returned to school after the holidays. While Mark was on the afternoon shift, Laura cooked dinner for the kids and watched them until Di returned home with Sarah, sometimes as late as 8 pm.

By early May, Sarah looked entirely different. In just two months, she had come to look like a confident pre-teenager. Her hair had grown back in thick curls and was much darker than before. She swept it back with a variety of purple clips and bands. When Sarah arrived for her appointment, I thought at first glance she was wearing raised heels. I called her into the doctor's room to measure her barefoot height and discovered she had grown 2 cm taller since the oral and IV nutritional support. Sarah's growth rate was staggering and she was rapidly attaining healthy above-average percentiles for height and weight. It seemed she would be spared the permanent growth stunting after all. She seemed so well that we drew a blood sample to determine her tumour marker levels.

Later, in the IV room, Sarah happily chatted with the others. Some time ago, she had stopped watching the door for caseworkers and was engaged in her own recovery process. Other patients shared the ups and down of their healing journeys, which inspired Sarah to reveal hers, including some traumatic memories of her incarceration. The other patients were moved to tears and became so protective that Sarah jokingly called them her extra aunts and uncles.

Each week Sarah's facial expression lightened as her burden lifted. A commanding personality emerged, her spiritual power becoming so vibrant that others in the room felt it. I began to realise that Sarah's strength was having a healing effect on others.

A young man with melanoma was a regular on the IV program for post chemotherapy nutritional support and glutathione treatment. He had been resentful of his disease and especially angry after his relapse following a long and gruelling course of chemotherapy. After each session at the clinic, he felt physically better, while emotionally he softened and looked more peaceful. He had come to his own level of acceptance by watching Sarah embrace each moment despite her grave illness.

Another woman with breast cancer came to the clinic on the days Sarah was there. She had been devastated when her family members had had trouble coming to terms with her illness and were unable to give her the support she needed. She always looked desperately sad and forlorn. After a few sessions, she started knitting a hat for Sarah. It was a simple act of kindness that helped her to finally let go and cry. Two other women in the room supported her with so much understanding that over the next few weeks she came to accept herself and no longer felt upset by her family's reactions – knowing she finally had the support she needed from other women who knew exactly what she was going through. She was at last able to feel gratitude for her life instead of focusing on what was lacking. Like Sarah, she started enjoying each day to the maximum. The woman's knitted hat turned out a masterpiece that inspired others to start their own handicrafts. Soon the women produced enough hats and scarves to supply various charities.

The IV room took on an exhilarating atmosphere of honesty, openness, and friendship between people who tried to make each day count despite their life-threatening conditions. For many it was a meditative experience – they came, sat down, and closed their eyes. They often left feeling deeply relaxed. The atmosphere clearly had a beneficial effect, not only on the patients, but also on the staff.

For me it was especially rewarding, a long-held vision realised. For years, I had wanted to create a clinic that gave my patients a chance to heal on all levels – body, mind and emotions. It saddened me that Sarah had never been offered this integrative way of healing before. It was hardly a way-out concept, since

Massachusetts General Hospital in the US has an entire clinical department devoted to mind–body medicine, and Harvard University has conducted extensive clinical studies that confirmed its efficacy. Although Sarah had been deprived of this option, it seemed that something was working for her at last. When Sarah's blood test results came back from the lab, it showed her tumour markers had levelled off. This meant the tumour growth had slowed down. Although it was not possible to say which factors had caused this, it was certain the supportive therapy had lowered Sarah's stress levels while the IV treatments had corrected a number of nutritional deficiencies and restored a degree of Sarah's general and immune health. At the very least, Sarah's positive response indicated that without a doubt the treatments had improved her life quality immeasurably. For a while, she was the energetic and happy child she had been before the department's intervention.

As good as this news was, however, we did not expect supportive treatment alone to hold off Sarah's aggressive cancer. For that, she required a form of cytotoxic treatment that would effectively target the cancer without destroying her life quality as the previous treatment had done. Since this was denied her, we could only offer Sarah a temporary improvement in her quality of life. This gave her a narrow timeframe in which to enjoy some of the things she had always wanted to do.

Since Sarah was feeling better, Ann Smith offered her a ride on her horses. Sarah had always wanted a pony, but had had to settle for Brutus the calf, who'd amazingly allowed her on his back. One Friday after clinic, Di and Ruth brought Sarah to Ann's farm where Sarah soon sat astride Ann's pinto mare, Treasure. Ann's granddaughter arrived later that afternoon. She was a champion rider and showed Sarah some dressage moves around the lunging yard. Sarah was delirious with excitement. Soon everyone, including the mare, beamed while Sarah realised one of her lifelong dreams. Ruth and Di were astonished at Sarah's natural horsemanship. She was a natural athlete with good balance and she wanted to ride on Treasure forever. By early evening, Ruth and Di barely managed to pull Sarah away from the horse to strap her into the seatbelt for the long drive home.

After waving goodbye, Ann had a feeling she might not see Sarah well enough to ride again. Ann's granddaughter, who was Sarah's age, still reminds her grandmother: 'Sarah and I could have been best friends'.

While Sarah was feeling well, Mark and Di took the whole family to Anna Bay during the winter school holidays. They rented a tiny cottage near the beach not far from the roar and spray of the Pacific Ocean. While Mark dropped a line in for a spot of fishing, Di took the kids for a walk on the beach. Despite the wintry weather, the sun warmed the air just enough for the kids to take a quick dip in the ocean. After the swim, Sarah collected sea shells along the beach with her sisters and little brother, Joshua. She reminded her mother of their last beach trip when the department had set the police in pursuit of them. Memories of that weekend, when the authorities were hunting them, were the most terrifying of Di's life. By contrast, this holiday was far more relaxed, but the kids still weren't game to stray too far from their parents, as their fear of caseworkers still haunted them.

Since Mark too would never forget that threat to his family, he had made preparations to prevent such a thing happening again. With one eye on the fish and the other on his family, he watched their every move. Mark was now far from the trusting person he had been before DoCS had entered their lives. He'd become savvy, battle hardened and uncompromising when it came to protecting his family and property. He would never allow another social worker near his children and he refused to speak to one without a lawyer or witness present. For the past few months, he'd kept an audio device at hand in case he encountered another caseworker. This was now in his shirt pocket ready to use at a moment's notice. Ever since DoCS had appeared in their lives last June, Mark had never been fully able to relax again, even on this sunny day.

Under her father's watchful eye, Sarah clambered around the beach with her siblings before sitting on a weathered rock peacefully gazing out to sea, digesting her own thoughts and feelings. Every lunchtime she ate her fill of fish and chips, calamari rings and prawns. In the afternoon, she returned to the cottage with her parents and siblings to laze in the hammock and watch the clouds go by before napping. She loved being around her family more than anything and her father was determined to give her that simple pleasure for as long as he could.

After the holidays, Mark and Di brought Sarah to the clinic once more. She looked like a fit and healthy teenager with a winter tan who was – incredibly – another centimetre taller yet again.

Dan Tyler had several unsuccessful tries at finding a suitable vein before we were able to insert the cannula and start the IV. Over the past month we'd had increasing problems accessing Sarah's veins due to scar tissue inside the veins resulting from frequent blood tests and cannulations. It was hardly surprising, after the hundreds of venipunctures Sarah had had during the course of her illness, but Dan was becoming concerned about the escalating problem.

While Sarah was having her IV, Dan took the parents into his office to ask their views about the possibility of inserting a permanent IV port into a larger, more central vein. Sarah would need the procedure done as an outpatient at the hospital, but it would guarantee easy IV access through the port any time without subjecting her to the ongoing trauma of cannulating a vein on each separate occasion. Both Mark and Di agreed that the treatments were doing Sarah a lot of good and even Sarah had told them she felt better since the treatments. The parents wanted the treatments to continue, and not be interrupted, since they were the only option that had not been blocked. On receiving the parents' consent to the procedure, Dan told Mark he would contact Dr Kotz's oncology registrar to discuss the procedure and hopefully set up an appointment for it at the hospital.

During Sarah's treatment that day, Di finished the needlepoint on the kids' matching cherry print outfits. Laura and another relative had helped with the smocking on the younger girls' dresses. Now she just needed a special occasion to show them off.

The following day was Saturday. While Mark was at work, Di convinced all six kids to try on their new clothes and walk up to Sarah's favourite hill to pose for some family photographs. Di's artistic streak made her an intuitive photographer. She took a series of shots of the kids on hay bales that turned out to be of professional quality. Sarah was restless during the photo shoot and threatened to take off across the paddock back home, but Di convinced her to pose for one more shot, which turned out to be the best of all. After barely holding still, Sarah was true to her word and bolted home. It was the last time the family saw her run that far.

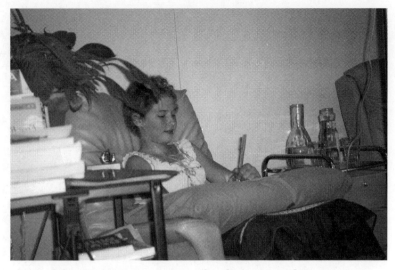

Sarah having IV treatment at the clinic around Easter 2004.

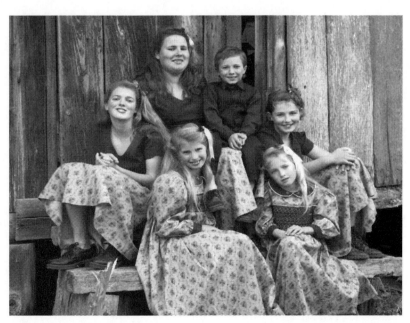

Di's picture of the kids wearing their new cherry print outfits. From top left; Clara, Laura, Joshua, Sarah, Leah and Hannah. July 2004.

TERMINAL BETRAYAL

> **Recognise the need for physical, psychological, emotional, and spiritual support for the patient, the family and Other carers, not only during the life of the Patient, but also after their death.**
>
> **AMA Code of Ethics**

By August, Sarah's treatment schedule at the clinic had come to a halt. Her veins were almost inaccessible from the many venipunctures she'd had during the course of her illness. Without further intravenous treatments, Sarah stood to lose the quality of life she had regained.

Between Sarah's clinic appointments, Dan made several attempts to phone Dr Kotz's registrar. When he finally got through to him, the registrar told Dan he would not assist him with the insertion of the port. Unfortunately, during Sarah's next appointment we were unable to gain vein access. After six attempts, Dan gave up and we promised to try again on the next appointment. The family was disappointed after travelling so far for the treatment. After that, Sarah missed a few appointments to allow her veins to rest.

In that short time, Sarah lost some of her energy and stopped going for walks. During the day, she spent more time on the couch.

Meanwhile, the parents took Sarah to another routine appointment at the hospital for a scan. Dr Kotz was surprised to see that Sarah had transformed into a tall teenager – all in the space of a few months. However, despite Sarah's fit appearance, the scan showed the tumour growing and the tumour markers in an upward trend again. Dr Kotz maintained that the only treatment he could offer was the same chemotherapy again, only this time, he offered much higher doses, which often proved lethal. Mark asked the doctor again why he was offering a repeat of a treatment that had failed miserably and destroyed Sarah's quality of life so completely. The doctor admitted, for the first time, that Sarah's prognosis was poor and because of that, he was willing to leave further treatment decisions up to the family. This only confirmed what Mark had suspected over the past year and it left him wondering why the doctor and the department would force treatments on a patient with a poor prognosis. However it did explain why the doctors had refused to give out much information and why they'd claimed to the court to be able to cure Sarah – to get the court orders they wanted. He suspected if he challenged the doctor on this he would only repeat his earlier claim of an 87% cure and that the doctor would never admit his claim was wrong. This was the first time the oncologist had given them a choice, but in reality, it was an empty offer: they still had no choices while Sarah remained a ward of the state and every decision was the subject of a court hearing.

By the end of the consultation, the oncologist still had not explained to the parents what they were likely to experience at the end of Sarah's terminal illness. They do not recall the doctor telling them about, much less offering, palliative care options or services. Some years later, they realised that the regional hospital did not even have a palliative care facility for children. It is best practice for doctors to be honest with terminal patients and inform them of palliative options that preserve quality of life. [41] The AMA ethically also requires doctors to 'try to ensure that death occurs with dignity and comfort'.

The following week, the parents took Sarah to the surgeon who had operated on her the first time, to explore if any surgical options were available. Dr Gilbert hadn't seen Sarah for over a year and, like Dr Kotz, was surprised to see her looking tall, confident and mature. However, he seemed sad when he saw her scans and read the imaging reports. When he gently tried to tell Sarah that she might not live for much longer, she didn't flinch. He seemed puzzled by her non-response, apparently unaware of the full extent of the torment Sarah had suffered during the forced treatment and the way it had affected her emotionally. She was suffering from the equivalent of battle fatigue. Sarah's situation differed radically from many other children, whose families can count on the unqualified support of health professionals while their child passes through the agonising terminal stages of their illness. By contrast, Sarah and her family felt betrayed by the medical profession. The parents were still struggling to keep their family together and safe from DoCS' threats to remove either Sarah or their other children, while still desperately trying to find last resort treatment options for Sarah, which the department had denied them throughout its involvement. The parents found it difficult to process the fact of Sarah's

---

[41] International Association for Hospice & Palliative Care.

terminal condition as long as their entire family's survival was at stake and while they had not explored every last option to help Sarah.

Sarah, however, had already been conditioned to the idea of dying, since staff at both hospitals had often told her she was certain to die without chemo. Now she heard that she was going to die despite having had the chemo forced on her. This irony confirmed her feeling that the medical profession had betrayed her. She had already told her parents that she thought all the professors, doctors and students who had gathered around her bed each day in hospital were only interested in her illness and not in her welfare as a person. In this, she had a reason to feel disregarded. The AMA Code of Ethics states:

> *Before embarking on any clinical teaching involving patients, ensure that patients are fully informed and have consented to participate.*

At no time did any doctor ask Sarah for permission to use her for clinical teaching. Sarah had lost all confidence in what doctors told her and, with the exception of a few health professionals, she thoroughly distrusted them. She was also well aware that DoCS and the doctors were denying her other cancer treatments. As far as she was concerned, she never wanted to see another caseworker or another oncologist again.

Dr Gilbert knew little of this, however, and he merely told the parents that he could offer no surgical options, before repeating the oncologist's offer of high-dose chemo. The family did not respond enthusiastically to the given options, and wondered why failed treatments were the doctors' only offerings when overseas patients had more choices.

The surgeon seemed genuinely sympathetic and left the decision up to the parents. However, even the well-meaning Dr Gilbert did not offer palliative care for Sarah at this time. The parents returned from their rounds of the specialists none the wiser about what to do next.

Sarah returned to the clinic on August 31 after missing several treatments. The parents brought Sarah's scans with them, and we were disappointed to discover that the cancer had spread. Even more than that, we were baffled that the doctors had apparently not offered the family supportive or palliative care for Sarah. We felt that while the supportive treatments had benefitted Sarah's general health over the last few months, in the terminal stages these measures would offer even more important benefits in the form of palliative care. Terminal ovarian cancer usually ends in bowel obstructions leading to faecal vomiting, dehydration and eventual starvation. We needed permanent venous access even more urgently, since without fluid hydration and nutritional support Sarah would have a rough time in her final days and weeks when she would be unable to keep down food or fluids. Although the parents knew Sarah might die, they did not want her death to be from the rigors of starvation and dehydration. They wanted her kept as comfortable as possible.

To ensure Sarah had access to such humane comfort measures, we had no choice but to persist with our attempts to arrange a permanent IV port through which to administer nutrition, hydration and pain relief when necessary. That meant we had to re-open discussions with Sarah's oncologist. If he refused our request again for permanent IV access, we planned to ask the surgeon for urgent help.

When Dan tried to cannulate that day, he was again unable to access Sarah's vein and he did not want to distress her with too many attempts. Since we could not administer any IV treatment, we discussed the options with Mark and Di instead. Sarah now needed palliative treatment and care. This included any reasonable measure that gave relief, comfort, and quality of life.

Incredibly, there still remained a one or two week window for salvage therapy, such as the type that had been given to Gina when she was already close to death from ovarian cancer in a hospital in Rome. Sarah was now in Gina's exact predicament when her oncologist in Rome offered her a final chance to buy time with metronomic chemotherapy and nutritional supplements. Gina in Italy was free to choose her medical treatment, whereas Sarah in Australia was not. Unlike Sarah, who was bound up in red tape that still prevented other treatment choices, Gina's cancer was arrested with the daily low dose of chemo. She was still enjoying full time work and an active social life while Sarah's family faced their final battle for their daughter's right to medical choices, comfort and dignity. At the end of the meeting, Mark said he was determined to free Sarah from the oppressive red tape once and for all. He wanted Sarah to have her last chance at treatment overseas. It was a long shot, but he would do whatever it took.

Meanwhile, Dan promised the parents he would continue to contact the oncologist and surgeon to ask for help with the IV access. [42]
Sarah's parents took her home that afternoon with a lot to think about. The next day was her birthday.

---

[42] Unfortunately this persistence would later pose a problem for us at the clinic since, after we'd stood in defence of the family in court, we had been subjected to heavy backlash from the authorities. Even some of our clinic patients told us that, for the sake of the other patients who relied on us, we should not have risked the authorities' wrath, but we nevertheless felt compelled to try to help the family.

The first of September 2004 was the first day of spring and Sarah's thirteenth birthday. That year it fell on an unremarkable Wednesday. A rain slick covered the sky and produced drizzle the entire day. For as long as Sarah could remember, her birthday had been warm, sunny and special, but this year no one felt like celebrating, and even the sky was gloomy.

In the morning, the kids sneaked into Sarah's room while she still slept. They decorated it with purple balloons before waking her up and surprising her with their homemade presents.

After breakfast, the children left for school while Mark prepared to check the fences before he was due at work that afternoon. Sarah wanted to go with him and refused to take no for an answer. Mark was unsure at first, but since she loved working outside with him, he relented. Muttley and Pooch wouldn't let Sarah out of their sights and eagerly hopped on the back of the utility. Together they headed up to Sarah's Hill to check the eastern fence-line. The paddocks seemed deserted without the cows and calves that had been sold to pay the barrister, but Mark still had to check the fences to ensure the neighbour's stock hadn't gone through them to get at the tall feed on his place. He had a feeling he should get things done on the farm sooner rather than later. For a while, he parked on top of Sarah's Hill, her favourite haunt in the carefree days before DoCS. They gazed toward the distant Barrington Tops while quietly mulling over their own private thoughts.

Being there reminded Mark of the terrible rainy day last June when they'd both sat in the utility on the same spot, watching the hawk. DoCS had called several times that day, forcing Sarah to answer morbid questions about how she felt about dying in the event she didn't have the oncologist's treatment. He'd felt terrible that day after spending a sleepless night reading the study Capewell had given him and making the grizzly discovery that those children in the study with Sarah's cancer had died despite the treatment the oncologists wanted to force on Sarah. He was convinced Sarah would have lived longer had she been allowed to go to a world-class cancer hospital for the personalised cancer treatment that best suited her needs. He believed the stress and trauma had shortened her life. Now she needed end of life care. If the clinic doctor couldn't get the oncologist's help to insert a permanent IV line, then where could they go?

Mark turned to Sarah. She had perched her feet on the dashboard and gazed wistfully at the homestead in the valley below. Occasionally she stared intently towards the mountains shrouded in mist, as if trying to burn the images into her memory.

'Jogue?' asked Mark.

'Yea, Dad'.

Mark chose his words carefully. 'The time might come when you need to go to the hospital'.

Sarah swung around and glared at her father. 'There's no way I'm staying at those two hospitals and I'm not seeing those two doctors again', she announced. 'No matter what', she added as she crossed her arms defiantly and returned to the scenery.

Mark knew she meant it and he honestly could not blame her. 'Okay Jogue. We'll figure something else out'.

When they returned to the house, Di was just turning out a freshly baked birthday cake from the oven.

At 2 pm, Mark left for work, and two hours later Sarah's siblings arrived home from school. That night Di and the kids made their best efforts to celebrate Sarah's birthday. After dinner, Laura played the piano and accompanied Sarah's sisters and little brother Joshua while they sang a medley of Sarah's best loved songs. Sarah lay on the couch and sang along with her all-time favourite: *My Heart Will Go On*. She belted out to her favourite lyrics: *Near, far, wherever you are, I believe that the heart does go on...*

She'd never really known what those lyrics meant until recently. In the past year she had learnt that it didn't matter where she was, her family was always safely in her heart – just as she was in theirs. She now felt certain the love in her heart would never disappear, but would always go on forever, no matter what bad things happened in the outside world.

Sarah slept soundly that night. From somewhere she had received a strong inner knowing that all would be well – no matter what.

The sound of a key in the French doors at 4 am jarred Di instantly awake. It was a fear reflex she had developed since the department had invaded their lives. To her relief, it was Mark who walked into the bedroom. He was home from the mine. In the dim hallway light, she saw his troubled face before he headed towards the shower. Di got up to put the kettle on; they both needed to talk. She set the cups and teapot out on the wooden table that had hosted so many joyful occasions over the years. It was barely 21 months before that Sarah had swung defiantly above it on the hardwood beam not long after her first operation. They'd all felt free then, until the caseworkers had sat at their table. They'd let trouble into their house that day and now she was afraid they would never get rid of it again.

Mark emerged from the bathroom in a tracksuit. 'How's Sarah and the kids?' he asked.

Di poured the tea and sat down. 'You should have seen the concert the kids put on for her. They were so good to her'. Di smiled. 'She loved it. But she's been getting weaker every day since those drips stopped'.

'I've noticed. They used to perk her up', said Mark, as he gulped a mouthful of hot tea. 'We've got to do something quick before she goes further downhill'.

'Haven't we already tried everything?' asked Di.

'Maybe. But while the clinic is trying to get her a permanent IV, we've got to make an emergency plan'.

'What else can we do?' asked Di.

Mark looked tired. 'While she's still well enough to travel, we've got to have another crack at getting her overseas for the salvage treatment. It's her last chance'.

Di slammed down her cup. 'Honestly, I'm getting fed up with this', she said angrily. 'How can you get our hopes up again?'

Mark stared out through the double doors. Outside was as dark as his mood.

Di's tears broke in a torrent. 'I couldn't bear it if they refused us again', she sobbed. In her pocket, she found a tattered tissue, 'It would be the last straw'.

Mark felt for Di, and he wished he could take her pain away, but he had his own worries that wouldn't ease up until there was an emergency plan to fall back on. Mark rubbed his red eyes. 'We have to make some serious decisions for Sarah right now. Is that something we want to leave to the social workers and caseworkers?'

Di blew her nose. 'You know the answer to that', she said thickly.

Mark leaned in. 'Right now they can keep forcing anything on her, right up to her last day. We've seen what happens when caseworkers become doctors. Not even the judge has reined them in. Don't ask me why, when plenty of other doctors were against it. This whole thing was wrong from the beginning. There's a lot that can't be explained'. Mark looked across the table. He saw fear in Di's eyes.

'Mark. You don't know what these people are capable of', said Di quietly.

'You're right about that', answered Mark. 'But we both know Sarah needs peace of mind and a chance to be with us again without the State owning her. She deserves proper care, dignity and a last chance at life. I'm going to court for one final try'.

The kitchen was silent except for the fridge motor purring softly before turning off with a shudder. While they grimly pondered their options, Di wondered what other choices they realistically had. She looked through the kitchen window into the dark, wondering if she would ever feel secure in her own home again.

'Maybe you're right' said Di. 'It can hardly get any worse than it's been. Remember what Sarah wanted last year on her birthday?'

'How could I forget?' replied Mark bitterly. 'She'd been in hospital detention all winter. She told me to tell the judge to make them stop tormenting her'. Mark pulled some lint from his tracksuit. 'You know I don't even believe in justice anymore. Not after last time in court when all the evidence was on our side and it still didn't matter'. He threw the lint on the floor. 'I just have to give it one more try; otherwise I couldn't live with myself'.

Di got up and wearily cleared away the teacups. It was nearly 5 am. The first light would soon wake the kids up – all except Sarah, who slept in late.

'I'm going to try for an hour's sleep', said Di as she headed for the bedroom.

'Do you still have those passport applications?' asked Mark.

'Yes. Why?'

'I want you to get them processed the minute I call you from the courthouse. But not a second before, or it'll raise the alarm. Then we'll take her to the American hospital while she's still well enough to travel. There's no time to waste'.

Di placed her hand on Mark's shoulder before heading off to bed. She didn't believe for a minute that they would be allowed to go overseas anymore, but she knew Mark had to give it one last try.

When the kids left for school, Mark got up. He was used to feeling seedy from lack of sleep and could not recall the last time he'd had six hours in a row. Di was in town food shopping. He made himself some breakfast and, after clearing away his dishes, started making phone calls. By midday, he had managed to arrange a court hearing for 9 September. He had told the department and the judge's associate that the matter was urgent, but this was apparently the first date they could offer him. He thought it unfair that while the department could get a court date within a few hours on some trivial pretext, he had to wait over a week to get a hearing for a gravely ill child. Now that Sarah's life was ebbing away, it seemed the bureaucrats were not in a hurry anymore.

Next Mark phoned the clinic to let us know the court date. This meant we would need to prepare a letter notifying the court why a permanent IV port was required. That afternoon Mark also started on his own affidavit for court, which he worked on until he left for work.

Over the next few days, we moved quickly at the clinic to come up with a plan to help Sarah. First, we prepared an affidavit informing the court that Sarah's condition had deteriorated and that we required the surgeon or the oncologist's help to insert a permanent IV port for the necessary fluids and medications. We were more than qualified at the clinic to manage this treatment since we constantly worked with oncologists and pain teams to treat many cancer patients, including some with complicated pain pumps that required regular reloading with pain-killing drugs.

Second, we persisted in trying to gather a team together to assist us with Sarah's palliative care, which we hoped could be administered while she was in her own peaceful home environment. Dan Tyler tried to contact the oncologist at the regional hospital again to request help. When Dr Kotz was continually unavailable, Dan got onto the oncology registrar again who told Dan that he was out of luck – nobody at the hospital would help insert the permanent central IV cannula.

After Dan's call, Dr Kotz composed a letter to the court, in which he stated:

> *Dr Tyler asked whether Sarah could be admitted under the [hospital oncology registrar's care] and if he was willing to put in a central line...he [the registrar] does not have admitting rights and refused.*

At the end of his letter, Dr Kotz added:

> *...if the family were willing to pursue more conventional therapy in the future then we would be willing to review Sarah again.*

To the parents it was obvious when they read the letter that the oncologist was prepared to administer only high-dose chemotherapy until Sarah's last day, and that he would not even consider any palliative or comfort measures.

Realising we could count on no help from the oncologist, we contacted the surgeon, Dr Gilbert. Dan explained the urgent need for the permanent IV access and added that we had administered IV vitamin C as a supportive treatment with good effect until venous access became impossible. The surgeon wanted Dan to provide him with studies indicating the efficacy of vitamin C against cancer. Unfortunately, although these studies do exist, only in hindsight was it clear the surgeon thought we were proposing an alternative cancer treatment rather than a supportive or palliative measure.

Over the years, confusion has persisted in the medical profession regarding the use of intravenous vitamin C on cancer patients. In several studies, late stage cancer patients have reported significantly better physical, emotional, and cognitive function after administration of vitamin C. On the other hand, terminal cancer patients have reported significantly less wasting, nausea, vomiting, and pain. (Chang 07, Padayatty 03, Gonzales 05). We also wanted the IV access to administer saline fluids to Sarah, who was by now becoming dehydrated.

Dan sent studies to Dr Gilbert and while we waited for a reply, valuable time was lost.

In a last ditch effort to buy his daughter more time, Mark appeared before the same Supreme Court judge on Thursday, 9 September. Mark boldly stipulated in his affidavit that he wanted Sarah released from DoCS' control in order to take her to a cancer hospital in the United States. At this point, he no longer had in mind the large teaching hospital that offered various cancer treatments as a curative measure; he now preferred an integrative cancer hospital with an excellent palliative care facility that offered metronomic chemotherapy as a last resort salvage therapy.

Mark then tendered Dan Tyler's affidavit, which had annexed to it the manufacturer's information on the proposed permanent port. Dan wrote:

> In the last two weeks, Sarah's health has dramatically deteriorated. She has poor appetite, is moderately dehydrated, listless and complains of abdominal discomfort. I am gravely concerned about her prognosis unless urgent action is taken. My recommendation is to provide a permanent venous access in the form of a PAS Port Mark 11 or similar as a matter of urgency.

While the judge reviewed the affidavits, Mark showed him clinical pictures of Sarah again. Mark explained that the forced treatment had been neither humane nor effective. He insisted that only he and Di, in partnership with a trusted doctor –and not a government department – should make such personal and important decisions about Sarah's health care. Now he wanted no more DoCS obstructions. Sarah deserved comfort measures and a last chance to have a treatment that might give her more time.

The judge read the evidence, including Dr Kotz's report in which the oncologist finally admitted that Sarah's prognosis was poor.

When he asked if there were any other issues that needed attention that day, Mark told the judge about the substantial expenses the department had imposed on the family through its constant demands, even though Sarah was technically a ward of the court. Mark added that the DoCS workers had guaranteed reimbursements and financial 'support', but had never honoured their promises.

The judge told Mark to make a list itemising their expenses and present it at the next court hearing, which he set for a week's time on 15 September.

Mark felt the familiar frustrations return. He was thwarted every way he moved, and it seemed to him no one really cared one iota about the welfare of his child or his family. The oncologist who had forced his unsuccessful treatment on Sarah was not interested in helping her now, even though it was obvious his treatment had not worked and that Sarah really needed palliative care. The department that had promised them 'help' and 'support' had nearly bankrupted them, not least by the way it had become tight-fisted when it came to compensating their out-of-pocket expenses. And now, for some inexplicable reason, justice would take a whole week to consider a matter of life and death. For anyone else a week was barely a blink of an eye, but for Sarah it was literally a lifetime. Where were all those who'd forced their will on Sarah because it was 'in the best interests of the child'? And why didn't they care now?

The next week crawled by. Mark accepted every overtime shift at work to finance the overseas trip. He planned to visit the bank manager again, and if the judge granted even a small amount of compensation, they might just be able to cover the medical and travel expenses.

On the hearing day, Mark was up before 5 am. While eating his toast on the run, he reminded Di to stand by for his call from the courthouse.

On the four-hour drive to Sydney, Mark mapped out the overseas trip in his mind. There were the fares, plane bookings and accommodation. He also planned to phone the US hospital when he got home to let them know they were coming. He and Di had told no one of their plans. The department had obstructed them so many times they decided to keep their trip under wraps for as long as possible.

Mark walked into the court building just before 10 am. He took the lift up to the Equity division and arrived just when the court was called into session. This time a different atmosphere prevailed. The judge seemed more than ready to dispose of the matter. For once, the Crown barrister had no objections to Mark's motion to get DoCS off their case. There was only one small stipulation, said the barrister. Dr Kotz had written the court a letter wanting Mark to agree to allow Sarah pain relief if or when she needed it. Mark wondered what on earth had prompted this proviso. When Sarah had been in agony during her forced chemotherapy at the regional hospital, staff had never offered her any pain relief other than a paracetamol tablet. When she'd had a 1 kg tumour pressing painfully on her internal organs, no one in three hospitals had offered her pain relief over the course of two agonising days. Meanwhile, Mark's sole reason for going to court was to ensure Sarah had relief from her symptoms, and he could not understand why the oncologist was refusing to help insert a permanent port that made it possible to administer pain medications.

Mark explained to the judge that he and Di had always wanted Sarah to have every comfort measure available – including pain relief – and that he was doing all in his power to make that possible. He then passed a list to the judge that itemised the expenses DoCS had imposed on them over the past 18 months.

On considering the expenses and after hearing Mark's undertaking, the judge ordered the revocation of Sarah's wardship and the restoration of Mark and Di's parental rights. But just as Mark was letting this good news sink in, the judge added that he would order no compensation or reimbursement for the expenses DoCS had imposed on the family. He did, however, leave a legal door open for Mark to make a claim in future. Mark had a feeling the judge had had enough of the case and wanted to wash his hands of it.

On the issue of the permanent IV port, the court was mute, leaving the oncologist's refusal as the final word.

Mark left the courtroom feeling empty. After 18 months of persecuting and brutalising his family, the system had simply disposed of them. The health care system had nothing to offer, just when they needed it most. Mark and Di had calculated they were over $300 000 out of pocket, while the taxpayer had already coughed up more than $150 000 in hospital fees and another $300 000 for forced chemotherapy. The taxpayer had also been billed for emergency air rescue craft and ambulances that weren't necessary, and yet this service had been denied on the two occasions Sarah had desperately needed them. Around 20 Supreme Court cases had kept scores of barristers busy, in and out of court, at $5000 per day, for months at a time. In the past 18 months the child protection department had spent over a million dollars and diverted an army of caseworkers just to prevent one 11-year-old child from having a cancer treatment personalised to her needs, while over 80 children in NSW, who had been reported to DoCS, had died of genuine abuse and neglect. Mark wondered why the state was happy to waste millions of dollars in this way, and yet could not now spare even a dollar to allow Sarah a peaceful and dignified end of life.

Mark emerged from the Supreme Court building feeling numb and shaky. He turned the corner to Macquarie Street and looked for a bench to sit on before his legs gave way. He had expected to feel elated on this day, but instead he was furious. The child protection authorities had certainly protected Sarah – from everything that might have helped her.

Mark sat for a while watching the lunchtime crowd emerge from their offices and head for the small eateries that lined the legal district. It was a sunny day with the temperature just reaching a perfect 23° C. His mind was still swimming in disappointment when he realised he had to exert control over his thoughts and make the next plan. He reminded himself that the State no longer controlled Sarah; she was free now, and there was not a second to waste. Tomorrow he had to ask the bank manager for $20 000. He opened his briefcase and dialled his home number. Di picked it up immediately.

'She's free', said Mark cheerlessly. 'But no compensation for what the mongrels put us through. You'll have to rush to get those passport applications in today', he added.

'I can't do that, Mark', said Di uneasily.

'What do you mean you can't do that?' Mark demanded loudly enough for passers by to turn their heads. 'We *have* to do it!'

'Sarah's not well. You'd better come home'.

Mark broke all the speed limits and arrived home four hours later, miraculously without a ticket. He rushed upstairs to find Sarah in bed with a vomit bowl beside her. For the first time, she'd vomited faecal matter, and had not kept down solids all day. He knew what that meant. The tumour was pressing onto her small intestine and partially obstructing it.

Despite feeling sick, Sarah cheered up when she saw her father.

Mark sat at the foot of Sarah's bed and announced the good news. 'Remember the date today, Jogue. September 15th is your lucky day. You're free'.

She held out her arms and hugged her father.

Mark felt suddenly teary and pulled away. He stood up and turned towards the window while wiping his eyes with the back of his hand. On the wall, he spotted Sarah's drawings of their family and pets. Above her bed, she'd taped her favourite drawing of a purple moonbeam butterfly.

Sarah's voice was hoarse. 'Dad, if they'd taken me away I would have come straight back home'. Sarah smiled weakly. 'Besides, I've always been free on the inside' she added.

Mark was startled at Sarah's clarity. At the age of thirteen, she already knew what most people spend a lifetime searching to discover: her mind was free no matter what the world did to her. Although the hospital staff had tried every trick to pressure her, Sarah had never once wavered from her own truth. How could she see through people so well? How could she resist the world's trickery? He realised what a special quality that was.

Mark picked up Sarah's favourite teddy from the floor and placed it on the pillow above her head. As a kid, she'd dragged it everywhere. Di even had to make regular repairs to it while Sarah was asleep. In the last few weeks, Sarah had started taking notice of it again, along with other things that held happy memories for her.

Mark opened his briefcase and took out a paper. 'For what it's worth Jogue, you're free on paper too', he said, as he proudly showed her a written copy of the court orders. 'And I'll make sure it stays that way'.

Sarah smiled and reached out for the paper. 'Thanks Dad. I need paper for my drawings'.

Mark chuckled as he drew back the document and returned it to his briefcase. He recalled the day the caseworkers had come to issue her with a summons. Stamped paper meant nothing to Sarah, and after the women had left, the summons went missing. A week later, Di had found it in Sarah's room covered with Sarah's drawings of the family and pets. Mark realised that in Sarah's beautiful childhood world, she only cared about her family. And it was the family's love –not pieces of paper – that had kept her spirit strong.

Mark smiled and closed the latch on his briefcase. 'You don't want that flimsy stuff. I'll get you some coloured cardboard instead'.

From downstairs wafted the smell of a roast dinner. Clara was on her way up the stairs with Sarah's dinner tray and Di was right behind her.

When Clara arrived with the steaming plate, Sarah dived for the vomit bowl and started retching. Clara made a face, turned on her heel, and left again, while Di rushed to support Sarah's head over the bowl.

Between Sarah's heaves, Di glanced at Mark. 'Dinner's on the table. I'll be a while. You'd might as well go downstairs and eat with the kids', she said.

After the children went to bed and Sarah was settled, Mark took Di's hand and led her outside to talk out of the children's earshot. For a minute, they stood on the veranda to get used to the dark, before inching towards the picnic table in the front yard. Mark had made the table and benches himself from timbers that grew on their property. It had hosted many happy family barbeques, and it was sad to sit there in the pitch dark to talk of such bleak issues.

'What do you think we should do tomorrow?' asked Mark.

'It's pretty clear she can't go on a long plane trip...' answered Di, '...if that's what you're asking'.

Mark covered his face with both hands. 'You're right', he muttered wearily. 'That was her last chance. They dragged their heels until it was too late'.

'I know. She went down fast without those drips. What do we do now?' asked Di.

Mark was tired of thinking up solutions. After the eight-hour drive and a gruelling day in court, he didn't know where he would find the courage or strength to carry on. Weren't the doctors supposed to read their medical journals, discover the latest overseas treatments, and then offer them to cancer patients in this country? Why did patients have to be forced into the same old cookie cutter, one-size-fits-all treatment? It was only today that Sarah had finally become too sick to travel, and yet Mark had seen letters from the oncologist in court that day admitting they hadn't had anything to offer Sarah for at least eight months. Shouldn't the department have released her months ago if that was the case? At any time this year, they could have taken Sarah to America, if only the doctors had been straight with them. Now not only was her last chance for salvage treatment gone, but the doctors were even depriving her of a permanent port for palliative care. Now what were they supposed to do?

Mark was so weary he could hardly move his face. 'The only chance we have left is the clinic. Let's hope they can convince the surgeon to put that permanent line in'. He tried to sound optimistic, but after today, he was not convinced that would happen.

The next day Mark phoned the clinic. From his update, we realised Sarah was in deep trouble and that we needed to step up our efforts to help her. Unfortunately, for the next week we were embroiled in futile academic discussions with the hospital doctors about the merits of vitamin C and whether or not its administration warranted the insertion of the permanent port – which the doctors still refused to carry out. This argument was completely irrelevant. Sarah urgently needed comfort measures: she was dehydrated, needed intravenous fluids, and we had begged the court to allow us to administer this and other basic comfort measures. Instead, while Sarah deteriorated daily, we were hindered and prevented from helping her in any way.

Each day the family felt their options further narrowing. Sarah adamantly refused to go to the hospital, quite justifiably fearing another DoCS intervention. The family had even lost trust in their local GP after discovering from court documents that his discussions with caseworkers and others had contributed to their being psycho profiled and the terrible course of events that had followed.

To make matters worse, in the final week of September, while still embroiled in the futile debate with the specialist about the IV port, something extraordinary happened to us. The clinic came under intense attack from the authorities, who wanted to enter the premises without giving a reason why. When we refused unless a reason was given, they suspended the clinic doctor's medical licence and demanded the clinic close its doors within three days. Even though my own professional licence remained unaffected, I could not continue to practise in a closed clinic.

Within three days, over 50 patients had their course of treatments interrupted. Several hundred other patients more were left stranded without the medical and health care the clinic had provided, while five staff members were suddenly out of work. We suspected it had something to do with our advocacy role in support of the family's rights, but this was impossible to prove. However, we were not the only ones affected in this way: two other health professionals who had treated Sarah and advocated for the family also encountered similar problems.[43] It seemed more than a coincidence; speaking out apparently came with serious risks. With the stroke of a bureaucrat's pen, all that I had worked for had disappeared overnight.

Meanwhile, Sarah was in an even worse position of course. She was about to lose her life, and yet not one of her hospital doctors would work with us to extend compassionate care to a terminal child. No one in Sydney offered palliative care to the family and there existed no such facility in the regional hospital. We wanted desperately to help Sarah but now found ourselves without a clinic, tied up in our own legal battle for survival and no longer in a position to help anyone.

---

[43] Those experts who gave evidence to the court in support of the family were, fortunately not affected.

For the next week, Sarah became sicker each day. Friday, 1 October was start of the Labour Day long weekend. Sarah had been vomiting daily and asked her parents if she could come to the clinic for an intravenous drip, claiming it had always made her feel better. Mark had the heartbreaking job of explaining it was impossible. Sarah spent the day on the couch sipping tiny amounts of juice while family and friends came to visit. It was Jim's birthday and Di put on a lunch. Sarah was unable to eat and instead disappeared into the garden for a few minutes. She shuffled towards the chook pen to visit the ducks she had caught last autumn, and was about to feed them when she suddenly felt sorry for the birds and opened the pen to let them go. At first, the ducks were hesitant, but when the drake led the way, the rest of the females followed and took flight toward the dam where they had lived before Sarah and her siblings had caught them. After that, Sarah was content and she went in search of butterflies for a few minutes. She returned to the house with an ice cream container filled with leaves and caterpillars. While the others ate, she took her tiny pets upstairs and slid the container under her bed. It was Sarah's last time in the garden.

That evening Sarah's siblings put on a concert for Jim and the family while Sarah lay on the couch. A neighbour filmed the kids' home-choreographed show. The lens captured Laura at the piano and the other kids performing their singing and dancing routines, before slowly lingering on Sarah in what turned out to be the last video images of her. On her face played a multitude of expressions as she sometimes wistfully sang along with her siblings.

When the guests left and the kids went to bed, Mark and Di stayed up to make a difficult decision.

Di was inconsolable about Sarah going downhill so quickly.

Mark sat down on the couch next to her. 'We've got to find someone to help us'.

'Who can we trust now the clinic has closed?' asked Di. 'She's terrified to go into any NSW hospital in case DoCS gets involved again. We can't even trust our local GP. We can hardly go to any other doctor without the whole mess blowing up again. With that mandatory reporting, who knows what will happen'.

Mark thought for a while. 'It's pretty obvious nobody in NSW is going to lift a finger. She really needs help now, not a bunch of caseworkers'.

'We can't go on like this. She's getting sicker by the minute', said Di.

Mark racked his mind for a solution. After a while, he grabbed Di's hand. 'Pack our bags tomorrow', he said. 'We're going'.

Di pulled away startled. 'You can't be serious. Where to?' she asked.

'Melbourne'.

'She's not fit to go anywhere', insisted Di.

'It's our last hope'.

The next morning Mark checked on Sarah and found her white. She had kept nothing down and was too weak to get out of bed. On her bedpost, a cocoon had attached itself by a slender thread. Sarah hoarsely explained it was one of the caterpillars she had picked up from the garden the day before. The rest were still in a container under her bed munching on leaves. The one on the post, she said, was a special one.

For the rest of the day, Mark and Di made preparations to leave with Sarah the following day.

The family awoke to the promise of a perfect, cloudless day, the kind that Sarah had always loved. From bed, Sarah took some time to check the cocoon on the bedpost before Di came up to get her ready.

Jim drove the sedan around the front to take Mark, Di, and Sarah to Newcastle airport. Ruth meanwhile gathered Sarah's siblings together. She would take them up to her house, thinking it was better to spare them the upset of watching Sarah leave in a car. That morning Mark and Di had told them their sister was gravely ill. They all cried when saying their goodbyes to Sarah. They knew by then they might never see their sister again.

When her siblings had gone, Mark carried Sarah down the stairs. She cast a final look around the old country kitchen and the adjoining dining room with its iron stove and wooden table where they'd sat each day as a family. Finally, she glanced up at the hardwood beam she had swung from to raise a stir. Mark carried her through the double doors before gently placing her into the backseat of her grandparents' car.

Minutes later, with all aboard, Jim inched down the drive. In the back seat, Sarah gazed through the rear window. She had a terrible pain in her tummy now, but it didn't stop her carefully scanning the homestead, the river and the rolling hills, as if making a mental picture. Muttley stood forlorn in the driveway with his tail hanging limp. The dog watched until the car disappeared from sight.

Two hours later, Jim delivered Mark, Di and Sarah to Newcastle Airport. After checking in, Mark carried Sarah across the tarmac and up the rear stairs into the aircraft. Di followed and paused briefly to give Jim a sad wave.

Jim stood outside the perimeter fence and watched the plane taxi down the runway before lifting off in a steep ascent. He knew Mark and Di had no choice but to take Sarah on a mercy flight to Victoria, but he was deeply upset that his family had to flee from their home in NSW in search of help.

Jim stood at the fence for a long time. He'd recently had his old glasses replaced with a new prescription and could track the plane in excruciating detail as it slowly disappeared into a south-westerly direction. He knew in his heart that he would never see Sarah again. Without that wild child – that free spirit – his life would never be the same. The old man took out his handkerchief and wiped his eyes before he headed back to the farm again.

LAST FLIGHT TO FREEDOM

Sometimes, even to live is an act of courage.
Seneca

He who is brave is free.
Seneca

The pilot banked the plane steeply out of Newcastle airport and set the flight path towards Melbourne. In the rear cabin, Sarah sat propped up in the middle seat. Her parents on both sides supported her. She usually loved flying and desperately had wanted to travel to America, but today her limbs would not obey even the simplest commands and sitting up was nearly impossible. She had a high fever and was bright yellow with jaundice. Her liver and other organs were failing and she was close to dying. Her mouth was too dry to form words and even if she had wanted to speak, the sadness of leaving her grandparents, sisters, and brother left her mute.

Unlike the last flight to Melbourne in December 2002, Sarah received no coloured pencils or in-flight children's meals this time. The attendants saw that the girl was ill and vomiting and discreetly left the parents alone to attend to their daughter. Sarah's condition had deteriorated alarmingly during the trip. The in-flight staff could not know the girl had only a short time to live.

The plane with its precious cargo touched down at Melbourne's Tullamarine Airport at lunchtime. By then, Sarah was in severe pain and unable to walk. Mark carried her off the plane and rushed her out of the terminal where Di urgently hailed a taxi. The parents' first stop was to Dr Milne, who took one look at Sarah and immediately arranged for her go to a nearby private hospital. She was to be admitted under Dr Billings, the Melbourne oncologist the family had consulted in 2002 for a second opinion.

Within the hour, Sarah was in the emergency department (ED), where the team of doctors immediately diagnosed severe dehydration and gave her an injection of morphine for the pain. They too had trouble accessing a vein, but were finally able to insert a special IV line that could be used multiple times. Sarah was severely dehydrated and required a litre of saline before she was fit to be transported, by gurney, to the X-ray department for abdominal scans. The images would show doctors the extent of the cancer and determine what, if anything, they could do.

Over the next several hours, the ED doctors tried to contact Dr Billings the Melbourne oncologist, but he never showed up. Finally, since Sarah's condition was deteriorating, doctors decided to transfer her to the Melbourne Royal Children's Hospital. The family never heard from Billings again.

A few minutes before midnight, an ambulance rushed Sarah and her parents through Melbourne's empty streets to the Royal Children's Hospital. By 12.05 am, Sarah lay semi-conscious on a trolley in the emergency medicine department. Her white fingers gripped the railings with each spasm of pain. Mark and Di sat next to their daughter looking nervously around the cubicle – the NSW problems always had a habit of following them.

When Sarah moaned, Di took her hand and gently stroked it.

'I just hope they will help her here'. Di said to Mark. 'I couldn't bear it if it happened all over again', she added in a whisper.

Mark was too tired to be reassuring. 'You're not wrong', he said grimly.

Both parents stayed alert for official-sounding footsteps outside the partially drawn curtains. The wall clock ticked loudly. It was 1.30 am. They hoped caseworkers were not around this time of night. In the distance, a baby cried and was quickly comforted. A suction device hissed faintly in a nearby cubicle. Nurses in crepe shoes padded softly around the unit. The murmur of friendly staff voices came from the nurse's desk. The fluoro lights glared into cubicles further along, but above Sarah, the light was dimmed. Just as Mark and Di started to wonder what this might mean, they heard footsteps approaching.

From behind the curtain, a nurse appeared with two cups of tea. When she held them out, the parents were too stunned to accept them at first. Not since the British nurse had any hospital staff member offered them this simple comfort. The parents reached out and almost wept at the thoughtful gesture.

The nurse had kind eyes. 'You must have gone through a lot before you came here and you're probably exhausted', she said. 'The doctors are just looking at Sarah's scans and they'll discuss them with you shortly. We have a few minor procedures to do before we get Sarah settled upstairs in the ward. After that you're welcome to catch some sleep when we find you a room'.

While sipping tea, Mark and Di watched as two nurses mixed up vials of antibiotics and slowly injected them into Sarah's IV tubing over a period of several minutes. Next, another nurse arrived with morphine in a syringe. After both nurses had double-checked the dose with her, she slowly injected the drug into the rubber bung of the IV tubing. Di held her breath. She had noticed over the past year that morphine made Sarah irritable and itchy, but she had not said another word about it after staff in the previous hospitals had practically accused her of not wanting Sarah to have any pain relief. Di hoped Sarah would not have a severe reaction to the drug, and to her relief, Sarah remained asleep.

The three nurses waited a few minutes for the drug to take full effect before they lubricated a long plastic tube and passed it down through Sarah's nose. They pushed it as far down as her stomach and instantly a rush of brown gastric fluid drained into a bag beside the bed. It would stop Sarah vomiting, they explained, by decompressing her stomach, since she had a partial bowel obstruction from the tumour. The nurses carried out this normally uncomfortable procedure almost without a flinch from Sarah.

Mark was relieved his daughter was finally getting the help she needed, but he was still worried that things could go off the rails. It was now 2.30 am. From the cubicle, he peered between the curtain edges down the corridor and saw only doctors and nurses quietly going about their business. From his recent experiences, he had come to associate social workers and caseworkers as coercive and strongly influential in hospitals. He was relieved to see – in this hospital at least – that the doctors and nurses made the decisions.

After the nurses placed Sarah on a pulse meter that measured her heartbeat, the emergency doctor came to discuss the X-rays with the parents. He invited them to a tiny side office and offered them a seat. From the tests, it appeared Sarah had several large tumours in her abdomen and liver. This had caused the jaundice. Some tumours had fulminated (become infected) and had caused a near fatal organ failure on top of the existing terminal cancer. She would require stabilising before any further plan could be made.

When the parents returned to Sarah's cubicle, Di broke down and wept. The nurse attending to Sarah pulled a box of tissues down from a shelf and placed her hand on Di's shoulder. 'Please don't worry. We'll take good care of Sarah', she said softly while handing Di a ball of tissues.

Di was shocked to hear no judgement or recrimination. This nurse focused on Sarah's needs and still had kindness left over for the parents. Why couldn't staff have been like this all along, she wondered.

Just before dawn, two nurses came in to transfer Sarah to the ward upstairs. Mark and Di followed behind the nurses as they wheeled Sarah into the lift. The overhead light cast deathly shadows on Sarah's face, causing the parents to wonder whether she would even survive the next 24 hours. Once the lift stopped at the upper floor, the nurses gave the parents a sympathetic smile and wheeled Sarah down the corridor into the hospital's cancer ward. There, she was allocated a private side-room with its own bathroom. After the ED staff left, the ward nurses settled Sarah into her new bed. They tried to wake her to let her know she had arrived in the ward, but Sarah moaned and blacked out again. The nurses told the parents they could stay with Sarah as long as they wished. Both Mark and Di were relieved to hear it. The nurses gave them a reassuring smile and before they left, turned on the soft night light to cast a reassuring glow around the room.

With their suitcases on the floor next to Sarah's bed, Mark and Di sat in a shocked daze until dawn. From the room's sixth floor window, they watched the sun light up the central business district of Melbourne and the parklands surrounding the hospital. Seeing the city come alive with cars and people made them realise how exhausted they really were. Perhaps they could relax now that Sarah was in good hands. She had barely stirred all night.

At 7 am, the morning staff arrived in the cancer ward and the night staff went off duty. A cheery morning nurse came into Sarah's room with another syringe of antibiotics in a kidney shaped dish. After she took Sarah's temperature and pulse, the nurse seemed pleased. She injected the antibiotics into the IV tubing and told the parents that Sarah's fever was coming down. She said she would be back later to give Sarah a sponge bath and a bedpan, but meanwhile offered to show the parents to their accommodation in a comfortable guest room two floors up. Mark asked how much it would cost, but the nurse assured him it was entirely free. This surprised him, since he had paid for it in NSW, including Sarah's halfway house accommodation.

The nurse smiled and showed them to their room two floors up before leaving them to rest and freshen up. They wearily put down their bags and looked around the top floor room with its picture window overlooking the city. For the first time since Sarah's diagnosis, they were in comfortable accommodation, able to spend unlimited time with their daughter and on the verge of being able to trust the medical staff.

After a hot shower and a quick breakfast in the hospital cafeteria, Mark and Di returned to the cancer ward to sit with Sarah. They were alarmed to see she had woken up irritated and was mumbling nonsense. Two nurses tried to calm her but Sarah was confused and uncharacteristically hostile. Di tried to restrain Sarah's flailing arms while explaining that this had not happened before. Di saw from Sarah's glazed eyes that she was not with it. One nurse rushed out to the nurses' station while the other stayed in the room to reassure the parents that this sometimes happened in the late stages. A few minutes later, at 8 am, the first nurse returned with a fresh dose of morphine. While she sterile-swabbed the rubber bung on Sarah's IV tubing she let the parents know that the hospital oncology team would soon be in to talk with them; they were still in the process of contacting the NSW hospital doctors to check on Sarah's medical history.

On hearing that, the parents gave each other worried looks.

'I'm sure this painkiller will settle her down', said the nurse as she injected the morphine slowly through the bung.

This worried Di even more. So far, Sarah seemed to have tolerated the previous two doses, but she was worried about her having it again.

As soon as the morphine hit Sarah's bloodstream, she turned deathly pale, cold and sweaty and slumped onto her pillow. The nurse who gave the injection rushed back to the office while the other checked Sarah's vital signs. Sarah's pulse raced, her blood pressure plummeted, and a crimson rash was starting to spread over her chalky white skin. Within minutes Sarah's face was covered in angry hives which, even in her delirium, she couldn't stop scratching.

To Di's relief the nurse meticulously charted Sarah's allergic reaction while the other nurse returned with the ward resident and some medication to counteract the side effects.

Mark had moved away to let the staff work and stared nervously out of the window with his back turned. Being around Sarah when she was uncomfortable and having procedures – even just injections–was never his strong point.

Within minutes of Sarah's allergic reaction to the morphine, two doctors from the specialist pain team arrived. By then the medication had settled some of the side effects, but she remained irritable. The team immediately diagnosed Sarah's long-standing sensitivity to morphine and found a solution to the problem – they replaced morphine with Fentanyl, a synthetic opiate. Within a few minutes, they expertly set up a continuous infusion with a calibrated pump that administered constant pain relief through the IV. Once the pain specialist started the Fentanyl infusion, Sarah's agitation disappeared and she stopped scratching the eruptions from the morphine allergy. It took only seconds for her to fall into a deep sleep.

Before they left, the pain team doctors told the parents they were available any time and promised to look in on Sarah regularly to ensure she had adequate pain relief.

After the staff had handled the crisis, they left the room to give Mark and Di time alone with Sarah. The parents had no idea the morphine problem they'd worried about for so long was so easily fixed by expert hands. No one had offered them alternative pain relief for their daughter before. Now Sarah lay comfortably in bed for the first time in weeks and the long-standing problem only took a couple of minutes to fix.

The parents were still enjoying their immense relief when, just before lunchtime, a neat but casually dressed young woman came into the room. When she introduced herself as the oncology social worker, Mark and Di froze. She told them she was there to help them and asked whether they required anything. They had heard the same phrases before and it terrified them. The parents looked stunned throughout the interview and said very little. Meanwhile the unsuspecting social worker left the room wondering what she had done to make the parents so apprehensive.

At 12.30, the lunches arrived on the ward, but none came for Sarah. Staff kept Sarah hydrated with saline, while the tube from her stomach drained the fluid backed up from the bowel blockage. She was now heavily sedated and clearly incapable of eating. With Sarah settled, the parents went down to the cafeteria for lunch. Neither ate very much. They worried about the phone conference between Dr Kotz and the Melbourne oncologists at the hospital. Over the past year, they had made a habit of not leaving Sarah alone for long and they were anxious to return to her room soon.

After lunch, the surgical registrar came into Sarah's room to speak with the parents. He led them to a small conference room at the end of the ward and offered them a seat. The young doctor, who was in his mid-thirties, spoke with the parents sympathetically. He had reviewed Sarah's scans and X-rays to decide whether any surgical interventions were possible. Now he shook his head and looked at them sadly. 'I'm so sorry to have to tell you that Sarah's cancer is inoperable. There is nothing we can do surgically to help her', he explained. 'The oncology team will be taking over her care from now on'.

Despite the surgeon's kindness, the parents were worried about his intention to hand Sarah's case over to the oncology team. They had heard it all before.

When Mark and Di returned to Sarah's room, two nurses were freshening Sarah up after they had toileted her on a bedpan. They had washed her back, face and hands and she looked comfortable under clean sheets. After weakly smiling at her parents, Sarah fell into a drugged slumber.

Later that afternoon the parents were relaxing with some light reading when the oncology team came to Sarah's room. It was the unit's head oncologist, an impressively intelligent man accompanied by the oncology registrar, Dr Katherine Davis. They introduced themselves and invited Mark and Di to the side office for a discussion. The parents were terrified as they followed the oncologists down the hall. The head oncologist opened the door to the office and invited everyone in. The parents sat down nervously on the two hospital-issue vinyl chairs provided. The two doctors sat directly opposite. It was a tiny office, the head oncologist was a large man, and suddenly Mark felt hemmed in.

The senior oncologist began the discussions. He told the parents that he and Dr Davis had spoken personally with Dr Kotz in NSW. Mark tensed, while Di cringed. The doctor went on to tell them that he and Dr Davis knew all about Sarah's history.

Mark stood up. 'Look, I'm not sure what you think you know, but–'

The oncologist interrupted. 'Please, Mr Westley. I know you and your wife have been through a lot'.

Mark interrupted the oncologist. 'You're not wrong and I'm not going to put my daughter through it again either'.

'Please just hear us out', insisted the oncologist as he motioned Mark to sit down again.

Mark sank slowly to his chair and glanced at Di.

The head oncologist leaned forwards. For a moment, he struggled with his thoughts, before he started hesitantly. 'First of all, I would like to repeat that we know about Sarah's medical history now'.

Mark and Di glanced anxiously at the door.

The oncologist looked mildly distressed. 'I want to reassure you both that we will not be involving outside authorities. As far as we are concerned, there is no place for outside parties in this matter. This is a private medical issue concerning your family. We realise it is a time of painful decisions and we will do everything we can to take your wishes and Sarah's into account'.

Mark and Di were dumbfounded.

Dr Davis had been watching the parents' reactions. Earlier that day she had reconstructed a chronology of Sarah's illness and found out that the girl had been in stage IV at the time she was being forced into treatments. Davis was in her early thirties. She had been a physician before starting her oncology training, and displayed unusual sensitivity and a talent for reading body language. She felt the parents needed further honestly and reassurance and took over from the senior oncologist.

Dr Davis reached out to touch Di lightly on the arm. 'This cancer is not your fault. There is nothing more you could have done', she said reassuringly. The doctor cast her eyes down and deliberately lowered her voice. 'But I'm so sorry to have to tell you that your daughter is in the terminal phase of cancer and there is nothing more we can do except offer palliative care'.

Mark spoke up. 'That comes as no surprise to us. You might have guessed by now that we've been put through the wringer and none of us have had the

Sarah's Last Wish

slightest chance of coming to terms with losing our daughter before today. All I ask is that you do not speak to Sarah about dying. She has heard enough about her death from the hospital staff in NSW over the past year'.

On hearing this, the senior oncologist raised his eyebrow and glanced at his colleague before reassuring the parents that this would not happen in his ward.

Dr Davis saw Di's eyes brimming with tears. She found a tissue in her lab coat pocket and offered it to her.

The head oncologist looked at Mark sympathetically. 'We realise that your experiences were out of the ordinary, which makes it more difficult for you to face such a terrible loss, but I promise you that Dr Davis and I will do everything we can to ensure you and Sarah are comfortable here. Is there anything you need right now?' he asked gently.

Mark glanced at Di and realised she was emotionally numb; he wasn't thinking straight himself either. 'This is a change of pace from our previous experiences and I think we need a minute to get our bearings', he replied.

Dr Davis stood up. 'In that case, we'll leave you alone for a while. We will look in on you and Sarah every day'.

The head oncologist held the door open for his colleague. 'Just let us know if you need anything', he told the parents before closing the door.

The parents sat silently for several minutes. After a while, Mark got up. In the corner was a hot water jug. He switched it on, took two teabags out of a jar, and filled two plastic cups with boiling water. He put a splash of milk in one and handed it to Di. 'Please tell me I'm not dreaming', Mark said.

Di took a tiny sip. 'Those two oncologists seem like real people with real feelings'.

Mark nodded in agreement. 'And they figured out by themselves Sarah got some rough treatment in the last couple of hospitals', he added.

Di shifted uncomfortably in her chair. Her leg was aching again but she didn't dare check it out. 'And they don't treat us like bad parents and Sarah like a prison inmate', answered Di.

'What do you think of the rest of the staff around here?'

Di thought about it for a while. 'It looks like they know what they're doing'.

That night, in the parents' accommodation, Mark and Di had their first uninterrupted night's sleep in months.

The following morning both oncologists arrived in Sarah's room to find her awake and asking for a vitamin C drip. Dr Davis looked puzzled until Mark explained that Sarah had felt better while having the drips at the Integrative

326

Health Clinic. She was also prescribed high potency vitamins, a complete mineral formula, glutathione, amino acids, and omega oils –all of which had kept her in surprisingly good condition for the better part of the year. Both oncologists were aware that many cancer patients used nutritional supplements and IV vitamin C for better life quality and that it alleviated unpleasant symptoms in the terminal stages. The senior doctor said, almost jokingly, that vitamin C was not standard issue in hospitals but if Mark could source pharmaceutical-grade intravenous vitamin C, he would be willing to administer it to Sarah, after the pharmacist approved it. As it happened, the wholesale pharmaceutical supplier was located not far from the hospital. Mark phoned us in NSW and it took only a phone call from us to arrange for a supply to be delivered to the hospital pharmacy. Once the hospital pharmacist checked it, the oncologist prescribed it on a special complementary medicine chart.

By late afternoon, Sarah was receiving vitamin C in an IV drip. Almost immediately, she brightened up and was able to sit out of bed in a chair. Sarah grinned at both oncologists when they dropped in to check on her. After she realised the doctors cared enough to actually listen to what she wanted for once, she enjoyed talking to them. In no time, she developed a special bond with Dr Davis, whom she called Dr Katherine from then on.

Later that evening, Nurse Margaret was on the late shift. After she had freshened Sarah up and tucked her in under clean sheets, she sympathetically stroked her forehead. The kind gesture caught Sarah by surprise. At first, she flinched until she looked up into a pair of kind brown eyes and realised the motherly paediatric nurse really cared. She had taken a special interest in the family and often went out of her way to make Sarah comfortable.

After Margaret settled Sarah for the night, the parents ventured upstairs to their room for a late supper. Mark left again in search of some food from the cafeteria downstairs, while Di set a makeshift table. Di suddenly realised she hadn't eaten much that day and grabbed an apple from the fruit-bowl. She lingered for a moment at the window to eat it. The familiar cityscape reminded her of her childhood years in Melbourne before she had met Mark. She was young and naïve and it was a different world from the nightmarish one they were living in now. The past year had forced them both to become persistent and thick-skinned just to navigate their way through the health system with Sarah.

Di pressed her forehead against the glass and peered several floors down. Below were parklands surrounding the hospital with playgrounds, wooden benches and walkways lined with flowers – a perfect setting for tomorrow when Ruth was due to arrive from NSW with their other children. She wondered if

Sarah was strong enough to withstand the excitement. Tomorrow was Hannah's eleventh birthday, and Leah's ninth was two days later. Sarah's Melbourne cousins were also due to arrive from Yarra Junction to visit Sarah at the hospital.

Di turned to throw the apple core in the bin when a pain shot through her left leg. This time she checked it to discover her leg was bright red and twice its normal size. The cellulitis had returned, along with the terrible memories of the last bout, in Sydney just after Sarah's splenectomy, when they'd nearly lost her. It was the last straw. Di collapsed on the bed and wept.

Mark wandered in with their meals to find his wife inconsolable. 'What's up?' he asked stunned.

'Why couldn't they have been this good to Sarah back home?' she sobbed.

Mark placed the tray from the cafeteria on the table. 'I don't know', he said cheerlessly. 'Maybe it was orchestrated, or maybe we just struck a whole mob of ice-cold mongrels. At least right now, she's in capable hands and we can enjoy some time with her. She might even pull through with all the good care she's getting here. Who knows?'

Di manoeuvred a pillow under her aching leg. 'She never wanted much. Why did we have to flee to another state just to find somebody who cares? Is this what's happening to other people – or just to us?'

Mark paced restlessly over to the window and glared into the darkness. 'It might be a long time before we get some answers', he replied. Mark's voice then took on a steely tone. 'But I can promise you two things for sure –I will never stop asking those questions. And I *will* get the answers'.

The next morning Di helped Nurse Margaret shower Sarah while Mark did the heavy lifting. Everyone who saw Sarah was astonished to see how much better she looked. Her deep yellow jaundice had diminished, the whites of her eyes were white again, and her allergic skin rash had faded into a mild case of spots.

After Sarah was settled, Di announced that she and Mark planned a food-shopping trip to the farmer's market near the hospital. She planned a luncheon for the rest of the family, who were due in from NSW in just a few hours. To everyone's amazement, Sarah felt perky and wanted to go with her parents. As usual, Margaret had a bright idea. In no time, the staff rigged up a wheelchair with an IV pole. Mark helped Margaret lift Sarah into the chair and surprisingly, she was able to sit up. The parents thought it was nothing short of a miracle, considering Sarah had been near death just two days ago.

Mark wheeled Sarah to the end of the ward and down the lift to the ground floor. Di had trouble keeping up. Her leg was throbbing.

Outside, Sarah squinted in the brilliant spring weather. She sat limp in the wheelchair, barely able to lift her arms, but determined to enjoy the outing. Mark wheeled her through the crowds, past the stands with Italian salami and German sausage hanging from hooks in the open air. She loved the smell of fresh-baked bread and olives marinating in brine. While Di rushed between stalls selecting fresh dips, cheese and olives, Sarah delighted in the food smells, the sun on her face and the fruit vendor's shouts. They returned Sarah to the hospital an hour later. By then she was more than ready for a nap.

After staff settled Sarah in bed again, Margaret couldn't wait to unveil her surprise for the parents. She led them next door to a huge family room, built to accommodate several families. Margaret had reserved it solely for the Westley family. When she showed them the sign she'd put up outside the door with their family name on it, Mark and Di were overwhelmed by her thoughtful gesture.

Ruth brought Sarah's five other siblings straight from the airport to the hospital. Margaret had prettied Sarah up before the family arrived. She was lying in bed with her hair swept up in a pony-tail when her four sisters and little brother walked in. The girls giggled nervously. They hadn't known what to expect, since Sarah had been at death's door the last time they'd seen her. They were shocked at first to see their sister looking so sick with spots still on her face from the morphine reaction, but happy she was alive after wondering if they would ever see her again the day she had left NSW on the plane.

The two birthday girls, Hannah and Leah, hugged their sister first. Clara hesitated at first before tiptoeing around the IV equipment. Next came Laura, who kissed Sarah on the forehead and then went straight to work decorating the kids with face-paint. Finally, Mark lifted Joshua up over the rail to hug his sister. After that, the boy hopped onto Mark's knee and stuck there like mud. Little Dude was happiest when his family was together in one place.

The staff arrived to temporarily disconnect the IV from Sarah. They capped the tubing and wrapped a crepe bandage around Sarah's arm to secure the cannula, allowing her more mobility while she was at the family gathering. Without the cumbersome IV pole and tubing, Laura and Mark easily transferred Sarah from the bed into the wheelchair. Finally, Mark wheeled Sarah next door to join the rest of the family who had meanwhile gathered in their specially designated room, which Margaret had festooned with balloons and streamers. Sarah's arrival sparked a rousing welcome with cheering and clapping. Ruth especially was relieved to see Sarah again after fearing she might not have survived the plane trip to Melbourne.

Soon Di's two brothers arrived with their families. It had been a long time since the Westley kids had spent time with their Melbourne cousins. Finally, Dude had a chance to hang out with boys his own age instead of his five older sisters.

Both Sarah's Melbourne aunts had brought tasty casseroles and finger foods to supplement Di's food from the markets. For dessert, Di cut up a watermelon into slices, and finally Laura and Clara lit the candles on the birthday cake.

From her wheelchair, Sarah hummed happy birthday to her sisters and clapped as Leah and Hannah blew out the candles. Sarah could stomach nothing but tiny sips of orange juice, but despite this, she clearly enjoyed herself as much as her condition allowed. Occasionally her head wobbled and she leant it on the wheelchair's high backrest. Sarah watched on as Hannah and Leah unwrapped their birthday presents. Both were artistic and each got coloured pencils and paper, which they immediately put to use making drawings for Sarah. Next, the family showered Sarah with presents. As much as she enjoyed the attention, all the excitement was too much for her and she asked to go back to bed. Mark and Laura returned Sarah to her room next door for a rest and soon after went back to finish eating. Meanwhile, Hannah sneaked into Sarah's room to steal some time with her sister.

The nurses had given Sarah a dose of pain medication and she was just drifting off when Hannah arrived. Sarah sleepily invited her sister up on her bed. Hannah hesitated at first, before climbing up and snuggling in.

Sarah put her arm around her sister. 'This reminds me of canoeing together on the dam', she murmured.

'I remember', said Hannah. 'Sometimes we'd tip it over and go swimming instead. We'd hold our breath and dive down to the bottom for clay, and make it into little balls'.

Sarah smiled weakly at the memory. 'And turf them at each other'.

Hannah interrupted. 'Yeah, and Mum would yell at us for coming home grubby'.

'That's why Dad always called you Grub', said Sarah dryly.

'That's why he called you Rogue!' retorted Hannah. 'And what about when we used to play schools?'

Sarah smiled weakly. 'Yeah. I was the teacher, and you were my teacher's aide. And Leah and Dude were our pupils'.

'How come you always got to be the boss cocky?' asked Hannah.

Sarah suddenly thought of something. She reached across to her bedside table, but was too weak to open the drawer. Hannah opened it for her and Sarah reached in to remove a small gadget the size of an egg, with a screen and three buttons. 'Mum bought me this Tamagotchi', Sarah explained as she offered her sister the electronic toy animal. 'You have to feed it, and it grows, and you have to clean up after it', she added.

Hannah sat up in bed and looked sternly at her sister. 'I can't take it – it's yours', she insisted as she pushed the toy back at her.

Sarah was unmoved. 'I want you to have it. You can be its mother now'. With that, Sarah lay back on the pillow exhausted. 'That makes you the boss cocky', she added with a weak smile.

Hannah accepted the tiny toy that made so many demands on its owner. For the next half hour, Hannah listened quietly as Sarah closed her eyes and wandered through their childhood memories.

The following day Di woke up with a fever and was unable to get out of bed. When Mark went downstairs to visit Sarah, he mentioned it to the nursing staff. They were instantly concerned and arranged for the oncologist to check on Di.

On seeing Di's leg, Dr Katherine made immediate arrangements to admit her to a nearby hospital. Di was ushered through the ED and admitted to the medical ward, where she spent the next two days on an antibiotic drip and strict bed rest. She was heartbroken to miss precious time with Sarah but she knew she couldn't continue pushing herself to the limit without breaking. Mark visited Di each day while Ruth and Laura stayed with Sarah. Meanwhile Di's brother and his wife were caring for the other Westley kids at Yarra Junction, and they drove the children to the hospital almost every day to visit their sister.

After a few days, the doctors discharged Di from the hospital in a wheelchair. She would have to stay off her feet for another day or two until she could bear weight on her leg again. For a while, both Di and Sarah were in wheelchairs.

Di returned to the children's hospital to find that Laura had been staying in one of the hospital's spare rooms and was spending each day with Sarah. She was pleased to find that Laura and Sarah had at last managed to get rid of every trace of their former sibling rivalry. It had started in childhood, when Sarah had flexed her strong personality and challenged her oldest sister almost daily–often deliberately irritating the more serious-minded Laura. Once Sarah had become ill, however, Laura had missed her sister sorely. The lack of information from the doctors had made it a confusing and lonely time for her, and on top of this, she had suddenly been burdened with the heavy responsibility of helping their relatives care for the younger kids while her parents were away for weeks at a time. This strain had persisted the entire 16 months that Sarah was in the last stage of cancer. Moreover, since the NSW oncologists had not admitted that Sarah was terminal until the very end, the family had never been given the chance to come to terms with losing her. The kids had known that their sister was seriously ill, of course, but they had thought she would one day recover. Meanwhile, the threat from DoCS had overshadowed any other issues.

Now, for the first time, Laura was able to spend quality time with her terminally ill sister. Laura's daily ministering of care to Sarah became a resolution for both of them and led to a strong bond of equals. Finally reunited, the two of them shared their precious family memories while they laughed and cried together. Ironically, this would make loosing Sarah more real and painful to Laura.

For the next week, the family appreciated the staff's kindness and consideration at the Melbourne Royal Children's Hospital.

Hannah describes the events best in her own words:

> *The Royal Children's Hospital was in the suburb-parklands, close to some shops and these big markets where they sold fresh fruits and vegetables, raw foods, meats and also clothing, toys and entertainment. The hospital was in a very attractive area, with lots of pretty trees and parks. Mum and Dad often took Sarah for walks in the wheel chair up to the pretty parks and sometimes to the markets but she was too sick to enjoy much.*

> *Sarah's room overlooked the other side of the hospital with another small picnic area under her window. She had a toilet but no shower in her room. Lots of visitors came to see her, mostly relatives and friends. The hospital was about 10 or 11 stories high and when the younger children got bored I would take them in a lift right to the top, stopping at every level. It kept them entertained.*

> *We used to go and see Sarah everyday in the hospital, some days we would have a picnic outside the hospital in the big park with*

our cousins. Also we would sit sometimes in a big room near Sarah's room with a pool table and table tennis.

Mum occasionally took Sarah down to the starlight room on the ground floor where there were lots of activities, games etc. The Starlight room was painted purple with stars and sparkles all over it, which brightened her up. The Starlight people were really nice to her and gave her a purple school bag, key rings, and things to share for the rest of the family.

I will never forget how kind the nurse, Margaret, was. She was a kind loving lady with a soft heart. Margaret was the nurse who held a party for Leah and I when it was our birthday.

The following week passed almost pleasantly despite the approaching loss. The Royal Children's Hospital housed the foremost children's cancer unit in the country, and its staff were highly trained in paediatric palliative care; they gave Sarah and her family expert care and support. The family found clarity in the staff's honesty, and comfort in their simple expressions of humanity and kindness. Most importantly, the two weeks the parents spent with their daughter while she was in safe hands, helped them at least to begin facing their impending loss.

Despite Sarah's two-week reprieve, however, she weakened each day and slept most of the time. One afternoon, while Ruth, Di and Laura were at the markets, Mark sat with Sarah. She snored softly for over an hour, but when she became restless and mumbled incoherently, Mark put down his newspaper.

'What is it Sarah?' he asked.

'Take me home Dad', she said without opening her eyes.

Mark searched frantically for a reply. 'You're too sick to go home Jogue', he said softly.

Sarah's eyes remained closed. 'Then take me home when I'm not sick anymore', she murmured before falling silent again.

When the women returned from their excursion, Mark went down to the nurse's station to ask for an appointment with the oncologist the following day. He had an idea that would allow Sarah to be even closer to her family.

The next morning Mark and Di had an appointment to see Dr Katherine. They told the oncologist that Sarah would surely enjoy spending whatever time she had left at Yarra Junction, where she could be with her siblings and close family. The oncologist was receptive to the idea and told them she would do whatever was necessary to make this possible. She promised to speak with the head of the cancer unit and with the pain team, who would change Sarah's pain medication to one that did not have to be administered intravenously. She told the parents that a palliative care team was available to visit each day and keep an eye on Sarah in a home environment. With a bit of luck, they could go as early as the day after tomorrow.

The following afternoon nurse Margaret breezed into the room with a broad smile and good news. She announced that Sarah would be allowed to leave the hospital tomorrow and, in preparation, she would remove Sarah's IV and replace it with trans-dermal adhesive patches that contained the same painkiller as the IV had delivered.

Mark told the nurse he would go downstairs to buy a paper and some ginger ale in the interim. Laura announced she was heading upstairs to check on her mother, who was upstairs resting her leg, and then she would start packing.

After making sure the door was shut, Margaret ran warm water into a sponge bowl to freshen Sarah up. She tried to mask the sadness she felt being around the terminally sick girl. Sarah's cancer was rapidly advancing through her lymphatic system, and her swollen legs made it a hopeless struggle to pull up the white surgical stockings. The girl's abdomen bulged with fluid from the bulky tumours. As a mother herself, she could only imagine what torment her parents were going through and what anguish still lay ahead of them in the next few days. Margaret gently rolled Sarah on her side and washed her back.

In the past two weeks, Sarah had enjoyed playing word games with Margaret. Now her mind computed slowly and her voice was thick. 'Your eyes remind me of my favourite chocolate', Sarah waited for a return volley.

'And your eyes remind me of two pools of mischief', replied Margaret as she towelled Sarah dry.

Sarah smiled weakly as Margaret powdered her back, straightened her draw sheet and rolled her on her back again. The nurse explained that she was about to remove Sarah's IV, beginning by gently peeling the micro-pore tape from the cannula. She then pulled the IV out with one gentle tug, before covering the puncture with a band-aid and pushing the drip stand with its drip counter and tubing into the corner. Next, Margaret showed Sarah an oblong analgesic patch and explained that from now on the patches would kill the pain just the same as the drip. When Sarah asked where she would stick them, Margaret lowered Sarah's gown a fraction to access the area below the clavicle. Sarah watched as the nurse removed the plastic tabs and stuck the painkilling patch to her skin.

Moments later, Mark returned to the room clutching a family-sized bottle of ginger ale. It was the only fluid Sarah could keep down – and then only in tiny sips.

Margaret wheeled the IV stand towards the door. 'Let me know if those patches don't take care of the pain and I can give her something extra', she said before leaving the room.

Mark thanked the nurse and settled back into the bedside chair. Sarah looked exhausted and he wanted her to rest. When she closed her eyes, he opened the newspaper and started reading. But Sarah was not asleep.

'Dad'.

Mark looked up from his paper, surprised. 'I didn't know you were still awake'. He opened the ginger ale and poured some into a glass for Sarah.

Sarah kept her eyes closed. 'You know how downstairs they said to make a wish?'

Mark searched the drawer of the bedside cabinet for a straw. 'You mean the other day when you were downstairs in the Starlight room?'

Sarah wet her lips before she could speak. 'Yeah. They said I could. Well, now I made a wish'.

Mark put the ginger ale with the straw up to Sarah's lips but she turned her head. What she wanted to say was far more important.

'What is it then?' Mark asked.

Sarah opened her eyes and focused on her father with unnerving clarity. 'You know what happened to me?'

'You mean the cancer?'

'No', Sarah said impatiently. 'I mean those ladies that came to our house and the doctors. The stuff they did to me –'.

'Yes', interrupted Mark. He did not want her to go on. He would never forget what they had done to his daughter.

'I want you to promise me something Dad', she insisted.

Mark realised this was a serious moment; he had never seen Sarah as lucid or as determined as she was right now. 'What', he asked gently.

Sarah fixed a determined stare on her father. 'What they did to me wasn't fair, and I want you to make sure that they can never do this to any other kid – ever again'.

Mark didn't know what to say. Did she know she would probably never live to see her wish come true? Did she know how difficult that wish would be to grant? It was not just up to him: hundreds, maybe thousands of other people needed to join together to make the changes that would prevent those things from happening again. He had no idea where to start, but how could he refuse her when he knew he had no choice but to try?

'Dad, I need you to promise me that', demanded Sarah.

'Yes, I promise', said Mark solemnly.

Sarah slumped back on her pillow and fell almost instantly asleep. Outside, dusk had fallen and the lights of Melbourne flickered on. She was now at peace and relieved of an unbearable burden, and it proved to be her last truly lucid moment.

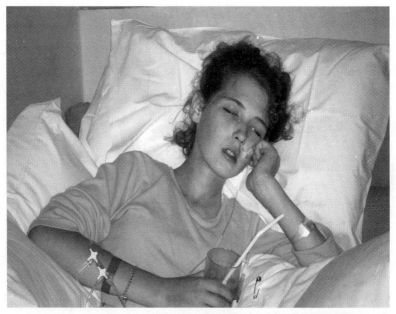

Sarah after she made her last wish on October 19, 2004.

GOING HOME

In my end is my beginning.

Mary Stuart

It was October 20, and the Royal Children's Hospital staff gave Sarah a warm send-off before the ambulance came to transport her to Yarra Junction.

Hannah writes in her own words:

> *Our Uncle and Auntie's House in Yarra Junction was very beautiful and peaceful. It was like Gloucester, very green, mountains, lovely calm waters and rivers. The small town of Yarra Junction was about the size of Barrington not far up the road, which Mum, Dad and Laura walked up there a few times to get out and have a break.*

> *It was a lovely drive to our Aunty and Uncle's house from where we younger children were staying. The colour of the house was similar to ours: maroon roof and cream walls – weatherboard, only one storey with a green vine on the verandah. The house was a long rectangle shape with a cream shed beside it. There was a small wooden cubby house out the back that the children played in and bikes to entertain them.*

> *Inside, the house was old style and very pretty. Our Aunty paints a lot and is very decorative. She made Sarah's room really nice, two white and gold beds – side by side. The wall was painted a dusty pink and she put lovely flowers in a vase beside her bed every day. Aunty made it gorgeous for Sarah. Sarah slept beside the window looking out over the lovely green view. Also, our Aunty put a bird feeder just outside her window and Sarah loved watching the small carefree birds twittering away and telling each other secrets.*

Sarah kept on telling us that she wanted to come home but we we-
ren't sure if she meant our house in NSW or at her cousin's house.
Sarah didn't complain about being at Yarra Junction because it was
finally like home – she had her family, Grandma Ruth, Aunty and
Uncle, a few cousins and friends with her. Also, our parents were al-
lowed to be with her all the time.

Di rode in the back of the ambulance with Sarah to Yarra Junction. The paramedics saw that Sarah was gravely ill and were very kind to Sarah and gentle with Di. They carried Sarah into the house and settled her into one of the single beds in the front bedroom. The other twin bed was reserved for family members, who took turns keeping vigil in Sarah's room each night. The paramedics wished the family all the best before leaving.

Every morning, after Ruth and Di washed Sarah; Mark carried her to the living room and placed her on the comfortable couch Laura had made up into a bed with sheets and pillows. Laura stayed with Sarah at Yarra Junction full time, while family friends who lived a half hour away, cared for the other children and brought them to visit Sarah for a short while each day. Though Sarah became sicker by the hour, she still held her hand out to her siblings and they were happy she still recognised them.

Over the next few days, the palliative care team from the hospital regularly visited Yarra Junction, to ensure the patches gave Sarah sufficient pain relief. A local doctor also called into the house daily, to check on Sarah and administer the occasional vitamin C drip and IV fluids. She too had trouble finding veins, but Sarah was taking strong painkillers, and the multiple attempts at venipuncture did not distress her. Sarah was vomiting several times each day – an indication that her bowel obstruction had worsened. The IV fluids were a humane measure that kept her hydrated and relatively comfortable. The nurses, oncologists and even the social worker at the Royal Children's Hospital kept in close contact with the family to see if they needed anything further. The staff sent regular comforting messages to the Westleys, and the hospital occupational therapist even took the trouble to find out about Sarah's life. She went on to compose a song about Sarah's lively personality and colourful antics, recording it on a DVD for the family.

By the fourth day, on October 24, Sarah's weakness had silenced her, and she spoke only occasionally. Di was sponging Sarah that morning and tried to engage her in small talk, but got no response. Di keenly felt the separation caused by Sarah's decline and wondered aloud whether Sarah still loved her.

'Why wouldn't I?' came Sarah's reply in a feeble voice.

The shock caused Di to jump. She realised that Sarah's personality was still intact and burst out laughing at her quick comeback. Sarah held out both her arms and Di enfolded her daughter in a long hug while all their unspoken love flowed wordlessly between them.

That same night, Laura kept vigil from 11 pm until dawn while Ruth slept in the twin bed next to Sarah. Laura had spent a tiring and emotional night as Sarah floated in and out of consciousness, evidently speaking with loved ones both living and long gone. By 5 am, Ruth woke up and readied herself to take over. Laura was exhausted and eager to catch some sleep. She had made herself a makeshift bed on the living room floor in an alcove just outside Sarah's room.

Ruth had just taken over when Sarah began humming the strains of an old song –*Sweet is the Rest that Comes with Dawn at Last*. Sarah looked blissful, as if seeing a wonderful sight right in front of her. She told Ruth about the bridge she could see. It was so beautiful she wanted to walk across it, but she knew that once on the other side, she would never return. She would cross it when the time came, Sarah said. Ruth stayed with Sarah, knowing that something profound was taking place inside her granddaughter.

By mid-morning, Di and Ruth had finished bed-sponging Sarah. Mark carried her to the living room couch as usual and there she dozed and snored loudly at times. Sarah's laboured breathing disturbed Di. She positioned the oxygen nasal prongs under Sarah's nose and turned on the oxygen to a low allowable level, but it made no difference to her breathing.

Around 10.30 am, Laura woke up tired and sore after only a few hours' sleep on the makeshift bed. After her shower, she helped Ruth and Di cut up fruit for morning tea. Laura brought Sarah small wedges of watermelon and tried to rouse her enough to eat it, but Sarah stared at it blankly and didn't seem to remember what to do with the fruit. Instead, Laura went to the piano and played Sarah's favourite song, *The Heart Does Go On*. She hoped for a faint sign of enjoyment from her sister, but Sarah was deeply asleep.

The next few hours passed peacefully. Mark, Di and Laura sat with Sarah and held her hand. They noticed she was too weak to return their grasp. The GP dropped in for a brief visit to check on Sarah's pain relief and hydration; she shook her head sadly when she saw Di had put the nasal oxygen prongs on Sarah. She took them off and reassured the family that Sarah could be without the extra oxygen – it would be all right for her to breathe room air. The doctor had no heart to tell Di that nothing she could do would save Sarah now.

By early evening, Sarah's breathing was even more irregular. She was white and impossible to rouse. It worried Di, and she replaced the oxygen prongs in the hope that Sarah's breathing would improve. When it made no difference, Di became alarmed and called the family friends to ask them to bring over their other children.

Within minutes of Di's call, the family friends gathered Sarah's other four siblings into the car and raced across town, only to be pulled over by a police officer. When the friend explained the grim circumstances, the officer seemed unmoved and issued him with a ticket anyway before allowing them on their way again.

The children arrived around sunset. They gathered around their sister and chatted to her as though she were awake. Surprisingly, Sarah in her semi-conscious state held out her hand to each of them while they took turns kissing and hugging her. Even then, the children clung to the hope Sarah would get through this crises, just as she had all the others. They had never seen their sister so weak and pale, but to them it was unthinkable they were saying their last goodbye. After sunset, the room darkened suddenly and Clara thought to turn on the top light, though it made no one's spirit any brighter.

Over the next few hours, Sarah's aunt and uncle kept the household running with dinner and cups of tea while the Westley family gathered around Sarah in the living room. Laura played hymns and Sarah's favourite songs on the piano while the family sang softly in accompaniment. After supper, the younger children became tired and wandered off in search of bed.

Mark and Di went outside for a break. They walked through the cottage garden and sat on the bench. Surrounded by fragrant tea roses, they felt nothing but grief.

'This can't be happening', murmured Di. 'Couldn't we take her to –'

'It's all too late', Mark interrupted.

Di turned on Mark angrily. 'Don't talk like that!' she shouted. 'She's got her whole life ahead of her. It's not fair!' Her anger turned to grief and she broke down in tears.

Mark held his wife and let her weep. He felt the first drop of rain on his face. Overhead a passing rain cloud blocked the moon's light and darkened the sky. Di shivered and pulled her cardigan around her. She looked towards the house where her daughter lay dying. From the windows came a soft glow that seemed the only warmth left in the world. Life was fragile and uncertain. Like a train-wreck, it sometimes veered off the rails and nothing could stop it.

'What kind of a world treats a little girl like this?' sobbed Di.

Mark wiped the rain from his forehead and took Di's hand into his.

'Sarah knows some people are cold and mean', he said despondently. 'But she still made people happy wherever she went'.

'Too bad so many let her down'. Di dissolved into fresh tears. 'Does she know how much we love her?'

Mark stared into the darkness. 'I think that's one thing she knows for sure'.

Mark wondered when the certainty had gone out of his own life. He'd always believed something good could come from terrible things, but lately he thought there might be exceptions. He was always the strong one but now he wondered if he could ever get over what happened.

When the rain started pelting down, they ran for shelter into the house.

By late evening, Sarah's breathing grew very irregular and Mark phoned the doctor at 11.30 pm. Di and Ruth had gathered around Sarah with Sarah's aunt and uncle. The youngest siblings had woken up and joined the group. They each took turns whispering in Sarah's ear and telling her they loved her.

Just before midnight, Sarah became restless and Mark thought she might need the commode. He gently slid his arms underneath Sarah and when he braced to lift her, she opened her eyes for the last time and put her arm around him. He saw that she was in perfect peace. 'We love you', he whispered.

Moments later Sarah took her last breath. Then there was an unearthly stillness. Mark carefully placed Sarah down, hardly believing that she had gone. For a few minutes, the room was hushed and Ruth felt a powerful and magnificent energy permeate the room.

The meaning of the silence suddenly hit Di, and she broke down in deep sobs. One by one, the children began to join her until they were all crying together. The only one who could not shed a tear was Mark, paralysed as he was by shock and grief. Ruth consoled Di and the children, taking the time to comfort each one separately.

The doctor and the palliative care nurse arrived shortly after midnight. Mark spoke with them for a while. On the couch, Sarah was in peaceful repose with her eyes closed. The doctor wrote out the death certificate while the nurse helped Mark and Di's brother carry Sarah back to the twin bed. There the nurse washed her and laid her out in her favourite dress, which turned out to be the cherry print outfit that Di had hand-made her while at the clinic.

Laura and Hannah took the younger two children to the garden to gather rose petals. Inside, Ruth helped Di place candles around the room. For the remaining night, Sarah rested on a bed of roses while the family kept their last vigil by candlelight.

Ruth recalls that no one slept that night. She was heartbroken and dreading having to tell Jim. Meanwhile, she comforted the little ones Leah and Joshua, who could not understand the finality of losing their sister. It had all been too confusing from the start.

Di remained grief-stricken while Clara clung to her for comfort. Hannah felt as if part of her had died with Sarah. All their childhood pranks and memories had been hers too and now she was the lonely keeper of those sisterly secrets. Hannah stayed close to Laura, who wore Sarah's dressing gown. It smelt of lavender soap and roses – their only comfort over the long night. Outside it rained as if Nature itself was in mourning.

Mark was numb that night. He knew only that he had to stay on autopilot. Sarah wanted to return home, and he would see to it she was returned to her rightful place.

Of the next day, Hannah recalls:

> *The day after Sarah died, all the family except Dad went for a drive up the road to a beautiful flowing mountain stream where we dropped flower petals and rose petals in the calm water. Down at the stream the nature was so beautiful and it was so quiet.*

While the rest of the family walked to the mountain stream, Mark stayed behind to make the necessary arrangements. By 10 am, two men in black suits from the funeral home came to collect Sarah. He could hardly bear to let them take his daughter away – so strong was his instinct to protect her. He felt cold and empty as he watched the hearse leave the driveway. His only consolation was that she was homeward-bound.

When the rest of the family came back from their walk, the family started packing. They thanked Di's brother and his wife for offering their home and support during the past agonising week.

By early evening, the Westley family boarded a plane at Melbourne airport bound for Newcastle.

A separate flight carried Sarah's precious remains in a mauve casket. She was returning to the place of her birth. She was finally free to come home.

HOME AT LAST

Saturday, 30 October was the day of Sarah's funeral. I drove up to Gloucester with Ann Smith and a couple of others from the clinic. The family had kindly marked the Barrington turn-off with a cluster of purple balloons to help us find the way to the property. Each bend of the road revealed the breathtaking valleys, hillsides and riverbanks where Sarah had grown up.

We found the homestead easily by following the convoy of other cars headed towards the property. It was the closest thing to a traffic jam the unsealed back road had ever seen. We turned into the driveway at the mailbox and followed the private road past the homestead and up the hill. This was Sarah's Hill, and an acre of it was now a temporary car park. A white marquee sat on the crest of the hill and behind it dozens of rows of folding chairs. On the spot where Sarah had often sat to pass the time was now a freshly dug grave, neatly shored up and protected with ornamental barricades. Sarah's mauve coffin stood braced on top of it. Mark had brought her home as she had asked him to, only last week. To carry out his promise Mark had had to overcome several obstacles posed by the local authorities, but after two days of negotiations, local officials had given permission. Sarah would be laid permanently to rest on the land of her forebears.

By early afternoon more than 100 cars had driven up the winding road to Sarah's Hill in a funeral procession. A dozen large men, including friends, relatives, and men from neighbouring farms stood guard around the property to keep out any uninvited visitors in government cars. Slowly, more than 550 close relatives and friends gathered on the hill and filled the seats. Meanwhile, the townspeople were gathering separately in Gloucester High school hall, where they'd organised a wake for the hundreds of people in the small community who also mourned Sarah's death.

Ann and I looked lost at first but Mark's brother soon ushered us to a seat in one of the front rows. Behind us were hundreds of close family and friends, while in front of us stood an open marquee where the family sat, all in a row, with Dude sitting on his father's lap. The children wore Sarah's favourite – the matching cherry print outfits that Di, Laura and a friend had made during

Sarah's brief respite. Mark and Di sat on one side of the children while Ruth and Jim sat on their other side. Mark and Di looked desperately sad while the children cried softly. A lay minister stood near the grave, preparing to deliver a simple, non-denominational service. In the seats behind us, people sobbed. He paused to wait for them to settle. Behind the minister opened a vast expanse of scenery, with the family homestead in the valley below and the Barrington Tops in the far distance. Standing next to Sarah's flower covered casket, the minister then began his moving eulogy, while the children listened quietly. It took all of Di's effort to remain composed. Mark, meanwhile, occasionally glanced down to the road. Even now, he could not relax; he still felt he needed to protect his family, even while burying his daughter. In the distance, he saw the reassuring sight of his neighbours, friends, and relatives still keeping watch by the mailbox.

In a photographic image that my mind has preserved in detail, I clearly recall that the weather that day was more beautiful than any summer's day in my memory. The vast sky was intensely blue, with white clouds drifting by. A warm silky breeze blew up from the gulley. In the distance, the Barrington Tops unleashed their full range of colours, including Sarah's favourite pinks and purples, while in the valley below, the sun glinted from the homestead's iron roof. Spring wild flowers covered the meadow, which teemed with bees and butterflies. Signs of Sarah's adventures were everywhere – the ducks she'd released swam on the dam with a new crop of ducklings, a few trees still bore her carved initials. On the dam grew prolific water lilies that had never before bloomed, and yet today a carpet of pink and violet blossoms covered the water. Ann and I felt Sarah all around us during the eulogy.

After the service, one relative released a flight of doves into the air. The white birds made a victory lap over Sarah's Hill before taking off on their freedom flight into the vast expanse. As the birds winged their way towards the Barrington Tops it seemed they were carrying news of Sarah's invincible courage out into the world with them. She had fought bravely for her right to live and die with dignity and now she was home to rest after her long walk to freedom.

After the doves had disappeared into the distance, close family members surrounded Sarah's grave. In a natural and innocent way, the children came forward to place toys and cards on top of the casket and other items that had special meaning to them. When the family then generously invited others to come forward to pay their respects, Ann and I came to place on the casket some flowers and the cards we'd written to Sarah. For the next half hour, the mourners mingled with the family, before being invited to Gloucester for the wake.

Epilogue

It was necessary to hold it in the school hall since half the town would have turned up to the funeral on the family property and there would have been no room for all of them.

Before leaving Sarah's Hill, I took one last look over the valley and it struck me again that I had never seen a more perfect October's day, or a sadder day than this.

Mark and Di invited us to spend some time at the homestead with the family before going into town. By now, Di was only just keeping herself from breaking down. Ruth was doing her best to lend support to everyone. To my surprise, Hannah and Leah showed me their drawings of Sarah and their family. Incredibly, in the upstairs room, the caterpillars Sarah had gathered three weeks before had all hatched. The girls had let a myriad of butterflies go free through the open window.

After a while, we headed into town to join the community wake for the family. I had never seen anything like it in the city. The community came out in the hundreds – teachers, pupils, friends, police, firemen, neighbours, and extended family – they filled the hall with home-cooking and baking that covered dozens of tables.

That day the people of Gloucester came out to take one of their own families into their hearts. That afternoon I glimpsed the real spirit of Australia. It was Sarah's true heritage.

EPILOGUE

The Westley family spent the next three years in deep mourning for the loss of Sarah. Their grief was made even more crushing by stresses imposed on the entire family during Sarah's illness. Mark felt the added responsibility of the promise he had made to his daughter before her death. It weighed heavily on him, and as soon as he was able, he intended to carry it out.

Many changes came over the family in the ensuing years. Sarah's five siblings are six years older now and some are young adults. Although they are still coming to terms with the past traumatic events, they have also come to know some of their strengths. They remain good-natured, talented, and free-thinking. All have matured into strong and resilient individuals who are aware of their identity and who know their rights and obligations as few members of society do.

Mark and Di have also emerged with renewed determination. Over recent years, Mark has lent his support to families in similar circumstances. He has also been a strong advocate for freedom of choice in healthcare.

Because of Sarah's Last Wish, beneficial changes are already occurring. These, Mark believes, are only the beginning. He is totally committed to the changes required to bring the health care and child protection system into line with human rights and freedom of choice.

For regular updates, extra resources, and a call to action, log onto:

www.sarahs-last-wish.com

For persons without computer access, written correspondence may be addressed to: Sarah's Last Wish, PO BOX 5165, NSW, 2261, Australia.

You can blow out a candle,
but you can't blow out a fire.
Once the flames begin to catch,
the wind will blow it higher.

Peter Gabriel

ABOUT THE AUTHOR

Eve Hillary lives in Sydney, Australia. She is a health practitioner, freelance journalist, and best selling author. Since 1996, she has written three books and a host of investigative articles on healthcare issues. She has explored the ways in which people recover from serious health challenges, and how current medical practices and systems can be brought into line with patients' human rights and freedom of choice, to offer the best outcomes for patients.

Eve holds a Bachelor of Health Science degree and has been a health practitioner for nearly 30 years, both inside and outside of the hospital system. Between 2001 and 2004, Eve co-founded and operated an integrative medical clinic. She is currently in private practice offering integrative health care that includes cutting-edge scientific breakthroughs in nutritional and complementary medicine. She assists people to more easily navigate through the health care system, and she also offers unique coaching that helps people to successfully identify and overcome barriers to healthy lifestyle changes, in order to bring lasting and beneficial changes to health.

For the past 15 years, Eve has made dozens of media appearances and has given over 200 seminars on health and wellness. She has taught thousands of people the skills and information that helped them successfully navigate through health crises.

Eve remains a strong advocate for freedom of choice in health care, children's rights, and family justice. She believes that lasting beneficial change can come through the power and magic of an inspiring story.

For book orders, appointments, or speaking requests, contact Eve at:

www.sarahs-last-wish.com

Email: sarahslastwish@gmail.com

REFERENCES

Adams, J. B., Baral, M., Geis, E., Mitchell, J., Ingram, J., Hensley, A., Zappia, I., Newmark, S., Gehn, E., Rubin, R. A., Mitchell, K., Bradstreet, J. & El-Dahr, J. (2009) Safety and efficacy of oral dmsa therapy for children with autism spectrum disorders: Part a--medical results. BMC Clin Pharmacol, 9, 16.

Anderson, R. (1981) Vitamin c and immune functions: Mechanisms of immunostimulation. IN Counsell, J. N. A. H., D. H. (Ed.) Vitamin c. London, Applied Science Publishers.

Andre, N., Rome, A., Coze, C., Padovani, L., Pasquier, E., Camoin, L. & Gentet, J. C. (2008) Metronomic etoposide/cyclophosphamide/celecoxib regimen given to children and adolescents with refractory cancer: A preliminary monocentric study. Clin Ther, 30, 1336-40.

Ashby, M. & Stoffell, B. (1991) Therapeutic ratio and defined phases: Proposal of ethical framework for palliative care. BMJ, 302, 1322-4.

Ashby, M. & Stoffell, B. (1995) Artificial hydration and alimentation at the end of life: A reply to craig. J Med Ethics, 21, 135-40.

Ashworth, A. (2001) Treatment of severe malnutrition. J Pediatr Gastroenterol Nutr, 32, 516-8.

Ayhan, A., Taskiran, C., Bozdag, G., Altinbas, S., Altinbas, A. & Yuce, K. (2005) Endodermal sinus tumor of the ovary: The hacettepe university experience. Eur J Obstet Gynecol Reprod Biol, 123, 230-4.

Baker, S. (2008) The metaphor of an oceanic disease. Integrative Med, 7, 40-5.

Banerjee, S. & Gore, M. (2009) The future of targeted therapies in ovarian cancer. Oncologist, 14, 706-16.

Barakat, L. P., Kazak, A. E., Meadows, A. T., Casey, R., Meeske, K. & Stuber, M. L. (1997) Families surviving childhood cancer: A comparison of posttraumatic stress symptoms with families of healthy children. J Pediatr Psychol, 22, 843-59.

Bennett, M. P. & Lengacher, C. (2009) Humor and laughter may influence health iv. Humor and immune function. Evid Based Complement Alternat Med, 6, 159-64.

Bertolini, F., Paul, S., Mancuso, P., Monestiroli, S., Gobbi, A., Shaked, Y. & Kerbel, R. S. (2003) Maximum tolerable dose and low-dose metronomic chemotherapy have opposite effects on the mobilization and viability of circulating endothelial progenitor cells. Cancer Res, 63, 4342-6.

Bocci, G., Francia, G., Man, S., Lawler, J. & Kerbel, R. S. (2003) Thrombospondin 1, a mediator of the antiangiogenic effects of low-dose metronomic chemotherapy. Proc Natl Acad Sci U S A, 100, 12917-22.

Bocci, G., Nicolaou, K. C. & Kerbel, R. S. (2002) Protracted low-dose effects on human endothelial cell proliferation and survival in vitro reveal a selective antiangiogenic window for various chemotherapeutic drugs. Cancer Res, 62, 6938-43.

Bray, T. M. & Taylor, C. G. (1993) Tissue glutathione, nutrition, and oxidative stress. Can J Physiol Pharmacol, 71, 746-51.

British Medical Assocation 1993. Medical ethics today: Practice and philosophy. London; BMA, 76.

Brooks, S. E. (1994) Preoperative evaluation of patients with suspected ovarian cancer. Gynecol Oncol, 55, S80-90.

Bunin, A., Filina, A. A. & Erichev, V. P. (1992) [a glutathione deficiency in open-angle glaucoma and the approaches to its correction]. Vestn Oftalmol, 108, 13-5.

Burnet, F. M. (1970) The concept of immunological surveillance. Prog Exp Tumor Res, 13, 1-27.

References

Burnet, F. M. (1971) Immunological surveillance in neoplasia. Transplant Rev, 7, 3-25.

Burnet, M. (1957a) Cancer; a biological approach. I. The processes of control. Br Med J, 1, 779-86.

Burnet, M. (1957b) Cancer: A biological approach. Iii. Viruses associated with neoplastic conditions. Iv. Practical applications. Br Med J, 1, 841-7.

Calabrese, V., Scapagnini, G., Ravagna, A., Bella, R., Butterfield, D. A., Calvani, M., Pennisi, G. & Giuffrida Stella, A. M. (2003) Disruption of thiol homeostasis and nitrosative stress in the cerebrospinal fluid of patients with active multiple sclerosis: Evidence for a protective role of acetylcarnitine. Neurochem Res, 28, 1321-8.

Calabrese, V., Scapagnini, G., Ravagna, A., Bella, R., Foresti, R., Bates, T. E., Giuffrida Stella, A. M. & Pennisi, G. (2002) Nitric oxide synthase is present in the cerebrospinal fluid of patients with active multiple sclerosis and is associated with increases in cerebrospinal fluid protein nitrotyrosine and s-nitrosothiols and with changes in glutathione levels. J Neurosci Res, 70, 580-7.

Cameron, E. & Campbell, A. (1974) The orthomolecular treatment of cancer. Ii. Clinical trial of high-dose ascorbic acid supplements in advanced human cancer. Chem Biol Interact, 9, 285-315.

Cameron, E., Campbell, A. & Jack, T. (1975) The orthomolecular treatment of cancer. Iii. Reticulum cell sarcoma: Double complete regression induced by high-dose ascorbic acid therapy. Chem Biol Interact, 11, 387-93.

Cameron, E. & Pauling, L. (1974) The orthomolecular treatment of cancer. I. The role of ascorbic acid in host resistance. Chem Biol Interact, 9, 273-83.

Cameron, E. & Pauling, L. (1978) Supplemental ascorbate in the supportive treatment of cancer: Reevaluation of prolongation of survival times in terminal human cancer. Proc Natl Acad Sci U S A, 75, 4538-42.

Canals, S., Casarejos, M. J., De Bernardo, S., Rodriguez-Martin, E. & Mena, M. A. (2001) Glutathione depletion switches nitric oxide neurotrophic effects to cell death in midbrain cultures: Implications for parkinson's disease. J Neurochem, 79, 1183-95.

Canfield, R. L., Henderson, C. R., Jr., Cory-Slechta, D. A., Cox, C., Jusko, T. A. & Lanphear, B. P. (2003) Intellectual impairment in children with blood lead concentrations below 10 microg per deciliter. N Engl J Med, 348, 1517-26.

Carlson, R. H. (2002) Metronomic timing adds antiangiogenic punch Oncology Times, 24, 32-4.

Carrington, B. M., Thomas, N. B. & Johnson, R. J. (1990) Intrasplenic metastases from carcinoma of the ovary. Clin Radiol, 41, 418-20.

Cascinu, S., Cordella, L., Del Ferro, E., Fronzoni, M. & Catalano, G. (1995) Neuroprotective effect of reduced glutathione on cisplatin-based chemotherapy in advanced gastric cancer: A randomized double-blind placebo-controlled trial. J Clin Oncol, 13, 26-32.

Ceriello, A., Giugliano, D., Quatraro, A. & Lefebvre, P. J. (1991) Anti-oxidants show an anti-hypertensive effect in diabetic and hypertensive subjects. Clin Sci (Lond), 81, 739-42.

Chen, Q., Espey, M. G., Sun, A. Y., Pooput, C., Kirk, K. L., Krishna, M. C., Khosh, D. B., Drisko, J. & Levine, M. (2008) Pharmacologic doses of ascorbate act as a prooxidant and decrease growth of aggressive tumor xenografts in mice. Proc Natl Acad Sci U S A, 105, 11105-9.

Chinery, R., Brockman, J. A., Peeler, M. O., Shyr, Y., Beauchamp, R. D. & Coffey, R. J. (1997) Antioxidants enhance the cytotoxicity of chemotherapeutic agents in colorectal cancer: A p53-independent induction of p21waf1/cip1 via c/ebpbeta. Nat Med, 3, 1233-41.

Chinta, S. J., Kumar, M. J., Hsu, M., Rajagopalan, S., Kaur, D., Rane, A., Nicholls, D. G., Choi, J. & Andersen, J. K. (2007) Inducible alterations of glutathione levels in adult dopaminergic midbrain neurons result in nigrostriatal degeneration. J Neurosci, 27, 13997-4006.

Clauson, J., Hsieh, Y. C., Acharya, S., Rademaker, A. W. & Morrow, M. (2002) Results of the lynn sage second-opinion program for local therapy in patients with breast carcinoma. Changes in management and determinants of where care is delivered. Cancer, 94, 889-94.

Conzen, S. D. (2008) Environmental stress and the neuroendocrine response: Is there a cancer connection?

Culine, S., Lhomme, C., Kattan, J., Michel, G., Duvillard, P. & Droz, J. P. (1997) Cisplatin-based chemotherapy in the management of germ cell tumors of the ovary: The institut gustave roussy experience. Gynecol Oncol, 64, 160-5.

Curtin, J. P. (1994) Management of the adnexal mass. Gynecol Oncol, 55, S42-6.

Dalhoff, K., Ranek, L., Mantoni, M. & Poulsen, H. E. (1992) Glutathione treatment of hepatocellular carcinoma. Liver, 12, 341-3.

Dallenbach, P., Bonnefoi, H., Pelte, M. F. & Vlastos, G. (2006) Yolk sac tumours of the ovary: An update. Eur J Surg Oncol., 32, 1063-75.

Deeb, K. K., Trump, D. L. & Johnson, C. S. (2007) Vitamin d signalling pathways in cancer: Potential for anticancer therapeutics. Nat Rev Cancer, 7, 684-700.

Del Carmen, M. G., Rizvi, I., Chang, Y., Moor, A. C., Oliva, E., Sherwood, M., Pogue, B. & Hasan, T. (2005) Synergism of epidermal growth factor receptor-targeted immunotherapy with photodynamic treatment of ovarian cancer in vivo. J Natl Cancer Inst, 97, 1516-24.

Di Monte, D. A., Chan, P. & Sandy, M. S. (1992) Glutathione in parkinson's disease: A link between oxidative stress and mitochondrial damage? Ann Neurol, 32 Suppl, S111-5.

Di Re, F., Bohm, S., Oriana, S., Spatti, G. B. & Zunino, F. (1990) Efficacy and safety of high-dose cisplatin and cyclophosphamide with glutathione protection in the treatment of bulky advanced epithelial ovarian cancer. Cancer Chemother Pharmacol, 25, 355-60.

Donnerstag, B., Ohlenschlager, G., Cinatl, J., Amrani, M., Hofmann, D., Flindt, S., Treusch, G. & Trager, L. (1996) Reduced glutathione and s-acetylglutathione as selective apoptosis-inducing agents in cancer therapy. Cancer Lett, 110, 63-70.

Dorfman, K. Understanding glutathione. New Developments, Winter 04-05. Vol 10, No 2.

Eltabbakh, G. H. (2004) Recent advances in the management of women with ovarian cancer. Minerva Ginecol, 56, 81-9.

Fairfield, K. M. & Fletcher, R. H. (2002) Vitamins for chronic disease prevention in adults: Scientific review. JAMA, 287, 3116-26.

Field, M. J. & Behrman, R. E. (2003) When children die: Improving palliative and end-of-life care for children. Institute of medicine of the national academies, Washington, DC, The National Academies Press.

Flagg, E. W., Coates, R. J., Jones, D. P., Byers, T. E., Greenberg, R. S., Gridley, G., Mclaughlin, J. K., Blot, W. J., Haber, M., Preston-Martin, S. & Et Al. (1994) Dietary glutathione intake and the risk of oral and pharyngeal cancer. Am J Epidemiol, 139, 453-65.

Frager, G. (1997) Palliative care and terminal care of children. Chil Adolescent Psychiatr Clin North Am, 6, 889-909.

Frei, B. & Lawson, S. (2008) Vitamin c and cancer revisited. PNAS, 105, 11307-8.

Fujita, M., Inoue, M., Tanizawa, O., Minagawa, J., Yamada, T. & Tani, T. (1993) Retrospective review of 41 patients with endodermal sinus tumor of the ovary. Int J Gynecol Cancer, 3, 329-35.

Gale Encyclopaedia of surgery: A guide for patients and caregivers IN Senagore, A. J. (Ed.) Detroit, USA, Gale Cengage, 2003.

Garcia, A. A., Oza, A. M., Hirte, H., Fleming, G., Tsao-Wei, D., Roman, L., Swenson, S., Gandara, D., Scudder, S. & Morgan, R. (2005) Interim report of a phase ii clinical trial of bevacizumab (bev) and low dose metronomic oral cyclophosphamide (mctx) in recurrent ovarian (oc) and primary peritoneal carcinoma: A california cancer consortium trial. J Clin Oncol, 23, 5000.

References

Garcia-Giralt, E., Perdereau, B., Brixy, F., Rhliouch, H. & Pouillart, P. (1997) Preliminary study of gsh l-cysteine anthocyane (recancostat compositumtm) in metastatic colorectal carcinoma with relative denutrition. European J of Cancer, 33, 171.

Gardiner, P., Dvorkin, L. & Kemper, K. J. (2004) Supplement use growing among children and adolescents. Pediatric Annals, 33, 227-32.

Gasparini, G. (2001) Metronomic scheduling: The future of chemotherapy? Lancet Oncol, 2, 733-40.

Gasparini, G., Longo, R., Toi, M. & Ferrara, N. (2005) Angiogenic inhibitors: A new therapeutic strategy in oncology. Nat Clin Pract Oncol, 2, 562-77.

Gately, S. & Kerbel, R. (2001) Antiangiogenic scheduling of lower dose cancer chemotherapy. Cancer J., 7, 427-36.

Giovagnoni, A., Giorgi, C. & Goteri, G. (2005) Tumours of the spleen. Cancer Imaging, 5, 73-7.

Giovanni, D. (2007) Current management stategies for ovarian cancer. Mayo Clinic Proceedings, 82, 751-70.

Gonzalez, M. J., Miranda-Massari, J. R., Mora, E. M., Guzman, A., Riordan, N. H., Riordan, H. D., Casciari, J. J., Jackson, J. A. & Roman-Franco, A. (2005) Orthomolecular oncology review: Ascorbic acid and cancer 25 years later. Integr Cancer Ther, 4, 32-44.

Hagen, T. M., Wierzbicka, G. T., Bowman, B. B., Aw, T. Y. & Jones, D. P. (1990) Fate of dietary glutathione: Disposition in the gastrointestinal tract. Am J Physiol, 259, G530-5.

Hauser, R. A., Lyons, K. E., Mcclain, T., Carter, S. & Perlmutter, D. (2009) Randomized, double-blind, pilot evaluation of intravenous glutathione in parkinson's disease. Mov Disord, 24, 979-83.

Herberman, R. B. (1980) Natural cell-mediated immunity against tumors, New York:, Academic Press.

357

Herberman, R. B. (1981) Natural killer (nk) cells and their possible roles in resistance against disease. Clin Immunol Rev, 1, 1-65.

Herberman, R. B. & Ortaldo, J. R. (1981) Natural killer cells: Their roles in defenses against disease. Science, 214, 24-30.

Hickman, M. P., Lucas, D., Novak, Z., Rao, B., Gold, R. E., Parvey, L., Tonkin, I. L. & Hansen, D. E. (1992) Preoperative embolization of the spleen in children with hypersplenism. J Vasc Interv Radiol, 3, 647-52.

Ho, P. I., Collins, S. C., Dhitavat, S., Ortiz, D., Ashline, D., Rogers, E. & Shea, T. B. (2001) Homocysteine potentiates beta-amyloid neurotoxicity: Role of oxidative stress. J Neurochem, 78, 249-53.

Hoffer, A. & Pauling, L. (1993) Hardin jones biostatistical analysis of mortality data for a second set of cohorts of cancer patients with a large fraction surviving at the termination of the study and a comparison of survival times of cancer patients receiving large regular oral doses of vitamin c and other nutrients with similar patients not receiving these doses. J Orthomolecular Medicine, 8, 1549-67.

Hoffer, L. J., Levine, M., Assouline, S., Melnychuk, D., Padayatty, S. J., Rosadiuk, K., Rousseau, C., Robitaille, L. & Miller, W. H., Jr. (2008) Phase i clinical trial of i.V. Ascorbic acid in advanced malignancy. Ann Oncol, 19, 1969-74.

Hulbert, J. C., Grossman, J. E. & Cummings, K. B. (1983) Risk factors of anesthesia and surgery in bleomycin-treated patients. J Urol, 130, 163-4.

Hunjan, M. K. & Evered, D. F. (1985) Absorption of glutathione from the gastro-intestinal tract. Biochim Biophys Acta, 815, 184-8.

James, S. J., Cutler, P., Melnyk, S., Jernigan, S., Janak, L., Gaylor, D. W. & Neubrander, J. A. (2004) Metabolic biomarkers of increased oxidative stress and impaired methylation capacity in children with autism. Am J Clin Nutr, 80, 1611-7.

James, S. J., Melnyk, S., Fuchs, G., Reid, T., Jernigan, S., Pavliv, O., Hubanks, A. & Gaylor, D. W. (2009) Efficacy of methylcobalamin and folinic acid treatment on glutathione redox status in children with autism. Am J Clin Nutr, 89, 425-30.

James, S. J., Melnyk, S., Jernigan, S., Cleves, M. A., Halsted, C. H., Wong, D. H., Cutler, P., Bock, K., Boris, M., Bradstreet, J. J., Baker, S. M. & Gaylor, D. W. (2006) Metabolic endophenotype and related genotypes are associated with oxidative stress in children with autism. Am J Med Genet B Neuropsychiatr Genet, 141B, 947-56.

James, S. J., Melnyk, S., Jernigan, S., Hubanks, A., Rose, S. & Gaylor, D. W. (2008) Abnormal transmethylation/transsulfuration metabolism and DNA hypomethylation among parents of children with autism. J Autism Dev Disord, 38, 1976.

James, S. J., Slikker, W., 3rd, Melnyk, S., New, E., Pogribna, M. & Jernigan, S. (2005) Thimerosal neurotoxicity is associated with glutathione depletion: Protection with glutathione precursors. Neurotoxicology, 26, 1-8.

Jenner, P. (1992) What process causes nigral cell death in parkinson's disease? Neurol Clin, 10, 387-403.

Jenner, P. (1993) Altered mitochondrial function, iron metabolism and glutathione levels in parkinson's disease. Acta Neurol Scand Suppl, 146, 6-13.

Jenner, P., Dexter, D. T., Sian, J., Schapira, A. H. & Marsden, C. D. (1992) Oxidative stress as a cause of nigral cell death in parkinson's disease and incidental lewy body disease. The royal kings and queens parkinson's disease research group. Ann Neurol, 32 Suppl, S82-7.

Jha, N., Jurma, O., Lalli, G., Liu, Y., Pettus, E. H., Greenamyre, J. T., Liu, R. M., Forman, H. J. & Andersen, J. K. (2000) Glutathione depletion in pc12 results in selective inhibition of mitochondrial complex i activity. Implications for parkinson's disease. J Biol Chem, 275, 26096-101.

Johannsen, P., Velander, G., Mai, J., Thorling, E. B. & Dupont, E. (1991) Glutathione peroxidase in early and advanced parkinson's disease. J Neurol Neurosurg Psychiatry, 54, 679-82.

Johnston, C. S., Meyer, C. G. & Srilakshmi, J. C. (1993) Vitamin c elevates red blood cell glutathione in healthy adults. Am J Clin Nutr, 58, 103-5.

Jones, D. P., Coates, R. J., Flagg, E. W., Eley, J. W., Block, G., Greenberg, R. S., Gunter, E. W. & Jackson, B. (1992) Glutathione in foods listed in the national cancer institute's health habits and history food frequency questionnaire. Nutr Cancer, 17, 57-75.

Joosten, K. F. & Hulst, J. M. (2008) Prevalence of malnutrition in pediatric hospital patients. Curr Opin Pediatr, 20, 590-6.

Julius, M., Lang, C. A., Gleiberman, L., Harburg, E., Difranceisco, W. & Schork, A. (1994) Glutathione and morbidity in a community-based sample of elderly. J Clin Epidemiol, 47, 1021-6.

Juretzka, M. M. & Teng, N. (2008) Adnexal tumors. IN Kavanagh, J. J. (Ed.).
        Kamen, B. A., Rubin, E., Aisner, J. & Glatstein, E. (2000) High-time chemotherapy or high time for low dose. J Clin Oncol, 18, 2935-7.

Kawai, M., Kano, T., Furuhashi, Y., Mizuno, K., Nakashima, N., Hattori, S. E., Kazeto, S., Iida, S., Ohta, M., Arii, Y. & Et Al. (1991) Prognostic factors in yolk sac tumors of the ovary. A clinicopathologic analysis of 29 cases. Cancer, 67, 184-92.

Kerbel, R. S. & Kamen, B. A. (2004) The anti-angiogenic basis of metronomic chemotherapy. Nat Rev Cancer, 4, 423-36.

Kerbel, R. S., Klement, G., Pritchard, K. I. & Kamen, B. (2002) Continuous low-dose anti-angiogenic/ metronomic chemotherapy: From the research laboratory into the oncology clinic. Ann Oncol, 13, 12-5.

Kidd, P. M. (2000) Parkinson's disease as multifactorial oxidative neurodegeneration: Implications for integrative management. Altern Med Rev, 5, 502-29.

Kleinman, I. (1991) The right to refuse treatment: Ethical considerations for the competent patient. CMAJ, 144, 1219-22.

Klement, G., Baruchel, S., Rak, J., Man, S., Clark, K., Hicklin, D. J., Bohlen, P. & Kerbel, R. S. (2000) Continuous low-dose therapy with vinblastine and vegf receptor-2 antibody induces sustained tumor regression without overt toxicity. J Clin Invest, 105, R15-24.

Koh, Y. S., Kim, J. C. & Cho, C. K. (2004) Splenectomy for solitary splenic metastasis of ovarian cancer. BMC Cancer, 4, 96.

Kurman, R. J. & Norris, H. J. (1976) Embryonal carcinoma of the ovary: A clinicopathologic entity distinct from endodermal sinus tumor resembling embryonal carcinoma of the adult testis. Cancer, 38, 2420-33.

Lam, T. K., Cross, A. J., Consonni, D., Randi, G., Bagnardi, V., Bertazzi, P. A., Caporaso, N. E., Sinha, R., Subar, A. F. & Landi, M. T. (2009) Intakes of red meat, processed meat, and meat mutagens increase lung cancer risk. Cancer Res, 69, 932-9.

Latorre, A., De Lena, M., Catino, A., Crucitta, E., Sambiasi, D., Guida, M., Misino, A. & Lorusso, V. (2002) Epithelial ovarian cancer: Second and third line chemotherapy (review). Int J Oncol, 21, 179-86.

Lenzi, A., Culasso, F., Gandini, L., Lombardo, F. & Dondero, F. (1993) Placebo-controlled, double-blind, cross-over trial of glutathione therapy in male infertility. Hum Reprod, 8, 1657-62.

Leung, P. Y., Miyashita, K., Young, M. & Tsao, C. S. (1993) Cytotoxic effect of ascorbate and its derivatives on cultured malignant and nonmalignant cell lines. Anticancer Res, 13, 475-80.
Liu, H., Wang, H., Shenvi, S., Hagen, T. M. & Liu, R. M. (2004) Glutathione metabolism during aging and in alzheimer disease. Ann N Y Acad Sci, 1019, 346-9.

Makar, T. K., Cooper, A. J., Tofel-Grehl, B., Thaler, H. T. & Blass, J. P. (1995) Carnitine, carnitine acetyltransferase, and glutathione in alzheimer brain. Neurochem Res, 20, 705-11.

Malogolowkin, M. H., Mahour, G. H., Krailo, M. & Ortega, J. A. (1990) Germ cell tumors in infancy and childhood: A 45-year experience. Pediatr Pathol, 10, 231-41.

Malvy, D. J., Arnaud, J., Burtschy, B., Sommelet, D., Leverger, G., Dostalova, L. & Amedee-Manesme, O. (1997) Antioxidant micronutrients and childhood malignancy during oncological treatment. Med Pediatr Oncol, 29, 213-7.

Man, S., Bocci, G., Francia, G., Green, S. K., Jothy, S., Hanahan, D., Bohlen, P., Hicklin, D. J., Bergers, G. & Kerbel, R. S. (2002) Antitumor effects in mice of low-dose (metronomic) cyclophosphamide administered continuously through the drinking water. Cancer Res, 62, 2731-5.

Mann, C. L., Davies, M. B., Boggild, M. D., Alldersea, J., Fryer, A. A., Jones, P. W., Ko Ko, C., Young, C., Strange, R. C. & Hawkins, C. P. (2000a) Glutathione s-transferase polymorphisms in ms: Their relationship to disability. Neurology, 54, 552-7.

Mann, J. R., Raafat, F., Robinson, K., Imeson, J., Gornall, P., Sokal, M., Gray, E., Mckeever, P., Hale, J., Bailey, S. & Oakhill, A. (2000b) The united kingdom children's cancer study group's second germ cell tumor study: Carboplatin, etoposide, and bleomycin are effective treatment for children with malignant extracranial germ cell tumors, with acceptable toxicity. J Clin Oncol, 18, 3809-18.

Merad-Boudia, M., Nicole, A., Santiard-Baron, D., Saille, C. & Ceballos-Picot, I. (1998) Mitochondrial impairment as an early event in the process of apoptosis induced by glutathione depletion in neuronal cells: Relevance to parkinson's disease. Biochem Pharmacol, 56, 645-55.

Meriwether, W. D., Ramsey, H. E. & Ward, S. P. (1971) Embryonal cell carcinoma of the ovary. Report of a case. Oncology, 25, 497-504.

Merrill, S. J. (1981) A model of the role of natural killer cells in immune surveillance--i. J Math Biol, 12, 363-73.

Merrill, S. J. (1982) Foundations of the use of an enzyme-kinetic analogy in cell-mediated cytotoxicity. Math. Biosci., 62, 219.

Moertel, C. G., Fleming, T. R., Creagan, E. T., Rubin, J., O'connell, M. J. & Ames, M. M. (1985) High-dose vitamin c versus placebo in the treatment of patients with advanced cancer who have had no prior chemotherapy. A randomized double-blind comparison. N Engl J Med, 312, 137-41.

Molloy, J., Martin, J. F., Baskerville, P. A., Fraser, S. C. & Markus, H. S. (1998) S-nitrosoglutathione reduces the rate of embolization in humans. Circulation, 98, 1372-5.

Morrow, C. P., Fleming, T. R., Creagan, E. T., Rubin, J., O'connell, M. J. & Ames, M. M. (1993) Tumors of the ovary: Classification of the adnexal mass. Synopsis of gynecologic oncology 4th edition. New York: Churchill Livingstone.

Moryl, N., Coyle, N. & Foley, K. M. (2008) Managing an acute pain crisis in a patient with advanced cancer: "This is as much of a crisis as a code". JAMA, 299, 1457-67.

Murata, A., Morishige, F. & Yamaguchi, H. (1982) Prolongation of survival times of terminal cancer patients by administration of large doses of ascorbate. Int J Vitam Nutr Res Suppl, 23, 103-13.

Murugaesu, N., Schmid, P., Dancey, G., Agarwal, R., Holden, L., Mcneish, I., Savage, P. M., Newlands, E. S., Rustin, G. J. & Seckl, M. J. (2006) Malignant ovarian germ cell tumors: Identification of novel prognostic markers and long-term outcome after multimodality treatment. J Clin Oncol, 24, 4862-6.

Nakashima, N., Nagasaka, T., Fukata, S., Oiwa, N., Nara, Y., Fukatsu, T. & Takeuchi, J. (1990) Study of ovarian tumors treated at nagoya university hospital, 1965-1988. Gynecol Oncol, 37, 103-11.

Nawa, A., Obata, N., Kikkawa, F., Kawai, M., Nagasaka, T., Goto, S., Nishimori, K. & Nakashima, N. (2001) Prognostic factors of patients with yolk sac tumors of the ovary. Am J Obstet Gynecol, 184, 1182-8.

Ozols, R. F. (2005) Treatment goals in ovarian cancer. Int J Gynecol Cancer, 15 Suppl 1, 3-11.

Padayatty, S. J. & Levine, M. (2000) Reevaluation of ascorbate in cancer treatment: Emerging evidence, open minds and serendipity. J Am Coll Nutr, 19, 423-5.

Padayatty, S. J., Riordan, H. D., Hewitt, S. M., Katz, A., Hoffer, L. J. & Levine, M. (2006) Intravenously administered vitamin c as cancer therapy: Three cases. CMAJ, 174, 937-42.

Pan, S. Y., Ugnat, A. M. & Mao, Y. (2005) Physical activity and the risk of ovarian cancer: A case-control study in canada. Int J Cancer, 117, 300-7.

Pawellek, I., Dokoupil, K. & Koletzko, B. (2008) Prevalence of malnutrition in paediatric hospital patients. Clin Nutr, 27, 72-6.

Pearce, R. K., Owen, A., Daniel, S., Jenner, P. & Marsden, C. D. (1997) Alterations in the distribution of glutathione in the substantia nigra in parkinson's disease. J Neural Transm, 104, 661-77.

Pectasides, D., Farmakis, D. & Pectasides, M. (2006) The management of stage i nonseminomatous testicular germ cell tumors. Oncology, 71, 151-8.

Perry, T. L., Godin, D. V. & Hansen, S. (1982) Parkinson's disease: A disorder due to nigral glutathione deficiency? Neurosci Lett, 33, 305-10.

Perry, T. L., Hansen, S. & Jones, K. (1988) Brain amino acids and glutathione in progressive supranuclear palsy. Neurology, 38, 943-6.

Perry, T. L. & Yong, V. W. (1986) Idiopathic parkinson's disease, progressive supranuclear palsy and glutathione metabolism in the substantia nigra of patients. Neurosci Lett, 67, 269-74.

Pietras, K. & Hanahan, D. (2005) A multitargeted, metronomic, and maximum-tolerated dose "Chemo-switch" Regimen is antiangiogenic, producing objective responses and survival benefit in a mouse model of cancer. J Clin Oncol, 23, 939-52.

Pietsch, J. B. & Ford, C. (2000) Children with cancer: Measurements of nutritional status at diagnosis. Nutrition in Clinical Practice, 15, 185-8.

Prasad, K. N., Kumar, A., Kochupillai, V. & Cole, W. C. (1999) High doses of multiple antioxidant vitamins: Essential ingredients in improving the efficacy of standard cancer therapy. J Am Coll Nutr, 18, 13-25.

References

Printz, L. A. (1988) Is withholding hydration a valid comfort measure in the terminally ill? Geriatrics, 43, 84-8.

Ramdath, D. D. & Golden, M. H. N. (1989) Glutathione in malnutrition. West Indian Med J. 31st Scientific Meeting of Commonwealth Caribbean Medical Research Council, Port of Spain, April 16-19.

Riederer, P., Sofic, E., Rausch, W. D., Schmidt, B., Reynolds, G. P., Jellinger, K. & Youdim, M. B. (1989) Transition metals, ferritin, glutathione, and ascorbic acid in parkinsonian brains. J Neurochem, 52, 515-20.

Riordan, H. D., Casciari, J. J., Gonzalez, M. J., Riordan, N. H., Miranda-Massari, J. R., Taylor, P. & Jackson, J. A. (2005) A pilot clinical study of continuous intravenous ascorbate in terminal cancer patients. P R Health Sci J, 24, 269-76.

Riordan, N. H., Riordan, H. D., Meng, X., Li, Y. & Jackson, J. A. (1995) Intravenous ascorbate as a tumor cytotoxic chemotherapeutic agent. Med Hypotheses, 44, 207-13.

Robison, L. L. (1993) Survivors of childhood cancer and risk of a second tumor. J Natl Cancer Inst, 85, 1102-3.

Rosai, J. & Ackerman, L. V. (1979) The pathology of tumors, part iii: Grading, staging & classification. CA Cancer J Clin, 29, 66-77.
Rose, E. A. (2000) The columbia presbyterian guide to surgery, New York:, St. Martin's Press.

Russell, D. J. (1995) The female pelvic mass. Diagnosis and management. Med Clin North Am, 79, 1481-93.

Rygaard, J. & Povlsen, C. O. (1976) The nude mouse vs. The hypothesis of immunological surveillance. Transplant Rev, 28, 43-61.

Saksela, E., Timonen, T. & Cantell, K. (1979) Human natural killer cell activity is augmented by interferon via recruitment of 'pre-nk' cells. Scand J Immunol, 10, 257-66.

Samaritani, R., Corrado, G., Vizza, E. & Sbiroli, C. (2007) Cyclophosphamide "Metronomic" Chemotherapy for palliative treatment of a young patient with advanced epithelial ovarian cancer. BMC Cancer, 7, 65.

Schipper, H., Goh, C. R. & Wang, T. L. (1995) Shifting the cancer paradigm: Must we kill to cure? J Clin Oncol, 13, 801-7.

Schmidinger, M., Budinsky, A. C., Wenzel, C., Piribauer, M., Brix, R., Kautzky, M., Oder, W., Locker, G. J., Zielinski, C. C. & Steger, G. G. (2000) Glutathione in the prevention of cisplatin induced toxicities. A prospectively randomized pilot trial in patients with head and neck cancer and non small cell lung cancer. Wien Klin Wochenschr, 112, 617-23.

Sechi, G., Deledda, M. G., Bua, G., Satta, W. M., Deiana, G. A., Pes, G. M. & Rosati, G. (1996) Reduced intravenous glutathione in the treatment of early parkinson's disease. Prog Neuropsychopharmacol Biol Psychiatry, 20, 1159-70.

Sen, C. K. (1997) Nutritional biochemistry of cellular glutathione. Nutr Biochem, 8, 660-72.

Senturker, S., Karahalil, B., Inal, M., Yilmaz, H., Muslumanoglu, H., Gedikoglu, G. & Dizdaroglu, M. (1997) Oxidative DNA base damage and antioxidant enzyme levels in childhood acute lymphoblastic leukemia. FEBS Lett, 416, 286-90.
Serov, S. F., Scully, R. E. & Bosin, L. H. (1973) Histological typing of ovarian tumors. International histological classification of tumours. World Health Organization, Geneva, Switzerland.

Serrou, B., Rosenfeld, C. & Herberman, R. B. (1983) Nk cells: Fundamental aspects and role in cancer (human cancer immunology) vol. 6., North-Holland, Amsterdam, Elsevier.

Shield, J. P. & Baum, J. D. (1994) Children's consent to treatment. BMJ, 308, 1182-3.

Sian, J., Dexter, D. T., Lees, A. J., Daniel, S., Agid, Y., Javoy-Agid, F., Jenner, P. & Marsden, C. D. (1994) Alterations in glutathione levels in parkinson's disease and other neurodegenerative disorders affecting basal ganglia. Ann Neurol, 36, 348-55.

Siebler, T., Shalet, S. M. & Robson, H. (2002) Effects of chemotherapy on bone metabolism and skeletal growth. Horm Res, 58 Suppl 1, 80-5.

Simone, C. B., Simone, N. L. & Simone, C. B. (1999) Nutrients and cancer treatment. International Journal of Integrative Medicine, 1, 20-4.

Sinha, R., Cross, A. J., Graubard, B. I., Leitzmann, M. F. & Schatzkin, A. (2009) Meat intake and mortality: A prospective study of over half a million people. Arch Intern Med, 169, 562-71.

Sink, J. D., Filston, H. C., Kirks, D. R., Ponzi, J. W. & Tayloe, D. T., Jr. (1982) Removal of splenic cyst with salvage of functional splenic tissue. J Pediatr, 100, 412-4.

Smyth, J. F., Bowman, A., Perren, T., Wilkinson, P., Prescott, R. J., Quinn, K. J. & Tedeschi, M. (1997) Glutathione reduces the toxicity and improves quality of life of women diagnosed with ovarian cancer treated with cisplatin: Results of a double-blind, randomised trial. Ann Oncol, 8, 569-73.

Sogut, S., Zoroglu, S. S., Ozyurt, H., Yilmaz, H. R., Ozugurlu, F., Sivasli, E., Yetkin, O., Yanik, M., Tutkun, H., Savas, H. A., Tarakcioglu, M. & Akyol, O. (2003) Changes in nitric oxide levels and antioxidant enzyme activities may have a role in the pathophysiological mechanisms involved in autism. Clin Chim Acta, 331, 111-7.

Sood, A. K., Abu-Rustum, N. R., Barakat, R. R., Bodurka, D. C., Brown, J., Donato, M. L., Poynor, E. A., Wolf, J. K. & Gershenson, D. M. (2005) Fifth international conference on ovarian cancer: Challenges and opportunities. Gynecol Oncol, 97, 916-23.

Sood, A. K., Bhatty, R., Kamat, A. A., Landen, C. N., Han, L., Thaker, P. H., Li, Y., Gershenson, D. M., Lutgendorf, S. & Cole, S. W. (2006) Stress hormone-mediated invasion of ovarian cancer cells. Clin Cancer Res, 12, 369-75.

Spina, M. B. & Cohen, G. (1989) Dopamine turnover and glutathione oxidation: Implications for parkinson disease. Proc Natl Acad Sci U S A, 86, 1398-400.

Stattin, P., Bjor, O., Ferrari, P., Lukanova, A., Lenner, P., Lindahl, B., Hallmans, G. & Kaaks, R. (2007) Prospective study of hyperglycemia and cancer risk. Diabetes Care, 30, 561-7.

Stutman, O. (1981) Immunological surveillance and cancer. IN Waters, H. (Ed.) The handbook of cancer immunology, vol. 7. New York, Garland Pub.

Syburra, C. & Passi, S. (1999) Oxidative stress in patients with multiple sclerosis. Ukr Biokhim Zh, 71, 112-5.

Teicher, B. A. & Ellis, L. M. (2008) Antiangiogenic agents in cancer therapy, Humana Press.

Testa, B., Mesolella, M., Testa, D., Giuliano, A., Costa, G., Maione, F. & Iaccarino, F. (1995) Glutathione in the upper respiratory tract. Ann Otol Rhinol Laryngol, 104, 117-9.

Thun-Hohenstein, L., Frisch, H. & Schuster, E. (1992) Growth after radiotherapy and chemotherapy in children with leukemia or lymphoma. Horm Res, 37, 91-5.

Tong, X., You, Q., Li, L., Cai, L., Wang, C. & Zheng, J. (2008) Prognostic factors of patients with ovarian yolk sac tumors: A study in Chinese patients. Onkologie, 31, 679-84.

Trickler, D., Shklar, G. & Schwartz, J. (1993) Inhibition of oral carcinogenesis by glutathione. Nutr Cancer, 20, 139-44.

Ueda, G., Abe, Y., Yoshida, M. & Fujiwara, T. (1990) Embryonal carcinoma of the ovary: A six-year survival. Int J Gynaecol Obstet, 31, 287-92.

Vargas, D. L., Nascimbene, C., Krishnan, C., Zimmerman, A. W. & Pardo, C. A. (2005) Neuroglial activation and neuroinflammation in the brain of patients with autism. Ann Neurol, 57, 67-81.

Vendemiale, G., Altomare, E., Trizio, T., Le Grazie, C., Di Padova, C., Salerno, M. T., Carrieri, V. & Albano, O. (1989) Effects of oral s-adenosyl-l-methionine on hepatic glutathione in patients with liver disease. Scand J Gastroenterol, 24, 407-15.

References

Vina, J., Lloret, A., Orti, R. & Alonso, D. (2004) Molecular bases of the treatment of alzheimer's disease with antioxidants: Prevention of oxidative stress. Mol Aspects Med, 25, 117-23.

Wang, S. T., Chen, H. W., Sheen, L. Y. & Lii, C. K. (1997) Methionine and cysteine affect glutathione level, glutathione-related enzyme activities and the expression of glutathione s-transferase isozymes in rat hepatocytes. J Nutr, 127, 2135-41.

Westphal, G. A., Schnuch, A., Schulz, T. G., Reich, K., Aberer, W., Brasch, J., Koch, P., Wessbecher, R., Szliska, C., Bauer, A. & Hallier, E. (2000) Homozygous gene deletions of the glutathione s-transferases m1 and t1 are associated with thimerosal sensitization. Int Arch Occup Environ Health, 73, 384-8.

White, A. C., Thannickal, V. J. & Fanburg, B. L. (1994) Glutathione deficiency in human disease. J Nutr Biochem, 5, 218-26.

Witschi, A., Reddy, S., Stofer, B. & Lauterburg, B. H. (1992) The systemic availability of oral glutathione. Eur J Clin Pharmacol, 43, 667-9.

Woltjer, R. L., Nghiem, W., Maezawa, I., Milatovic, D., Vaisar, T., Montine, K. S. & Montine, T. J. (2005) Role of glutathione in intracellular amyloid-alpha precursor protein/carboxy-terminal fragment aggregation and associated cytotoxicity. J Neurochem, 93, 1047-56.

Yeom, C. H., Jung, G. C. & Song, K. J. (2007) Changes of terminal cancer patients' health-related quality of life after high dose vitamin c administration. J Korean Med Sci, 22, 7-11.

Yorbik, O., Sayal, A., Akay, C., Akbiyik, D. I. & Sohmen, T. (2002) Investigation of antioxidant enzymes in children with autistic disorder. Prostaglandins Leukot Essent Fatty Acids, 67, 341-3.

Young People and informed consent project. Joint publication of the australian medical association and medical practitioners board of victoria. Victoria 2002.

Zhang, X., Zhu, H. & Xu, J. (1995) [clinical trial of oral etoposide in the treatment of malignancies]. Zhonghua Zhong Liu Za Zhi, 17, 454-7.

Sarah's Last Wish

References